MENTAL HEALTH
Psycho-Social Pespectives

VOLUME ONE: Issues and Interventions

The details of the forthcoming volumes are:

Volume 1: Issues and Interventions

Volume 2: Multigroup Analysis

Volume 3: Strength of Human Resources

Volume 4: Therapeutic Applications

About the Editors

Aradhana Shukla is Prof. and former Head Department of Psychology, Kumaun University Campus, Almora Uttarakhand. Currently she is Campus Dean (Arts) at Kumaun University Campus, Almora. She has served in Department of Pediatrics of Banaras Hindu University, Post Doctoral fellow (U.G.C.) at University of Gorakhpur and has been serving here for last 27 years. She has published 100 research papers of national and international repute, ten books in which nine are published by national agencies and one from Germany (LAP). She has carried out 4 major projects from ICSSR and UGC and co-worked in UNICEF and GFATM-round 7 projects. She has guides 45 Ph.D. students and prepared 26 psychological tests. Moreover, she has attended 40 Seminars of national and international repute and organized 4 seminars in her department. Her major thrust areas are: developmental psychology, personality psychology, cultural psychology, environmental psychology and mental health care system.

Anubhuti Dubey is Associate Professor of Psychology at Department of Psychology, DDU Gorakhpur University, Gorakhpur. Her research interest includes Health Psychology, Applied Social Psychology, Gender and health and Counselling. She had published a book entitled "Psychological Perspectives on Chronic Illness". She had also completed a research project sponsored by ICSSR on "Psychological Dynamics of Health and Illness in Women of Eastern Uttar Pradesh." She had published 25 research papers in journals of national and international repute and also contributed 11 chapters in different edited volumes. Four students had been awarded their Ph.D. thesis under her supervision. She had received university gold medals at under-graduate and post-graduate levels. She is also a Master Trainer and Supportive Supervisor for Training HIV/AIDS counsellors under GFATM-Round 7 programmes.

MENTAL HEALTH
Psycho-Social Perspetives

Volume One
Issues and Interventions

Edited by
Aradhana Shukla
Anubhuti Dubey

CONCEPT PUBLISHING COMPANY PVT. LTD.
NEW DELHI-110059

ISBN-13: 978-93-5125-173-6 (Series)
ISBN-13: 978-93-5125-169-9 (Vol. I)

First Published 2015

Published and Printed by

Concept
Since 1974

Concept Publishing Company Pvt. Ltd.
A/15-16, Commercial Block, Mohan Garden
New Delhi-110059 (India)
T: 25351460, 25351794, *F*: 091-11-25357109
E: publishing@conceptpub.com, W: www.conceptpub.com
Editorial Office: H-13, Bali Nagar, New Delhi-110 015, India.

Cataloging in Publication Data--Courtesy: D.K. Agencies (P) Ltd. <docinfo@dkagencies.com>

Mental health : psycho-social perspectives / edited by Aradhana Shukla, Anubhuti Dubey.
volumes 1-2 cm
Contributed articles.
Includes bibliographical references and indexes.
Contents: volume one. Issues and interventions -- volume two. Multigroup analysis
ISBN 9789351251736 (Series)
ISBN 9789351251699 (Vol. I)
ISBN 9789351251705 (Vol. II)

1. Mental health--Social aspects--India. 2. Mental health--Social aspects. I. Shukla, Aradhana, editor. II. Dubey, Anubhuti, editor.

DDC 300.72 23

Preface

We desire to live a healthy and happy life. It is a common and well accepted fact that everyone desires to live a healthy life. The mind and bodily functions are closely embedded hence, the relative significance of mental health along with physical wellness cannot be denied. As mind and bodily functions are closely embedded we cannot deny the relative significances of mental health a long with physical wellness. Mental health is an integral part of health, mental health is more than the absence of mental illness, and mental health is intimately connected with physical health and behaviour. Mental health is the foundation for well-being and effective functioning for an individual and for a community. Good mental health is a sense of well-being, confidence and self-esteem. It enables us to fully enjoy and appreciate other people, day-to-day life and our environment.

Mental health is the sheer responsibility of a person himself. The mental health field aims to deal with (1) mentally ill people, (2) people at risk, and (3) promoting mental health of normal people so that their normality can be sustained.

If we go back into the history of mental health we can see that it was treated either as "boon of God" (good or positive mental health) or "curse of God" bad or negative mental health). Both the Eastern and Western evidences support the notion. Not only in abroad but our ancient evidences also support this notion. The Western literatures on mental health were seen hallucinations as communication of humans with bad souls, ghosts and witches. Moreover, in the ancient Indian literature of Ayurveda, Mental disorders are represented as various forms. The aetio-genesis of these disorders was thought to be endogenous because of provoked humours like *Vat*, *Pitta* and *Kaph*. Exogenously the causes were attributed to sudden fear or association with ill influence of certain mythological gods or demon. *Charak Samhita* listed Psychiatry as *'Bhuta Vidya'*. Psychotherapy was known as *Ilaj-I-Nafsani* in Unani Medicine. But time never remains stable. Years and years were passed and the outlook of people towards mentally ill people become more and more aversive and they were treated like an undesirable social being for whom only such behaviour was required that was only meant for animals or criminals. Even with the advent of modern scientific methods and practical thoughts, the stigma and discrimination against mentally illnesses prevail the society. However, the advocates of Psychology started to cola soft touch and healing approach for the mentally ill people. Again it took decades to develop behaviour and psycho-therapies against tying mentally ill people with iron chain, and treat them like prisoners. A complete soft and medico-human environment under single roof was constructed for them and it was termed as asylum or mental hospital. Psychologists attempted such patients to get out from the boundaries and from the trap of *ojhas, neem-haquims* and other such traditional healers and placed them at asylum. The patients were properly medicated along with different psychotherapies and many of them got complete recovery. At first the asylums were established in abroad but in India the first asylum was established in 1787 by Surgeon Kenderline in Calcutta and thereafter many asylums were made. This period was relatively longer but it opened the doors of a new era for the support and care of mental ill-health. They not only paid attention to treat the mentally ill people but also concentrated on maintaining and nurturing public health, and trying to eradicate the stigma and discrimination faced by people with mental disorders. Psychologists and mental health care professionals are still trying to launch innovative programmes for the same. The focal theme of these developmental programmes are the utilization of community resources for mental health care. These programmes have given new vision to the mental health care professionals to prevent mental disorders and promote mental health. This also needs a greater role for the non-medical mental health care professionals and better utilization of cultural resources in terms of belief, practice and important social institutions like family and community groups. The contemporary world's realization about mental health and mental illness has come to a point where we find passionate discussions and caring mental health professionals to deal with mental disorder and promote well-being.

Keeping these views into consideration the innovative thought of this series appeared in our mind and we decided to pool the thoughts of psychologists and health care professionals regarding various concerns of mental health. The basic aim of this series was: (i) to bring concepts, issues, strengths and treatment in a single jacket, (ii) bring a sense of mental health awareness in people so that they can make their health safe with additional attention on social health, (iii) to carve the research competence in young researchers, and (iv) to put forth the mental health policies before the readers, so that a better understanding of mental health can be developed.

About the series Mental Health: Psycho Social Perspectives

It is a series on the psychology of mental health and we have tried to cover as many areas as possible and we could justify its name, i.e. rethinking. Many traditional notions of mental health have been reconceptualised and many concepts in a new framework have been introduced. This series has four volumes:

1. ***Mental health: Psychological Issues and Interventions:*** In this volume we have covered various issues that foster or hamper mental health. Also, strategies to minimize negative mental health and improve positive mental health are discussed.
2. ***Mental health: Multigroup Analysis:*** This volume covers the conceptual background and psycho-social perspective of mental health in various social settings.
3. ***Mental health: Strength of Human Resources:*** In this volume we have tried to throw light on the promotional strategies of mental health following which a person can be relieved from negative mental health.
4. ***Mental Health: Therapeutic Applications:*** This volume covers a range of behavioural therapies which were found effective to minimize or overcome mental ill health.

We have exercised our best attempt to seek out as many experiences as possible and we also anticipate that this will open new foresight for the researchers. However, we will be highly blessed to obtain the healthy and critical comments from our colleagues, seniors and friends and we will appreciate them from the bottom of our hearts.

Aradhana Shukla
Anubhuti Dubey

Acknowledgements

We, the editors, feel immense pleasure to present our series on mental health before the august readers. We hope that it will be admired by you all and the comments will be highly appreciated.

We feel our deep sense of gratitude and thankfulness to our respected contributors. It was only their support that the volumes came in the shape. We are thankful to Mr. Abhishek and Mr. Pankaj Tewari for computer task.

Last but not least, we are thankful to Mr. Ashok Mittal, M/s. Concept Publishing Company Pvt. Ltd., New Delhi to shape our dreams in concrete form.

15 January 2015
Makar Sankranti

Aradhana Shukla
Anubhuti Dubey

Contents

Introduction

The concept of mental health was commenced from when a person started to act, respond or behave. Recent advances made in the areas of neurophysiology and group and individual dynamics opened a new door for non-medical professionals to rethink over this concept and provide the ways of interventions to meet with the mental health problems.

As defined by the researchers of psychology, mental health may be described as a state of psychological presence of well-being, complete social and physical state and absence of diseases or infirmity. WHO, however, in the first 30 years stressed highly on specific illness (Tuberculosis, Malaria) and not so much as health. In 1978 Alma Ata Conference was made and health was considered as the 'individuals' own responsibility not the matter of others'. It clearly reveals that it is our responsibility that we make us healthy physically as well as mentally, but it must not be done on the cost of others' disregard. It means to say that we should make a balance between us and others. (आत्मवत् सर्वभूतेषु यः पश्यति सः पश्यति).

Our balanced behaviour is the most important indicator of mental health which explains that we must not do any injustice for ourselves and for others as well. This balanced behaviour is also paralleled by positive behaviour, alertness and making bond even with negative conditions but no one can always be happy and cheerful. Many times we face such type of situations that shake us entirely and as a result we loose our temper, become depressed or become isolated from the society. But if it is temporary it cannot be considered our situation based on bad or ill mental health.

The ground of mental health is adaptability, balanced behaviour desirable behaviour and satisfaction. They serve as the hazards of poor mental health and make person healthy. The other important variable that helps to maintain the magnitude of mental health is the awareness of own's limitation we become disturbed only when we cross our limit and situation becomes is out of control. So self-awareness is an important facilitation of mental health.

There is one more truth that needs to be thought. Mental illness or mental circumstances are not common for all. Every segment of society had its own problems, own worry and own way of solution, whether rich or poor, child or adolescents, old or young, male or female. Persons living in joint or neuclear femily are surrounded by their own problem(s) and they have their own way to get rid of.

One strange situation which we have seen is the oscillation of person between illness and health. We are not ill but we are not healthy. It is impossible some times but true. We have no time to take care about us. We just take us to meet with the demands of daily life and people think that we are absolutely fine, but the situation is entirely reversed. We suppress our disease and prefer the other priorities of life because we think them more important than us. This is a major cause that affects our mental health. As the time and situation appears they show their signs in us.

It is a common fact that variation of mental health is shared by people living in various societies and economic standard. It has generally observed that curable and costly diseases are shared by affluent while incurable diseases most often shared by the poors. When the poor finds that any disease by which he or his family members are surrounded is more expensive than his pocket. He becomes anxious and this anxiety influences his mental health. This notion has similarly been investigated in India and abroad.

Although similar attempts have been made in India and abroad to study concept, etiology and promotion of mental health yet in India it is being studied till the ancient time. Indian psychology stress more on the positive aspect of mental state that being happy and balanced in every circumstances and converting negative into positive is the best sign of mental health. *Atharva Veda* states the causes and remedy of mental disorder. The aim of this Veda is to guide the humanity to universe welfare.

Atharva Veda states three mental attributes of mental health. They are: *Satogun, Rajogun* and *Tamogun*. They provide mental balance and purity (*Satogun*), dominance and work orientedness (*Rajogun*) and anger and mental retardation (*Tamogun*). All the sort of treatments is based on meditation and atharvanic therapy, Kausik tantra, transference, consolation, desensitization, tap and divya, havan. *Yoga* has also become successful to maintain and cultivate positive mental health. *Hathyoga*,

Mantrayoga, Bhaktiyoga, Ayanyoga, Karmayoga, Layagyoga are the main schools of yogi science. In addition, Abhidhamma theory of Buddhism also focuses on mental health and describes it through two factors, namely skilled factor and unskilled factor. Both are necessary for proper development and a person feels good mental health by making a balance between these two factors.

A close perusal of the notions discussed above reveal that classic approach of Indian school is worth to be appreciated and then implemented.

As already has been mentioned mental health is caused by many positive factors. They need to be maintained and their nurturance is very important for good mental health. But, there are some factors that hamper the flow of mental health. They are like, poverty, race discrimination, deprivation/disadvantage, physical or mental handicap or many more about which there is a need to think. They serve as the issues of mental health and intervention is required for them.

This notion was kept in the cognition of the editors when they thought to pen. This appeared in terms of "Mental Health: Psycho-social Perspectives", this volume aims to seek out the main issues of mental health that act as a challenge for it and provides the ways of interventions to promote the magnitude of mental health. We have also tried to put forth the young talents of psychology and we are blessed by the blissful articles of our senior professionals. This volume is comprised Twenty-Two articles. They are review based or empirical articles.

The first article of Aradhana Shukla and Anubhuti Dubey is an introductory chapter in which they have laid their views on the concept and issues of mental health. Mental health of women has been viewed by Khushbu Rani and S.C. Tiwari. Chandra Bhal Dwivedi has discussed subjective well-being in Hinduism by adhering through a spiritual style. Anubhuti Dubey and Kamini Mani Tripathi have explored the distress and quality of life in women suffering from diabetes and cancer. Laxmi Vajpeyi has also studied women's mental health with special reference to sexual assault. She has also presented an ecological model. Parenting type and problem behaviour of children and childhood technololism are the good papers regarding the mental health of children. They are presented by Ruchi Kakkar and Aradhana Shukla and Shivali Sharma and Supriya Chaturvedi. Neelam Verma has shed light on child abuse and suicide ideation of children and adolescents and dyslexia management is presented by Anubhuti Dubey and Shalini Gupta. Sarita Joshi and Aradhana Shukla have explored the impact of parenting on the emotional disturbance of children. The concern of parenting has also been extended by Pragya Tripathi, and Anubhuti Dubey. They have taken run away children in consideration. The concept of emotional disturbance in developmental perspective has been experimented by Pooja M. Galiakoti and Aradhana Shukla and they have taken residential locale, gender and family type of the participants as affectors. Muniram and Arun Kumar have studied suicide risk with mental health and etiology of stress and burn out in doctors is explored by Anubhuti Dubey and Darshana Shahi. Jyotsana Shukla studied environmental toxin as a threat to mental health and Akbar Husain has related mental health to mediation. Tanu Shukla's paper deals with the organizational effectiveness and organization health relation.

Navya Pande has compared eastern and western models of existential anxiety and identity crisis through Advaitic Vedanta and Reeta Chauhan, Poornima Awasthi and Saroj Verma have explained health and well-being as an outcome of proactive coping. Neelam Verma raised the health issue of child and adolescent mental health. Anjali Bhatia has made a study in classroom setting to provide primary prevention and empowerment of teacher training.

Last but not least is the paper of Aradhana Shukla. It is the concluding remarks of volume and she has described the challenges and interventions. She has also provided some strategies to recover mental health and cope with mental health problems.

I have made a sincere endeavour to provide as many aspects of mental health as I can but if anything remains I will try my best to cover it in future. I request the esteemed readers to provide healthy comments on the volume and it will be highly solicited.

Aradhana Shukla
Anubhuti Dubey

List of Contributors

Akbar Husain is Coordinator, UGC-SAP (DRS - I) Department of Psychology, Aligarh Muslim University, Aligarh, Uttar Pradesh.
Email: profakbar6@gmail.com, a.husain.py@amu.ac.in, akbar6h@yahoo.co.in

Anjali Bhatia is Lecturer, ICFAI University, Dehradun and Life Skills Trainer, Eupsychia, Dehradun, Uttrakhand.
Email: bhatia.amali.82@gm.ail.com

Anubhuti Dubey is Associate Professor of Psychology, DDU Gorakhpur University, Gorakhpur. Email: anubhutiddu@rediffmail.com

Aradhana Shukla is Professor of Psychology and Dean (Arts) Kumaon University Campus, Almora. Email: aradhana.shukla5@gmail.com

Arun Kumar is Project Fellow, Department of Psychology, M.D. University, Rohtak, Haryana.

Chandra Bhal Dwivedi is Former Head and Professor of Psychology, Department of Psychology, Banaras Hindu University, Varanasi.
Email: cbd_bhu@rediftmail.com

Darshana Shahi is Ph.D. in Psychology from DDU Gorakhpur University, Gorakhpur.

Jyotsana Shukla is Assistant Professor of Psychology at Amity University, Lucknow. Email: jsreena@ gmatl.com

Kamini Mani Tripathi is Ph.D. in Psychology from DDU Gorakhpur University, Gorakhpur. Email: kaminimanitripathi@rediffmail.com

Khushbu Rani is Post Doctoral Fellow, Department of Geriatric Mental Health, King George's Medical College, Lucknow. Email: drkhushbu 10@gmail.com

Laxmi Vajpeyi is Assistant Professor & Head, Department of Humanities, Babu Banarasi Das National Institute of Technology & Management, Lucknow. Email: laxmi.vajpeyi@gmail.com

Muniram is Research Scholar, Department of Psychology, M. D. University, Rohtak, Haryana.

Navya Pande is Research Scholar, Department of Psychology, Kumaun University Campus, Almora, Uttrakhand.
Email: pandenavya.banasthali@gmail.com

Neelam Verma is Clinical Psychologist, Child and Adolescent Guidance Clinic, Noormanzil Psychiatric Centre, Lucknow, Uttar Pradesh.
Email: neelampsycho. 86@gmail.com

Pooja M. Gailakoti is Research Scholar, Department of Psychology, Kumaun University Campus, Almora, Uttrakhand.
Email: pmehta3Q10@gmail.com

Pragya Tripathi is Research Scholar, Department of Psychology, DDU Gorakhpur University, Gorakhpur, Uttar Pradesh.
Email: pragyatripathi24@yahoo.com

Purnima Awasthi is Assistant Professor in Department of Psychology, Banaras Hindu University, Varanasi, Uttar Pradesh.
Email: awasthip9@gmailcom

Reeta Chauhan is Research Scholar in Department of Psychology, Banaras Hindu University, Varanasi.

Ruchi Kakkar is Research Scholar, Department of Psychology, Kumaun University Campus, Almora, Uttrakhand.
Email: kakkarharsh2001@gmal.com

S.C. Tiwari is Professor and Head, Department of Geriatric Mental Health, King George's Medical College, Lucknow, Utttar Pradesh.

Sarita Joshi is Assistant Professor of Home Science, S.V.P. University of Agriculture and Technology, Meerut, Uttar Pradesh.
Email: saritajoshi156@vahoo.com

Saroj Verma is Professor, Department of Psychology, Banaras Hindu University, Varanasi, Uttar Pradesh. Email: saroj_vrma@rediffinail.com

Shalini Gupta is Counsellor and Technical Assistant, Community Engagement for JE/AES Prevention and Control, BRD Medical College, Gorakhpur, Uttar Pradesh. Email: shalinig335 @gmail.com

Shivali Sharma is Senior Lecturer, Amity University, Lucknow, Uttar Pradesh, Email: shivalil374@gmail.com

Supriya Chaturvedi is Assistant Professor and Head, Department of Psychology, Mahavidyalaya Bhatawali Bazar, Goakhpur, Uttar Pradesh.
Email: supriyachat@rediffmail.com

Tanu Shukla is Assistant Professor of Psychology, Department of Humanities and Social Sciences, BITS, Pilani, Rajasthan.
Email: tanushukla8@gmail.com

1

Mental Health

Concept and Issues

Aradhana Shukla and *Anubhuti Dubey*

These days many psychologists of India and abroad have focused their attention to seek the courses of negative mental health and best possible ways to improve and try to feed positivity in people. This endeavour has appeared in terms of a new branch of psychology named Health Psychology. This field has obtained a relative recognition in the reader's professionals and practitioners of psychology. The researchers working in this area have also focused upon demographic variables, like age, role and socio-economic class as determined by the adoption and practice of health and positively rotate it with the status (Varying or Static) of mental health.

Mental health is a fundamental component of health which can be realized by a person (or by the others) about his own cognitive affections and relational abilities and healthy mental dispositions allows coping well with life's challenges to wake productively and to wake a positive contribution to one's community mental health has been reported as an important factor influencing individuals' various behaviours, activities, happiness and performance. It can be defined as the ability to adjustment to the environment on the plane of reality.

Mental health is not just the absence of mental disorder. It is defined as a state of well-being in which every individual realizes his or her own potential, can cope with the normal stresses of life can work productively and fruitfully, and is able to make a contribution to her or his community (WHO, 2008). This most acceptable definition was also influenced by the earlier definitions of WHO (2008). "Health is the state of complete physical, mental and social well-being not merely an absence of disease or informity."

In most countries, particularly low and middle income countries, mental health services are severely short of resources—both human and financial. Of the health care resources available, most are currently spent on the specialized treatment and care of the people with mental illness, and to a lesser extent on an integrated mental health system. Instead of providing care in large psychiatric hospitals and develop community based mental health services. Even less funding is available or mental health promotion, an umbrella term that covers a variety of strategies, all aimed at having a positive effect on mental health well-being in general. The encouragement of individual resources and skills and improvements in the socio-economic environment are among the strategies used.

Mental health promotion requires multi-sectoral action involving a number of government sectors and non-governmental or community based organizations. The focus should be on promoting mental health throughout the lifespan to ensure a healthy start in life for children and to prevent mental disorders in adulthood and old age.

Mental health deals with our feelings about our oneself about others and our ability to meet with the demands of life. There may be some confusion in people's minds as to the difference between mental ill health and mental illness. Mental ill health refers to the kind of general mental health problems, we can all experience in certain stressful circumstances; for example, work pressures can cause us to experience poor mood swing and sleep disturbance.

Such problems are usually of temporary nature, are relative to the demands a particular situation makes on us and generally respond to support and reassurance.

All of us suffer from mental health problems at times, and such temporary problems do not necessarily lead to mental illness. However, being mentally unhealthy limits our potential as human beings and may lead to more serious problems.

Mental illness can be defined as the experiencing of severe and distressing psychological symptoms to the extent that normal functioning is seriously impaired.

In this way it is surely fair to say that mental health makes the mind a capacity to participate in social network, playing the role according to situation time norms, standards and everything else that is decided by society and the person believes it as good and desirable for him and for the society. It means that mental health is a balance between personal feeling and society.

Thus, mental health is a nebulous concept at the best of times. In a broad sense it is a rubric, a label which covers different perspectives and concerns such as the absence of incapacitating symptoms, integration of psychological functioning, effective conduct of personal and social life, feelings of ethical and spiritual well-being and so on (Kakkar, 1984). How this concept is best interpreted in the provision of mental health services in a multicultural context is complicated. Clearly, we need to look carefully at differences in the way mental health is seen in the diverse (cultural) traditions that comprise British society in broad terms, Asian, African, Caribbean, and European. But there are important reservations to this approach. Similarities (between cultural traditions) should never be under-estimated and generalizations (about cultural traditions) have dangers, they may be taken up as stereotypes of people who are seen as 'belonging' to one or other cultural group because of the way they 'look' or to be used to reduce a specified culture having one or two meanings and realities of basic tenets in most instances misleading, if not downright erroneous. Notwithstanding these problems, we can see any other way of exploring cultural diversity in this instance except by comparisons between 'western and eastern'. However, by doing so, one not implying that east and west are any more than traditions from the past current states of mind rather than geographical regions (Kakkar, 1982).

(1) **Mental health in India:** One way of simplifying a complex held is to see cultures (in relation to mental health) as being on a sort of continuum divided into eastern tradition and the notion of mental health was not new in Indian setting whereas in western approach it was studied quantitatively in India was started since long and the approach was sheer qualitative. The Indian advocates of health psychology, namely G. Mishra, Sudhir Kakkar, R.L. Kapoor, Radhakrishna Nidu, Satwant Pasricha etc. have very intensively studied the concept of health in qualitative perspective and their approach is totality based on Indian treasure.

As already stated studies on health in India had long been studied the desire of leading a normal and long life was experienced by all (*Jivem Shraddha Shatam*). Also, it was desired that the life should be full of courage, vigour, longevity and enthusiasm means active till the last breath. Health was considered good for persons only by following the main pathways of life, i.e. *Dharma*, *Artha*, *Kama* and *Mokshs*. They are the conduct cores and they had to make the life disciplined. But it was also observed that health was also flourished with the rules of harmony, evolution and connectivity across life span. It is mainly decided by the society in which the person is surrounding. In *Upanishad* the concepts of *Panch Kosh* (*Annamaya, Pranmaya, Manomaya, Vigyanmaya, Anandmaya*) was given and it was termed as multi-sheath organization which articulate human existence. These 5-health theory operates following the principies of complementarily inter-dependence. Sharing and reciprocity between self and other like environmental surrounding. We can consider *parmanand* or *sattchitanand* (*Sachchidanand*) as the positive self. In this way mental health was defined as "total journey of self-discovery" by Indian psychologists so there is a need to peep inside and discover our self if we want to be healthy but when we are not healthy and unaware about our internal we will never be healthy because self (and to awareness) always helps the person to accept and follow the truth and avoid or reject the false.

Ayurveda is the treatment aspect of psychophysical health which is highly famous for health management and provides various skills to promote health. It is based on three *doshas* (*Vat*, *Pitt* and *Kaugh*) and the rostcome of all diseases lies here. Due to disturbance in these *doshas* whole body is effected. The mental setup is organized by three *gunas* namely *Satva* (*Satogun*), *Tamas* (*Tamogun*) and *Rajas* (*Rajogun*). The other and equally important is *Charak Samhita* which deals a disease by regularizing metabolic system, dietary system and daily routine system.

Even today when allopathic has become a central foci of attention in present society due to its very quick relief technique yet the importance of Indian approach of health cannot be denied because our Indian approach make a fine balance in mind body system.

Emerging issues: The discussion made earlier clearly reveals the relative significance of mental (and physical) health and it has made a solid ground of research in psychology. Researches are being conducted in this area but there is still so many issues that are to be studied and they are as follows:

Impact of Mental Health Condition on Development and Social Integration

As it is appeared that mental health conditions have a significant impact across a wide range of developmental outcomes and thus opportunities of social integration limits. One area that can be implemented for mental health conditions in adolescent and early adulthood is the development of safe and healthy relationship with parents, peers and teachers. As, the period of adolescence is critical for identity formation and role taking especially with peers many mental health conditions affect adversely on youth's ability to form supportive and healthy relationship and manage conflict within these relationships. For example, many adolescents complain the system of depression, irritability, anger and avoidance of social interaction (Kessler, 1997). There negative tendencies make them rejected from their peers.

The other negative mental health of youth is hyperactivity. Thus attention deficit emerges and this alteration deficiency and hyper activity of adolescents and youth make item too for their pro-social peers (Stomshak, Bierman, Brushchi, Dodge and Cole, 1999). They make their linkage with delinquent peers and disengaged from the academic affairs and it also generates behavioural and mental conditions (Lynne Landsman, Bradshaw and Ialongo, 2010; Patterson, De Baryshe and Ramsay, 1989).

The other common mental health concern among youth is substance use. In a study it was found that substance use was strongly correlated with repeating in school grade and varieties of other negative outcomes title physical injury crime, sexual violence and risky sexual behaviour (Reddy *et al.*, 2010).

Mental health conditions also affect youth's self-esteem, social interaction and harming to them outs and the others (Bradshaw, Rebok and others, 2012). It causes many academic obstacles like learning disability discipline poor attendance and even school dropout. The opportunities for the social and economic integration we look forward the youth and we find that mental health conditions are very restricted. This restriction of mental health impact their development and stands their quality of life. Poor mental health conditions, not only, lower the self-esteem of youth but also limit their social interactions and academic performance. Also, their economic potential and wider engagement with their communities has also been ceased or at least, restricted. The overall disease burdens on mental health conditions expressed on the number of years lost due to ill-health, disability or early death, known as Disability Adjusted Life Years (DALYs) has been on the rise. Thus, it is clear that young people are at the greatest risk of a range of mental health conditions from childhood to adulthood (Kessler *et al.*, 2005). It goes a long way and disturb the whole life when an adolescent becomes an adult.

Cultural and Contextual Considerations

When we talk above the mental health of global society we cannot avoid the cultural setup from where they have originated and where they are living. Culture affects mental health by providing content for its expression yielding different for us of expression in different cultures even for the same mental health conditions, thereby influencing prevalence and incidence rates across cultures. Culture should thus, have an impact on the seduce solution and adaptation of appropriate prevention and intervention strategies (Lewis-Fernandis and Khennman, 1994; Mascolo Misra and Rapisardi, 2004; Ban *et al.*, 2012).

Culture also plays an important role with respect to mental health conclusions. It is important during the period of later adolescence and early adulthood for understanding the difference between appropriate relevant social functioning roles and social behaviour, and those considered problematic. It is a fact that metal health conditions often sit on the social lines between the normal and abnormal.

Cultural and contextual conditions also influence the mechanism by which different risk factors affect prevalence course and outcome of different mental health conditions and the ways in which cultural conditions create circumstances that promote mental health. The most important way through which culture has and direct impact on mental health conditions is in its interaction with factors like gender, age, marital status and poverty. These demographic factors act as a predictor across cultures for variations in mental illness but there are some more variables which emerged from the local ground and influence directly.

Poverty and Mental Health

In 2010 the World Health Organization (WHO) has shed light on the risk of a cyclical relationship between vulnerability and mental health. In this relationship with people and varying mental health conditions are vulnerable.

Group subject stigma, discrimination, violence marginalization and other violations of their group right. There contextual factors on one wide deteriorate mental health, increase this decline on the other and create more health and emotional problems later on.

Similarly, the relation between poverty and poor mental health appears to be cyclical in both high and low resource settings. People living in poverty experience higher rate of stress. Social exclusion and nutrition and poor health care cause mental disorders.

Homeless Street-involved Youth and Mental Health

Homeless youth fall more in mental health problems as compare to those counterparts who live in their homes. They face many types of problems like poverty, discrimination, disability, lack of emotional attitude and educational opportunities. Once a youth leaves the home and comes on the road he is trapped in the attraction of such people who in spite of convincing him, make his life hell. Scanlon, Tomkins Lynch and Scanlon (1998) and Wernham (2004) have stated that homeless youth are considered as plague for the society.

West (2003) has stated that homeless youth face many types of problems while establishing their sly and form their identity. They are not expert in employing coping strategies. They use maladaptive coping hebaviour, anti-social behaviour, life time drug use. Substance use is associated with other health problems that is positive HIV status, physical complaint and depletive symmphtac (Embelton, Wangi, Vreeman Ayuku and Braistein, 2013).

Gender role and contextual factors influence the plight and outcome of homeless and stateyath. A. Ptekar and Ciano Federoff (1999) have stated that street boys are more adjusted than girls but most of their basic needs are fulfilled by the strangers. Street life snatches the childhood, laughter and emotion of youth. As they don't have parents so they build their relationship in social site and become isolated from their home.

Juvenile Justice

A large number of young offensive suffer from same mental health condition, that is highly influenced by their experience in the Juvenile system (Glaser *et al.*, 2001). Almost all researches in youth have been done in middle and high SES group and Low SES has only been taken as a comparing variable. In addition intact families are more studied that the distorted families Juvenile justice facilities in low and middle income setup presents a number of circumstances that would lead to increasingly poor outcomes for incarcuates youth with poor mental health conditions. In many low resource setting, youth particularly marginalized and/or home less experience frequent negative interaction with the justice system from police harassment on the streat (e.g. corruption, abuse) to abuse in detention and inadequate support for reintegration upon release (Wernham, 2004).

Such type of incarnated youth are regularly subjection to violence, intimidation, exploitation and inhumane conditions like lack of adequate nutrition, hygiene or mental care (Wernham, 2004).

In a number of low and middle income countries inadequate or non-esixtent juvenile facilities have resulted in youth being housed with older inmates when they may be subjected to above, exploitation and/or degrading treatment (UNICEF, 2006). In many such settings, mental health concerns are not prioritized and even if they were, there would be too few mental health professional to address the level of real and good practice would be happened by the lack of resource.

Mental Health Care System

The lack of mental health professionals and modern medication or treatment options means patients are housed in over crowded, long term, in-patient facilities but little attempt has been made towards rehabilitation and/or social integration. So people deprived of getting proper nutrition and medicines and sometimes the patients are very badly treated by the family members because they have been bared due to the long illness of the patient.

Victims of HIV/AIDS

In many low and middle income countries specific experience of youth lay its significant impact on mental health conditions. They are exposed to armed conflict, female genital mutilation, child labour and orphaned by HIV/AIDS come from low resource setting predominantly. The experience of youth orphaned by HIV/AID is post-traumatic stress and depression (Benjet, 2010). Such types of experience is appeared from poverty, loss of care gives risk of internalizing problems, depression, anxiety anger, hopelessness and sometimes suicidal thought as compared to those who are orphans but not victimized by HIV/AID.

Stress and Management

Stress and stress management are such issues which are highly highlighted by India as well by abroad yet they read more to be explored. In a plethora of studies stress researches were conducted on life event perception, coping behaviour, and other significant management devices, but psychologists have diverted their attention towards variation of people in stress experience, eventual description management device and personal control systems.

Dalal and Misra (2002) have viewed the need of Indian devices of stress management like meditation and relaxation and they have also stated that sometimes experience of stress is necessary for personal growth.

Pranic Healing Practices

Pranic healing is an energy that is developed by maser Chog Kok Sui stutiliza prana or life forces to heal ailments in the body by manipulation of the energy of the person. Being a science pranic healing is developed based on techniques on techniques and principles and could be learnt, studied experimentally and then validated. Although in India subjective and quantitative interpretable has being make by Neki (1973), Kakkar (1982) and Joshi (1988, 2000) have laid a solid foundation for this stress of work to build on but there is a read to study healing, spirituality and *yoga* in ineregenous perspective and implant it.

Health psychologist read to wake in union with health preditions of both traditional and medical variety. Although we know a lot about the causes of ill mental health yet many related aspects like mortality, psychosocial and cultural dimensions of morbidity conditions are still to be explored.

Well-being

Well-being is the ultimate good of life and leads to the psychological state and experience that lead a good life. Well-being has been studied very widely in India and in abroad yet there are many variables that need to be correlated or experiments as per the need of the study life, happiness, effort self-esteem, gratitude, attachment, emotional attachment positive strength, etc. on the whole there are many aspects that need to be explored.

All these issues that are discussed are posing a new challenge and provide new opportunities for resources. All there notions pertaining to the challenges can be met through proper understanding and handling as well.

There are many other factors which not only hamper the developments but also a need for today. They directly influence the child and disturb his mindset. It appears in terms of bullying and peer rejection, repression of traumatic experience from early childhood, post-conflict condition. They also serve a stress for lifetime and people have to suffer it like a curse. There are many issues that should be worth concern. They are described as following.

Bullying as per Rejection

Bullying may be deprived as international and many times repeated act of aggressions that take physical (heating, beating), verbal (abuse by word, harassment, threats, name calling and relation (spreading rumors, theft, influencing social relationship), Olweus (1903) has stated that bullying occurs maximum when there his a status gap the high income students generally feel superiority complex try to suppress their those counter-parts. Those students who are built by them face many worries and problems relating to them face many worries and problems relating to them or relating activities.

Although there is a growing body of research across the globe suggesting that frequent involvement in bullying can be pervasive, long tasting effect on children's socio-emotional functioning (Nausad *et al.,* 2001) including internalizing and externalizing problems (O Brenan, Bradshaw and Sawyer, 2009). Here effect tends to vary as a function of the Gants pattern of involvement in bullying.

Traumatic and Adverse Events in Children and Youth

There are many researches which make a link between adverse life events and varities of mental health conditions (Jordanava *et al*., 2007) cross-sectional and longitudinal studies both are associated with mental health conditions (Kessler, 1997). Adverse life events like physical assault, death of a close relative, unemployment or break-up in romantic relationship are found to be associated with severe depression (Lewinsohn *et al.,* 1988). Such type of events occur more in children and adolescents and they do not have any effect of any other demographic variable like, age, gender or SES. Traumatic events may include natural deserter, catastrophe, human error or equipment failure, physical or sexual assault, rape, robbery/imaging, serious accident, witnessed violence, injury or death, combat, torture or imprisonment threat or harm to self or loved ones, domestic violence and physical abuse fire or burn survivors and life threatening etc. (Giaconia *et al.*, 1995; Sulleiman *et al.*, 2009; Finchan *et al.*, 2009). Trauma, most often experienced by young children and these "adverse childhood events" imprints throughout the life (Anda *et al.*, 2006). Moreover, males feel more trauma than (Foster *et al.*, 2004). But some studies have not shown this (Giaconia *et al.*, 1995). This is an important concern to be studied.

Post-Conflict Mental Health

Many studies of mental health conditions have focused on post conflict or disaster setting. Exposure to was and conflict remain one of the greatest risk factor for PTSD and other mental health conditions (Ballany, 2005). Trauma faced here is found entirely different and have been found to include combat and situation, being forced into the role of child soldier, fleeing or being forced from their homes and loss of parents or caregivers (Machel, 1996; Suliman *et al.*, 2009) children who are affected by conflict and either remain in their own country or are displaced to another low or middle country often have few option for care services due to continued political limitability and/or lade of resources or funding for mental health care (World Health Organization, 2008). Although, quite a number of programmes are running in this field yet it can be studied as an important issue is be studied.

Requisition of Rethinking: Thus, it is appearent that there are many issues related to mental health celeritous. Although, they have been studied widely yet the importance of nation, terms and atmosphere cannot be avoid. They are already emerged still in consideration and should be studied in future.

References

Aptekar, L. and Ciano-Rederoff, LM. (1999). Street children in Nairobi: gender difference in mental health, *New direction for Child and Adolescent Development*, 85, 35, 46.

Ballany, C. (2005). *The State of the World's Children 2005 Childhood under Threat.* New York: UNICEF.

Bass, J.K.; Eaton, W.; Abramawitz, S. and Sartorius, N. (2012). Global Mental health issues culture and Psychopathology. In W. Eaton (ed.) *Public Mental Health.* New York.

Benjet, C. (2010). Childhood adverties of population living in low income countries prevalence characteristics and mental health consequences, *Current Opinions in Psychiatry* 23(4), 356-362.

Bradshow, C.P.; Rebok, G.; Zabltsky, B.; La Flair, L.; Mendelson, T., and Eaton W. (2012) Models of stress and adapting to risk. In W. Eaton (ed.) *Public Mental Health,* pp. 269-302. New York: Oxford.

Dalal, A.K. and Misra, G. (2010). (Eds.) *New Directions in Health Psychology*, New Delhi. Sage Publications.

Embleton, L.; Mwangi, A.; Vreeman, R. Ayuker, D. and Braiststein, P. (2013). The epidemilogy of substance use among street children in resource constrained setting: Systematic review and meta-analysis. Addiction (Epubin) *Advances of Publication* do I: 10.111/add.12252

Fincham, D.S.; Altas, L.K.; Stein, D.J. and Seedat, S. (2009). Post-traumatic stress disorder symptoms in adolescents: Risk factor versus resilience moderation. *Comprehensive Psychiatry*, 50(3), 193-199.

Gia Conia, R.M.; Reinharz, H.Z.; Silverman, A.B.; Pakiz B.; Frost, A.K. and Choen, E. (1995) Trauma and post traumatic stress disorder in a community population of older adolescents. *Journal of the America population of older adolescents/Journal of the America Academy of Child and Adolescent Psychiatry*. 34(10). 1369-1380.

Glaser, B.; Calhour, G.; Broadshaw, C.; Batis, J. and Socherman, R. (2001). Multi-observer assessment of problem behaviour in adjudicated youth. Pattern of discrepancies. *Journal of Child and Family Behaviour, Therapy* 23(2) 33-45.

Glasser, W. (1976). *Positive Addiction*, New York: Harper and Row.

Joshi, P.C. (1998). Traditional medical system in the Central Himalaya. *The Eastern Anthropologist*, 41, 77-86.

Joshi, P.C. (2000). Relavance and utility of traditional medical system (TMS) in the context of a Himalayan tribe. *Psychology and Developing Societies*, 12, 5-29. *http://data.worldbank.org/about/couning.classifications*)

Kakkar, S. (1982). *Shamans, Mystics and Doctors*, New Delhi: Oxford University Press.

Kessler, R.; Berglund, P.; Demler, O.; Jin, R. and Wallaers, E.E. (2005). Lifetime prevalence and age of onset distribution of DSM disorders in the national comorbidity survey replications. *Archfemine of General Psychology*. 62, 593-602.

Kessler, R.C. (1997). The effect of Stressful life events on depression. *Annual Review of Psychology*, 48, 191-214.

Lewinrohn, P.M.; Hoberman, H.M. and Rosebaum, M. (1998). A Prospective study of risk factors for unipolar depression. *Journal of Abnormal Psychology*, 97(3), 251-264.

Lewsi-Fernandis, Robert Khennman, Aruther (1904). *Culture, Personality and Psychopathology*, 102, 67-71.

Lynne-Landsman, S.D.; Bradshaw, C.P. and Ialongo, N.S. (2010). Testing a development cascade model of adolescent substance use trajectories and young adult adjustment development and psychopathology. *American Psychologist*, 44(2), 329-335.

Machel, G. (1996). *Promotion and protection of the right of children: Impact of armed conflict on children, United Nations*.

Mascolo, F.; Misra, G. and Rapisaradi, C. (2004). Individual and relational conceptions of self in India and the United States. In M.F. Mascolo and Jin

Li (Eds.), *Culture and Developing Selves: Beyond dichotomization,* Sam Fransico Jasey-Boss.

Nausad, T.R.; Ovedrpeak, M.; Pilla, R.S.; Ruan, W.J.; Simmons Mortor, B. and Scheidt, P. Bullying behaviour among united states youth prevalence and association with psychosocial adjustment. *Journal of the America Medical Association.* 285, 2094-2100.

Nek, J.S. (1973) Guru-Chela relationship: The personality of a therapeutic paradigm. *American Journal of Orthopsychiatry,* 43, 755-66.

O'Breman, L.; Bradshaw, C.P. and Samyer, A.L. (2009). Examining developmental differences in the social emotional problems among present bullies victims and bully/victims. *Psychology in the Schools,* 46(2), 100-115.

Olwus, D. (1903). *Bullying at School,* Oxford England Blackwell.

Reddy, S.P.; James, S.; Sewpaul, R.; Koopman, F.; Funoni, N.I.; Sifurda, S.; Jusie, S.; Masuka, R.; Kambaran, N.S.O.; Mardien, R.G. (2010), *Unthentle Uhlaba Usanila: The South African Youth Risk Behaviour Survey,* 2008. Cape Town: South African Medical Research Council (Online) at: *http://www.healthpromotion/healthpromotion.htm.*

Scanlon, T.J.; Tomkins., Lynch, M.A. and Scanlon, F. (1998). Street Children in Latin America. *British Medical Journal,* 316, 1596.

Stormashak, E.; Bierman, K.; Bruschi, C.; Dodge, K. and Cole, J.D. (1999). The relation between behaviour problems and peer preference in different classroom context, *Child Development,* 70(1), pp. 169-182.

Suliman, S. Mkbile, S.G.; Fincham, D.S.; Ahmed R.; Stein, D.J. and Seedat, S. (2009). Commutative effect of multiple trauma on symptoms of post-traumatic stress disorder, anxiety and depression in adolescents *Comprehensive Psychiatry,* 50(2), 121-127.

Tordanova, V.; Stewart, R.; Goldberg. D.; Babbington, P.E.; Brugha, T.; Singetton, N.; Meltzer, H. (2007). Age variation in life events and their relationship with common mental disorder in a national survey population, *Social Psychiatry and Social Epidemiology,* 42(8), 611-616.

UNICEF (2006). Juvenile Justice in South Asia: Improving protection for children in conflict with the law. (online) from: *http://www.unicef.org/rasa/juvenilejustice in south Asia*.pdf.

UNICEF Nations (2006). Convention on the rights of person with disabilities. (online) *http://www.un.org/disabilities.conventions/conventionfull.shtm.*

Wernham, M. (2004). An outside Chance: Street Children and Juvenile justice: an international perspective. Consortium of street children. (online) from *http://www.crin.org/resourceinfordata.*

West, A. (2003). At the margins: Street Children in Asia and the Pacific. Asian Development Bank No. 8 (online) from *http://www.adb.org/publications/marginsstreet-children-asia and pacific.*

World Health Organization (2008). *Mental Hhealth Policy and Development and Implementation in South Africa Situation Analysis.*

World Health Organization (2008). Mental health policy and implements in South Africa: A information analysis. Geneva Retrived.

2 Mental Health Issues of Women

Khushbu Rani and *S.C. Tiwari*

Mental health is a state of emotional and social well-being that allows an individual to cope with the normal stresses of life and achieve their occupational potential. A mental health problem interferes with a person's cognitive, emotional and social abilities, but to a lesser extent than a mental illness. Mental health problems are more common and less severe than mental illnesses, and generally of shorter duration.

In this review, a gendered, social model of health is used to investigate critical determinants of women's mental health with the overall objective of contributing to improved, more effective promotion of women's mental health, that is grounded in research evidence. Adverse factors for mental disorder as well as for good mental health are addressed and where possible, a clear distinction has been made between the opportunities that exist for individual action and individual behaviour change and those that are dependent on factors outside the control of the individual woman.

It is essential to recognize how the socio-cultural, economic, legal, infrastructural and environmental factors that affect women's mental health are configured in each country or community setting. Only by responding to the complexities and particularities of women's lives' can health promotion strategies hope to increase the opportunities women want and need to control the determinants of their health.

Common Psychiatric Problems in Women

Mental illnesses affect women and men differently—some disorders are more common in women, and some express themselves with different symptoms. The common mental disorders affecting women include the following:

Anxiety Disorders, (including OCD, Panic, Social Phobia, and Generalized Anxiety Disorders)

In general, women are more likely than men to suffer from anxiety disorders, and anxiety symptoms may increase during periods. Some women who have a diagnosed anxiety disorder, like obsessive-compulsive disorder, may notice even more severe anxiety during their periods than at other times during the month. Other women may only experience anxiety symptoms when they get their periods.

Women are twice as likely to experience anxiety disorders as men. About 60 per cent of the people with phobias or obsessive compulsive disorder are women. Phobias affect about 22 in 1,000 women, compared with 13 in 1,000 men (http://www.mentalhealth.org.uk).

Anxiety disorders are mental health conditions that involve excessive amounts of anxiety, fear, nervousness, worry, or dread. Anxiety that is too constant or too intense can cause a person to feel preoccupied, distracted, tense, and always on alert. Other women may only experience anxiety symptoms when they get their menstrual periods. Menstrual disorders often manifest by a combination of physical, psychological, and emotional symptoms related to menstrual process.

Bipolar Disorder

Bipolar Disorder (also known as manic depression) causes serious shifts in mood, energy, thinking, and behaviour—from the highs of mania on one extreme, to the lows of depression on the other. More than just a fleeting good or bad mood, the cycles of bipolar disorder last for days, weeks, or months and unlike ordinary mood swings, the mood changes of bipolar disorder are so intense that they interfere with your ability to function. During a manic episode, a person might impulsively quit a job, charge up huge amounts on credit cards, or feel rested after sleeping two hours. During a depressive episode, the same person might be too tired to get out of bed, and full of self-loathing and hopelessness over being unemployed and in debt. The causes of bipolar disorder aren't completely understood, but it often appears to be hereditary. The first manic or depressive episode of bipolar disorder usually occurs in the teenage years or early adulthood.

Bipolar Disorder, or manic-depressive illness, is a type of mood disorder characterized by recurrent episodes of highs (mania) and lows (depression) in mood. These episodes involve extreme changes in mood, energy, and behaviour.

Depression is one of the most common and recurrent disorder that affects people today. It affects a person's physical, emotional, social and psychological well-being. People those suffer from depression experience a low mood, profound and persisting feelings of sadness or despair, decreased self-esteem and confidence, loss of interest in things that were pleasurable in the past, as well as appetite and sleep disturbances.

More women than men experience depression. One in four women will require treatment for depression at some time in their life, compared with one in 10 men. The reasons for this are unclear, but are thought to include social factors such as poverty and isolation and biological factors such as the hormonal changes experienced by women. However, some researchers dispute the relatively low depression rate for men.

Major depressive disorder is the most common mood disorder and is ranked fourth in the list of the most urgent health problems worldwide by WHO with the life time prevalence of depressive disorder of around 10-25 per cent for women and 5-12 per cent for men (Kaplan, H.I., Sadock B.J., 1998).

The World Health Organization has ranked depression as one of the most disabling disorder in the world since depression can have a negative impact on one or both aspects of a person's life: the intrapersonal level and the interpersonal level (family life, social life, work setting). In addition to its prevalence, depression also has a high rate of recurrence. The recurrence rate may be associated with (i) Genetic vulnerability, (ii) early symptoms onset, (iii) poor diagnosis and treatment, and (iv) inadequate prevention.

Postpartum depression: Postpartum depression (PPD) is temporary depression related to pregnancy and childbirth. It comes in two forms: early onset commonly referred to as the "baby blues," and late onset. The early onset type is mild and may affect as many as 80 per cent of women after they deliver. It starts after delivery and usually resolves within a couple of weeks without medical treatment. The later onset form is what most people think of as postpartum depression. This more severe form is usually recognized several weeks after delivery. Overall, it affects about 10 per cent to 16 per cent of women.

Symptoms of mild PPD include sadness, anxiety, tearfulness, and trouble sleeping. These symptoms usually appear within several days of delivery and go away 10 to 12 days after the birth. Usually the only treatment needed is reassurance and some help with household chores and care of the baby. About 20 per cent of women who have postpartum blues will develop more lasting depression. It is very important to let your health care provider know if you experience "blues" that last longer than two weeks (*http://as.webmd.com/html.ng.*). Studies report prevalence rates among women from 5 per cent to 25 per cent. Focusing on depression in expectant and new fathers the prenatal and postpartum depression not limited to mothers. Postpartum depression usually begins in the first few months after childbirth.

Post-traumatic stress disorder (PTSD): Post-traumatic stress disorder (PTSD) is a mental health condition that is triggered by a terrifying event. Symptoms may include flashbacks, nightmares and severe anxiety, as well as uncontrollable thoughts about the event.

Many people who go through traumatic events have difficulty adjusting and coping for a while. But with time and taking care, such traumatic reactions usually get better. In some cases, though, the symptoms can get worse or last for months or even years. Sometimes, they may completely shake up your life. In a case such as this, you may have post-traumatic stress disorder.

Post-traumatic Stress Disorder (PTSD) is an emotional illness that that is classified as an anxiety disorder and usually develops as a result of a terribly frightening, life-threatening, or otherwise highly unsafe experience. PTSD sufferers re-experience the traumatic event or events in some way, tend to avoid places, people, or other things that remind them of the event (avoidance), and are exquisitely sensitive to normal life experiences. Worldwide, more women are affected by PTSD than men, largely because women are exposed to more sexual violence. The risk of developing PTSD after any traumatic event is 20.4 per cent for women and 8.1 per cent for men (http://www.mentalhealth.org.uk).

Specific Psychiatric Problems in Women

Schizophrenia is a chronic, severe, debilitating mental illness that affects about 1 per cent of the population, more than 2 million people in the United States. With the sudden onset of severe psychotic symptoms, the individual is said to be experiencing acute schizophrenia (http://www.medicinenet.com/alcohol). Schizo affective disorders appears to be more common in women (Alcoholism and Alcohol Abuse) (Alcohol Use Disorder, 2014).

Mental handicap mentally handicapped persons is not able to learn or develop skills at the same rate as most other people because they have a problem with their brain. It is now considered more polite to say that someone is learning disabled or that they have special needs or learning difficulties. It is more common in males (M:F = 4:3) with intellectual and developmental disabilities.

Alcoholism

Alcohol abuse and dependence, now both included under the diagnosis of alcohol use disorder, is a disease that is characterized by the sufferer having a pattern of drinking excessively despite the negative effects of alcohol on the individual's work, medical, legal, educational, and/or social life. It may involve a destructive pattern of alcohol use that includes a number of symptoms, including tolerance to or withdrawal from the substance, using more alcohol and/or for a longer time than planned, and trouble reducing its use. Alcohol abuse, on the less severe end of the alcohol use disorder spectrum, affects about 10 per cent of women and 20 per cent of men in the United States, most beginning by their mid-teens. Alcohol, especially when consumed in excess, can affect teens, women, men, and the elderly quite differently. Risk factors for developing a drinking problem include low self-esteem, depression, anxiety or another mood problem, as well as having parents with alcoholism (Sadhu & Malik, 2003). However, alcoholism is 8 times more common in men.

Substance Abuse in Women

In India, the Hindu scriptures condemned the social use of alcohol and other drugs but encouraged their use in religious ceremonies. *Bhang* was and still used in worship while *charas* and *ganjas* have been used to facilitate meditation by priests for centuries. Some Indian *sadhus* use *dhatura*. Other religions like Islam clearly prohibit the use of intoxicants, particularly alcohol (Sadhu, & Malik, 2003).

Despite the absence of reliable statistics, the overwhelming consensus, based on the available information, indicates that the number of women, especially in urban areas, resorting to alcohol and drugs is on the increase. NIMHANS noted a fourfold increase in the number of women registering their alcohol-related problems over the last ten years. The use of heroin has also increased among women in different cities throughout India. A rapid assessment survey conducted in 14 cities in India in 2000-01, showed that women substance abusers represented a mean of 7.9 per cent of the sample and the heroin, alcohol, cannabis and painkillars were the dominant substance of abuse. Female substance users were generally single, educated and employed, had an early onset of substance use, and engaged in unsafe practice such as early initiation into sex and sharing injecting equipment (Sharma, 2009).

Excessive partner alcohol use increased the risk for substance use disorders two to threefold. Partner violence and alcohol-related problems each partially mediated the association between partner excessive alcohol use and these mental disorders. Women's own violence-related attitudes were also independently associated with them (Nayak, Patel, Bond & Greenfield, 2010). Peer pressure, a need for excitement and stress appear to operate as initiators into drug use. High levels of drug use in the household, early sexual experience, financial independence all appear to increase the vulnerabilities (Sharma, 2009).

Premenstrual Dysphoric Disorder

Premenstrual syndrome (PMS) is a combination of emotional, physical, psychological, and mood disturbances that occur after a woman's ovulation and typically ending with the onset of her menstrual flow. The most common mood-related symptoms are irritability, depression, crying, oversensitivity, and mood swings with alternating sadness and anger. The most common physical symptoms are fatigue, bloating, breast tenderness, acne and appetite changes with food cravings.

A more severe form of PMS, known as premenstrual dysphoric disorder (PMDD), also known as late luteal phase dysphoric disorder) occurs in a smaller number of women and leads to significant loss of function because of unusually severe symptoms. The American Psychiatric Association characterizes PMDD as a severe form of PMS in which anger, irritability, anxiety and tension are especially prominent. The Clinical features of PMS includes—Recurrence of symptoms between ovulation and menstruation—subsidence during; menstruation, and absent between menstruation and ovulation. The Physical symptoms related to PMS are feeling bloated, weight gain, tender breasts, headache, backache, and cramps. In addition to physical symptoms the psychological changes germinated by PMS includes tension, irritability, depression, tiredness and forgetfulness.

Social Disadvantage and Mental Health

Poor educational status, the lack of specialized vocational training, starting work at a young age, early marriage, and a lack of social support are the social disadvantages. These factors become particularly important in periods of rapidly changing roles and lifestyles and when people are suffering from specific vulnerabilities (Sharma, 2009).

Sex Violence and Mental Health of Women

Women experience various forms of discrimination in public and private life. One of the biggest results of discrimination is violence. Women's mental health is affected by gender-based violence is a serious violence of women's human rights. Yet little attention has been paid to the mental health of women and girls. Women who have experienced physical, sexual, or psychological violence suffer a range of health problems, often in silence. Abortions can result in chronic pelvic pain, vaginal bleeding or discharge, vaginal infection, painful menstrual discharge, sexual dysfunction, fibroids, pelvic inflammatory disease, urinary tract infection and infertility. Rates of depression are high in women attending gynaecological clinics and qualitative studies demonstrate a strong relationship among vaginal discharge, weakness, psychosomatic symptoms and psychosocial stress. In sex selective abortion cases, women generally suffer from depression, post-traumatic stress disorder, sleep difficulties and emotional distress. The best way of preventing the sex selective abortions is the economic empowerment and education of women. Women should be encouraged to engage in economic activities and to earn their own living so that they are not considered to be a burden on the family (Sharma, 2009).

Psychosocial Factor of Mental Health in Women

Disruptive, negative life events that cannot be controlled or evaded are most strongly related to the onset of depressive symptoms. An increase in the number of such events is paralleled by an increase in the numbers of women becoming depressed. The size of the contribution made by these events to common mental disorders is evident from a number of studies on women's mental health carried out over recent years in different countries.

Severe, disruptive negative events could involve loss or danger but other features were more important in initiating depression. The experience of humiliation, defeat and a sense of entrapment, often in relation to a core relationship, were found to be more important than the actual loss. Almost three quarters of the severe events occurring in the six months prior to the onset of depression involved entrapment or humiliation whereas just over one-fifth involved loss alone and only 5 are concerned danger alone (Brown, Harris, & Hepworth, 1995).

Gender and Co-morbidity

The multi-country WHO studies on psychological problems in general health care also found that current panic attacks and a diagnosis of panic disorder were frequently associated with the presence of a depressive disorder. Women predominated in all three disorders panic attacks, panic disorder and depressive disorder. The combination of these disorders results in a long lasting and severe disorder that was linked to a higher rate of suicidality (Lecrubier & Ustun, 1998).

Previous study examined gender differences in a range of lifetime psychiatric disorders in a sample of 272 offenders newly admitted to a prison substance abuse programme. Although these men and women did not differ in severity of substance use in the six months prior to incarceration, women were significantly more likely than men to report a lifetime psychiatric disorder and a lifetime severe disorder. Furthermore, gender differences emerged in the pattern of lifetime psychiatric comorbidity. Women reported greater lifetime major depression, post-traumatic stress disorder, eating disorder, and borderline personality disorder; men were more likely than women to meet criteria for antisocial personality disorder. Additionally, female offenders were found to have a higher degree of internalizing disorders than male offenders, but there were no gender differences in degree of externalizing disorders (Zlotnick, Clarke, Friedmann, Roberts, Sacks, & Melnick, 2008).

Professional Therapies

The professional therapies can be of four types in order to treat and give help to the client—psychotherapy, behaviour therapy, yogic therapy and drug therapy. The kind of approaches generally in the context of helping women with mental health problems in all the three above mentioned therapies is given below:

Psychotherapy

Cognitive Therapy is about the negative thoughts and beliefs, low self-esteem and lack of confidence that individuals may be experiencing, and learning to replace those negative thoughts and beliefs with positive ways of thinking.

Client-centred Psychotherapy aids individuals in finding their own solutions to their problems. Individuals are encouraged to discuss their experiences and express their feelings. The purpose is to allow individuals to arrive at solutions to their problems by examining their own thoughts. Individuals can then decide for themselves in what ways they need to change.

Solution-focused Brief Therapy is a specific type of Brief Therapy that focuses on what clients want to achieve through therapy rather than on the presenting problem(s) that prompted them to seek help.

Behaviour Therapy

Behaviour therapy is focused on helping an individual understand how changing their behaviour can lead to changes in how they are feeling. The goal of behaviour therapy is usually focused on increasing the person's engagement in positive or socially reinforcing activities. Behaviour therapy is a structured approach that carefully measures what the person is doing and then seeks to increase chances for positive experience. Common techniques include:

Self-Monitoring: This is the first stage of treatment. The person is asked to keep a detailed log of all of their activities during the day. By examining the list at the next session, the therapist can see exactly what the person is doing.

Schedule of Weekly Activities: In this technique patient and therapist work together to develop new activities that will provide the patient with chances for positive experience.

Role Playing: This is used to help the person develop new skills and anticipate issues that may come up in social interactions.

Behaviour Modification: In this technique the patient wiil receive a reward for engaging in positive behaviour (*http://psychcentral.com*).

Yogic Therapy

Sudarshan Kriya yoga emphasizes slow and modulated breathing (*ujjayi*, *bhastrika*, and Sudarshan Kriya yogic breathing) thought to alleviate anxiety, depression, everyday stress, post-traumatic stress, and stress-related medical illnesses. The mechanisms in Sudarshan Kriya yoga thought to contribute to calmness include increased parasympathetic drive, calming of stress response systems, and the reduction of neuroendocrine release of hormones, such as cortisol (Brown, R.P., Gerbarg, P.L., 2005).

During meditation, parts of the brain known to be involved in attention and in the control of the autonomic nervous system are activated, providing an anatomic and neurochemical basis for the effects of meditation on various physiologic activities (Cohen, S.; Doyle, W.J.; Turner, R.B. *et al.*, 2003). Meditation has been shown in one study to produce significant increases in left-sided anterior brain activity, which is associated with positive emotional states (http://nccam.nih.gov/health/whatiscam/#mindbody).

Patients with menstrual irregularities having psychological problems improved significantly in the areas of their well-being, anxiety and depression by learning and applying a programme based on Yogic intervention (*Yoga Nidra*) (Rani, Tiwari, Singh, Agrawal, Ghildiyal, Srivastava, 2011). The patients with mild to moderate anxiety and depressive symptoms improve significantly with '*Yoga Nidra*' intervention. There is no significant improvement in the patients with severe anxiety and depressive symptoms (Rani, Tiwari, Singh, Singh, Srivastava, 2012). *Yoga Nidra* appears to be a promising intervention for psychosomatic problems. It is cost-effective and easy to implement. The results indicate that somatoform symptoms in patients with menstrual disorder can be decreased by learning and applying a programme based on Yogic intervention (*Yoga Nidra*) (Rani, Tiwari, Singh, Agrawal, Srivastava, 2011). However, these studies were not randomized, controlled trials and, therefore, more research is needed to assess possible negative effects of meditation for individuals with mental illness.

Drug Therapy

Antidepressant and anti-anxiety drugs: Depression is commonly treated with antidepressant medications. Antidepressants work to balance some of the natural chemicals in our brains. These chemicals are called neurotransmitters, and they affect our mood and emotional responses. Antidepressants work on neurotransmitters such as serotonin, norepinephrine, and dopamine. The most popular types of antidepressants are called Selective Serotonin Reuptake Inhibitors (SSRIs). These include: Fluoxetine, Citalopram, Sertraline, Paroxetine, Escitalopram and Fluroxemine to name a few. Other types of antidepressants are Serotonin and Norepinephrine Reuptake Inhibitors (SNRIs). SNRIs are similar to SSRIs and include venlafaxine, desvenlafaxine, muneciprem and duloxetine. Another antidepressant that is commonly used is bupropion (Wellbutrin). Bupropion, which works on the neurotransmitter dopamine, is unique in that it does not fit into any specific drug type. SSRIs and SNRIs are popular because they do not cause as many side effects as older classes of antidepressants. Older antidepressant medications include tricyclics, tetracyclics, and Monoamine Oxidase Inhibitors (MAOIs). For some people, tricyclics, tetracyclics, or MAOIs may be the best medications.

Mood stabilizers: Mood stabilizer usually refers to a drug that treats and prevents both mania and depression, the up and down mood swings experienced by people with bipolar illness, also known as manic-depressive illness. Mood stabilizers can also treat depression, even if the person has never been manic. When used to treat depression, mood stabilizers are commonly combined with antidepressants. This either enhances the effect of the mood stabilizer or protects against a manic episode. Sometimes mood stabilizers are used alone to treat depression. The best-known drug in this category is lithium. Two other drugs, valproate and carbamazepine also have become established mood stabilizers. Other commonly used drugs are: Lithium, Valproate, Carbamazepine and Lamotrigine (*http://www.intelihealth.com/IH/ihtIH/W/9273/9273.html.*).

Antipsychotic drugs: Antipsychotic medications are used in those with bipolar disorder as a short-term treatment to control psychotic symptoms such as hallucinations or delusions or mania symptoms. Some also treat bipolar depression, and several have been demonstrated long-term value to prevent future episodes of mania or depression. These symptoms may occur during acute mania or severe depression. In people with bipolar disorder, antipsychotics are also used "off label" as sedatives, for insomnia for anxiety and for agitation. Often, they are taken with a mood-stabilizing drug and can decrease symptoms of mania until mood stabilizers take full effect. Some antipsychotic drugs may also help lessen bipolar depression (*http://www.webmd.com/drugs/index-drugs.aspx.*).

Conclusion

Working women in India continue to face a plethora of problems, most of which pertain to the family and the working environment. The attitude of the family should improve thus accepting working women sans homemaker as a single package, rather than sticking to the demands of traditional roles. Works place should be made as comfortable as possible to avoid any undue stress among working women. Reduce the stress of women should choose healthy life style good dietary habits, calcium and vitamin, adhering to an exercise regimen at least 2 or 3 times a week, practicing stress relaxation techniques, and avoiding alcohol and caffeine.

References

Alcoholism and Alcohol Abuse (Alcohol Use disorder). (2014). Medicine Net, Inc.21/01/2014. http://www.medicinenet.com/alcohol.

Antipsychotic Medication for Bipolar Disorder. Bipolar Disorder Health Center. http://www.webmd.com/drugs/index-drugs.aspx

Brown, G.W., Harris, T.O., Hepworth, C. (1995). Loss and depression, a patient and non-patient comparison. *Psychological Medicine*, 25, 7-21.

Brown, R.P.; Gerbarg, P.L. (2005). Sudarshan Kriya yogic breathing in the treatment of stress, anxiety, and depression: part I—neurophysiologic model. *J. Altern Complement Med.*; 11(1): 189-201.

Cohen, S.; Doyle, W.J.; Turner, R.B., *et al.* (2003). Emotional style and susceptibility to the common cold. *Psychosomatic Medicine,* 65(4): 652-657.

Kaplan, H.I., and Sȧdock, B.J. (1998). *Synopsis of Psychiatry* (8th edition). Waverly Ltd., New Delhi.

Lecrubier, Y., Ustun, T.B. (1998). Panic and depression, a worldwide primary care perspective. *International Clinical Psychopharmacology*, 13, Supplement 4, 7-11.

Madhabika, B. Nayak, Vikram Patel, Jason, C. Bond and Thomas, K. Greenfield. (2010). Partner alcohol use, violence and women's mental health: population-based survey in India. *BJP*, 196: 192-199.

Michael Herkov. About behaviour therapy. http://psychcentral.com.

Mind-body medicine. (2011). National Institutes of Health National Center for Complementary and Alternative Medicine. May 3, 2011. http://nccam.nih.gov/health/whatiscam/#mindbody.

Mood Stabilizers. Medical content reviewed by the faculty of Harvard Medical School. http://www.intelihealth.com/IH/ihtIH/W/9273/9273.html

Postpartum Depression Health Center. (2005-2014). http://as.webmd.com/html.ng

Paulson, J.F. (2010). "Focusing on depression in expectant and new fathers: prenatal and postpartum depression not limited to mothers". *Psychiatry Times*, 27(2).

Rani, K., Tiwari, S.C., Singh, U., Agrawal, G.G., Ghildiyal, A., Srivastava, N. (2011). Impact of *Yoga Nidra* on psychological general well-being in patients with menstrual irregularities: A randomized controlled trial. *International Journal of Yoga*; 4: 20-5.

Rani, K., Tiwari, S.C., Singh, U., Singh, I., Srivastava, N. (2012). *Yoga Nidra* as a complementary treatment of anxiety and depressive symptoms in patients with menstrual disorder. *International Journal of Yoga*; 5:52-6.

Rani, K., Tiwari, S.C., Singh, U., Agrawal, G.G., Srivastava, N. (2011). Six-month trial of Yoga Nidra in menstrual disorder patients: Effects on somatoform symptoms. *Indian Psychiatry Journal*; 20: 97-102.

Sadhu, D.S. and Malik, R. (2003). Ethnocultural background and substance abuse treatment of Asian Indian Americans in Straussner, S.L.A. (ed.). *Ethnocultural factors in substance abuse treatment*. (pp. 368-392). Guildford Press: New York.

Sharma, I. (Ed). (2009). Women Mental Health. Indian psychiatric society and Indian Medical Association—BHU in collaboration with BHU, Varanasi.

Schizophrenia. (2014). Medicine Net, Inc. 21/01/2014. http://www.medicinenet.com/alcohol.

Specific psychiatric problems in women.www.trickcyclists.co.uk.

Women and Mental Health. Mental Health Foundation. http://www.mentalhealth.org.uk.

Zlotnick, C., Clarke, J.G., Friedmann, P.D., Roberts, M.B., Sacks, S., Melnick, G. (2008). Gender differences in comorbid disorders among offenders in prison substance abuse treatment programmes. *Behavioural Science and the Law*; 26(4): 403-12.

3
Inculcating Subjective Well-Being in Hinduism by Adhering to a Spiritual Life Style

Chandra Bhal Dwivedi

Introduction

Style of life was brought into main realm of Psychology by Alfred Adler (1929). Style of life as conceived by Adler is the system principle by which the individual personality functions; it is the whole that commands the parts. The Hindu style of life, however, cannot be understood from that yardstick because Hinduism is considered more a style of life than a religion. It is very difficult to separate the living and religion in the life of a devout Hindu. Both are so intricately interwoven into one another that one cannot be conceived of without considering the other. Both complement each other. Spirituality and religion are part and parcel of a Hindu's life.

Hinduism attached so much importance to spirituality that it had made it the ultimate goal of life and attempted to visualize spirituality in every walk of life. Opening *śloka* of the *Iśāvāsyopaniṣad* states:

Iśāvāsyamidam sarvam yatkiñca jagatyāñjagat
Tena tyaktena bhuñjīthāh mā gridhah kasya svid dhanam

It means that whatever is there in this world is the abode of the Lord. Realizing that this all is His you make use of it without greed, for whose wealth is it after all. This approach towards sacredness in everything inculcates spirituality in a person. The conceptualization of human reality in the indigenous Indian tradition has been undertaken at several levels.

These levels place human beings in their total eco-systemic context, which encompasses the material, the socio-cultural, as well as the spiritual worlds together. It construes human existence as a part of the universal order which is perceived as natural. In the Western view the terms—mind, spirit, and consciousness—are all synonymous indicating the main characteristics of the being. There it is thought to be an immaterial substance. In contrast to this, ancient Indians put it in most unambiguous terms that mind is something material and different from consciousness. More specifically, mind according to Indian point of view is a metabolic energy that has a tendency to stabilize itself in the uppermost part of the body, presumably the heart *Śiva samkalpa sūkta* of the *Śukla Yajurveda* tells us—

> *Suṣārathiraśvāniva yanmanuṣyān nenīyate'bhiśubhirvājina iva Hṛtpratiṣṭham yadajiram javiṣṭham tanme manah śiva samkalpamastu* (34/6)

"May that mind of mine, which guides living beings from one place to another, as a good charioteer does with horses, and controls them by reins, which resides in the heart and is never old, which is very fast, be of auspicious resolutions"—Tr. Ramesh Kumar Pandey (1997). The indigenous Indian approach emphasizes a continuous relationship between man and nature. It places *man in nature* against the Western approach of *man over nature*. The harmonious and non-separate relationship between man and nature leads to inculcating spirituality across all life forms. This realization is reflected in Hindu daily practices. Immediately as a Hindu gets up in the morning he recites these *ślokas:*

> *Karāgre vasate lakṣmih karamadhye sarasvati*
> *Karamūle to govindah prabhāte karadarśanam*

"*Lakṣmī* resides at the tips of the fingers, *Sarasvatī* in the middle of the hand, and *Lord Govinda* at the roots of the palm. Thus the hand must be seen in the morning"—Tr. Ramesh Kumar Pandey (1997). This is followed by the recital of a *mantram* seeking permission and forgiveness from Mother Earth for treading on it:

> *Samudravasane devi! parvatastanamaṇdite*
> *viṣṇupatni namastubhyam pādaspaṣrśam kṣamasva me*

"O Devi! (Mother Earth), wife of Lord Viṣṇu, whose clothes are the ocean, whose breasts are the mountains, I salute you and beg your forgiveness for placing my feet on you"—Tr. Ramesh Kumar Pandey (1997).

Spirituality is now being considered inseparable from all walks of life including psychotherapy (*see* Miller, 2012; Pargament, 2011) though one cannot fail to notice that there are many different views on what it means to be spiritual. In modern usage it includes such a wide range of human experience—traditional religious practices, personal mystical experience, ecstatic meditational experiences, and the quest for meaning in life—that researchers have not been able to agree on a universal definition that can be applicable for all those phenomena. There is no one clear and comprehensive definition of spirituality in the literature. Partly for this reason, nearly all the research on spirituality and health measures religious commitment or practices and labels them as relating to spirituality.

Spirituality appears to be a multidimensional construct in which a few core constructs repeatedly emerge. Spirituality implies that there is a deeper dimension to human life an inner world of the soul. It assumes that humans are fundamentally spiritual in their pure consciousness. It is noticeable that in the modern usage "spirituality and consciousness are at the extreme end of ambiguity. Even the notion of science with its intrinsic implication of objectivity has gone through a bewildering array of disputations. To further compound the confusion, the concepts of science and spirituality are conceived in the Western tradition as polar opposites that are hermetically sealed in the tightly compartmentalized behavioural loops. However, in the classical Indian tradition, the dichotomies such as science and spirituality are less sharp permitting their possible coexistence in a holistic conception of human nature" (Rao, 2011a, pp. 14-15).

Rolland (1960), while comparing the Western and Indian knowledge, described Western knowledge as the "science of facts" and spirituality as "the science of the soul, a peculiarly Indian science" (p. 91). While attempting a psychological analysis of the concepts of the *Bhagavadgîta*, Dharam Bhawuk (2011) noted that "a major difference between philosophy and spirituality, or for that matter religion and spirituality, is that spirituality, as practiced in India, has an action bias over and above cognitive (thinking or thoughts) or value (considering something important concerns. Spirituality has been valued in the Indian culture from time immemorial, and it is no surprise that many innovations in the field of spirituality originated in India" (p. 25).

In this context Akbar Husain, Moazziz Beg and Chandra Bhal Dwivedi (2013) very pertinently noted that "the spiritual heritage of India is one of the world's standing miracles. It would rank among its greatest human achievements. It is more like a reception—the opening of a people to receive, through inspiration the Vedas or the Breath of the Eternal; for the outbreathing of the Eternal is what India has taken truth of the Veda to be. It was Truth Itself—truth that had become incarnate in the tradition that sustained them; inasmuch as the truth is so subtle, so abstruse that knowing it fully merges with being. Only when discerned in a life that is living it—a life that incarnates it in its outlook, moods, and conduct—that the truth of this order becomes fully convincing. If we see the Vedas in this light, as apertures through which the Infinite entered conscious human awareness, what word of the Infinite do the Vedas impart? First the warning that on this topic words are unequal to their task; a fundamental Vedic understanding concerns the limitations of words themselves when directed towards the Infinite. In this kind of knowing words do not cause understanding; at best they can occasion it as from spirit to spirit communion leaps" (p. 126).

The Meaning of Spirituality

The word 'spirituality' is more frequently described in a variety of ways than defined operationally. The word derives from the Latin *spirare*, which means, to breathe. In the modern usage it includes such a wide range of human experience that the researchers have not been able to offer any universally agreed definition for measuring this inner experience. Koenig, McCullough and Larson (2001), in their *Handbook of Religion and Health*, point out the inadequacy of dictionary meanings of religion and spirituality and list several distinguishing characteristics of each of these. According to them, religion is community-focused, observable, measurable and objective, whereas spirituality is individualistic, less visible and measurable, and more subjective. Similarly, religion is organized, behaviour-oriented and involves several outward practices, while spirituality is less formal and systematic, and more inward-directed.

Koenig *et al.* (2001) described religion as 'an organized system of beliefs, practices, rituals and symbols' and spirituality as 'the personal quest for understanding answers to ultimate questions about life, about meaning and about relationship to the sacred or transcendent…' (p. 18).

Empirical studies have almost unequivocally shown religion and spirituality as overlapping constructs and Miller and Thoresen (1999) have even pointed out that "the field of religion is to spirituality as the field of medicine is to health" (p. 28). According to Peter Hill and Kenneth Pargament (2003), "the sacred, which includes the divine and the transcendent, is the common denominator of religious and spiritual life. Spirituality is a search for the sacred, a process through which people seek to discover, hold on to, and, when necessary, transform whatever they hold sacred in their lives" (p. 65). It becomes apparent that in the West spirituality is considered as a concept of an immaterial reality. It is considered as an inner path enabling a person to discover the essence of one's being or the deepest values and meanings by which people live. As such spiritual practices including prayer, meditation and contemplation have been included in spirituality to develop an individual's inner life.

It was in that spirit that Akbar Husain (2011, pp. 24-43) attempted to describe and operationalise spiritual knowledge and practice. The spiritual knowledge domain according to him includes sacredness, positive energy, intellect, reasoning, inner experience, transcendence, universalism, awareness, life force, intuition, transformation, and yearning. On the other hand, the spiritual practice domain includes the aspects of sacraments, purification, initiation, renunciation, illumination, temperance, unity, awakening, love, imagination, tranquillity and yoga.

Spirituality in Hinduism

Since time immemorial a spiritual aspiration has been the governing force or the core of thought and ruling passion of Hinduism. Every Hindu follows *sanātana dharma* which may be roughly translated as the Eternal Path or Code. It has its own peculiarity in that *sanātana dharma* was not founded or revealed by any particular historical person. It had made spirituality its highest aim of life and it tried to turn the whole of life towards spirituality. It is seen in the importance attached by the Hindus to the four *puruṣārthas*, viz., *dharma, artha, kāma,* and *mokṣa.*

Dharma is derived from root *dhṛ* meaning to hold or support. Thus, *dharma* is what maintains and supports life and universe; it is the way of life that supports life, which without the way, will be dissipated and destroyed. The *Vaiśeṣika Sūtra* defines *dharma* as "*dharma* is that by which one attains righteous advancement in life as well as release from the bondage of rebirth"[1]—Author's translation. In the same spirit the Karṇa Parva (ch 69/58) of the *Mahābhārata* defines *dharma* in these words:

"Rendered into English, it means *Dharma* sustains the society, *dharma* maintains the social order, *dharma* ensures well-being and progress of humanity, *dharma* is surely that which fulfils these objectives"[2]—Author's translation.

Thus *dharma* is what maintains and supports life and universe. The second *puruṣārtha* of *artha* is meant for acquiring worldly materials to adequately mange one's *dharma*. The third *puruṣārtha* of *kāma* is the desire for attaining mundane and spiritual knowledge. These three *puruṣārthas* are only meant for preparing oneself towards the last *puruṣārtha* of *mokṣa* which shows the inherent spirituality in the Hindu mindset. The fact that *mokṣa* was considered as the most important *puruṣārtha* becomes apparent when we see the four *āśramas* that were proposed for pursuing each of these four *puruṣārthas* in an orderly sequence. The *āśramas* are– *brahmacarya, gārhasthya, vānaprastha* and *saṁnyāsa*.

K. Ramakrishna Rao (2011b) has suggested that "there is a general consensus between the Indian and Western perspectives that the common ground between religion and spirituality is the sacred. The sacred may refer to different things such as god, divinity, ultimate reality and so on. The common denominator of all of them, it would seem, is transcendence. Transcendence implies going beyond what is given in one's normal sensory experience. In the spiritual traditions of India, whether Hindu or Buddhist, there is an overwhelming emphasis on transcendence as a state of being that goes well beyond sensory awareness. Spiritual pursuit is an exercise for transformation of the human condition to achieve transcendence" (p. 9).

Moreover, the Indian approach to spirituality is unambiguous. The Sanskrit equivalent word of spirituality is *adhyātma*, which is obtained by combining the prefix *adhi* with the word *ātma* (or self). It denotes subjectivity (*ātmānam adhikṛtya*) as well as *ātmano viṣayakam jñānam* or the transcendental knowledge pertaining to the Self. The fundamental idea of Hinduism is one common to the highest thinking everywhere. It maintains that the supreme truth of all that is apparent is a Being or an existence beyond the mental and physical appearance. There is a firm belief in the Hindu mindset that beyond mind, life and body there is a Spirit and Self-containing all that is finite and infinite surpassing all that is relative, an Eternal and Supreme Absolute, from which all transient elements originate and which supports them all.

Hinduism did not set a single narrow path of manifesting that spirituality in man. Unity in diversity has been its greatest virtue. It has maintained that the same truth can be realized by following the path of one's own choice. But whatever be our way of reaching that Truth, the one important reality of spiritual experience is that He is in the heart and centre of all existence and all existence is in Him and to find Him is the greatest self-finding. Differences in creedal belief and dogmas are to the Hindu mind nothing more than various ways of actualizing and realizing the one Self and Godhead in all. Self-realization has been always regarded as the highest goal of life. To open to the inner Spirit, to live in the Infinite, to seek after and discover the Eternal, to be in the union with God is the common idea and aim of Hinduism. That indeed has been the sense of spiritual salvation, the living truth that fulfils and releases. This dynamic following after the highest spiritual truth and the highest spiritual aim are the uniting bond of Hinduism. That approach is also visible in the practices of self-restraints (*yamas*) and self-observances (*niyamas*). In the present paper I will briefly elaborate these practices as aids in inculcating spirituality in Hinduism.

Sri Aurobindo (1972) has contended in *The Foundations of Indian Culture* that "Indian religion placed four necessities before human life. First, it imposed upon the mind a belief in the highest consciousness or a state of existence universal and transcendent of the universe, from which all comes, in which all lives and moves without knowing it and of which all must one day grow aware, returning towards that which is perfect, eternal and infinite. Next, it laid upon the individual life the need for self-preparation by development and experience till he or she is ready for an effort to grow consciously into the truth of this greater existence. Thirdly, it provided it with a well-founded, well-explored, many-branching and always enlarging way of knowledge and of spiritual discipline. Lastly, for those not yet ready for these higher steps it provided an organisation of the individual and collective life, a framework for personal and social discipline and conduct, of mental and moral and vital development by which they could each move in his own limits and according to one's own nature in such a way as to become eventually ready for the greatest and highest existence. The first three of these elements are the most essential to any religion, but Hinduism has always attached to the last also a great importance; it has left out no part of life as a thing secular and foreign to the religious and spiritual life" (p. 124).

What is Meant by Self-Restraint (*Yama*)?

Self-restraints and self-observances are foundational to all yogic thoughts.

Dwivedi (1967) (and more recently Husain, Beg and Dwivedi, 2013) has shown that *Yoga* is practical psychology. Apart from *Yoga* it is also seen that to inculcate spirituality several observances and restraints have been suggested in almost all religious systems. Most of these are shared universally by Jews, Christians, Buddhists, Jaina, Muslims, Sikhs and others. However, in most of these systems they have been described as observances to be followed in order to avoid punishment; in Hinduism they have attained prominence with regard to the inculcation of spirituality in an aspirant. *Yama* has been defined by Raja Radhakant Deva (1857/1967) in his encyclopaedic dictionary the *Śabdakalpadruma* (Volume 4, p. 19), as "that which controls and directs sense-driven activities is *yama*"[3] (Author's translation). *Yama* is derived from root *yam* which when attached with suffix *ghaiñ* makes the word *yama.* It means control. *Amarakośa* (3.9.18) has similarly defined *yama* as "—*yama* is control in one's actions by resorting to ideals and principles"[4] (Author's translation). Śaṅkarācārya while commenting on *śloka* 13.149.30 of the *Mahābhārata*[5], i.e., has defined *yama* as "that by which one conducts one's journey within is *yama*"[6] (Author's translation).

Yama is rooted in the notion of developing a positive personality. It defines the attributes to be practiced by a spiritual aspirant. Adhering to the observation of *yama* means sticking to one's ideals and principles. It is about the development of positive traits that will transform the human nature into a divine nature and annihilate cravings and negative qualities. About the absolute necessity of *yamas* and *niyamas* Sri Aurobindo (1971) has stated in the *Synthesis of yoga* that "It (Rājayoga) does not start with *Āsana* and *Prāṇāyāma*, but insists first on a moral purification of the mentality. This preliminary is of supreme importance; without it the course of the rest of the *Rājayoga* is likely to be troubled, marred and full of unexpected mental, moral and physical perils. This moral purification is divided in the established system under two heads, five *Yamas* and five *Niyamas*. The first are rules of moral self-control in conduct such as truth-speaking, abstinence from injury or killing, from theft, etc.; but in reality these must be regarded as merely certain main indications of the general need of moral self-control and purity. *Yama* is, more largely, any self-discipline by which the rajasic egoism and its passions and desires in the human being are conquered and quieted into perfect cessation. The object is to create a moral calm, a void of the passions, and so prepare for the death of egoism in the *rajasic* human being. The *Niyamas* are equally a discipline of the mind by regular practices of which the highest is meditation on the divine Being, and their object is to create a *sattvic* calm, purity and preparation for concentration upon which the secure pursuance of the rest of the *Yoga* can be founded" (pp. 516-217).

Techniques of Self-Restraints (*Yamas*)

In *Yoga-Sūtra* self-restraints (*yama*) and self-observances (*niyama*) have been described in Book II, aphorism 29 as the first two limbs of Yoga and Vyāsa while commenting on this aphorism states that "they must be performed in succession"[7]—Translation James Woods (1914/2007, p. 178). The next aphorism mentions their names. "Abstinence from injury and from falsehood and from theft and from incontinence and from acceptance of gifts are the abstentions"[8]—Tr. Woods, (1914/2007, p. 178). *Haṭhayoga Pradīpikā* and different *Purāṇās* have described ten *yamas* and there exists difference in their enlisting also. For example, *Haṭhayoga Pradīpikā*[9], *Skanda Purāṇa* (5.91)[10] and *Garuḍa Purāṇa* (chapter 109)[11] have enumerated *yamas* in a different manner.

Pooling these lists we come across so many kinds of *yamas.* Limiting them to five or ten was not the purpose of the Hindu spiritual teachers. Surendranath Dasgupta (1922/1991) explains the purpose of enlistment of *yamas.* "The purpose of *Yoga* meditation is to steady the mind on the gradually advancing stages of thoughts towards liberation, so that vicious tendencies may gradually be more and more weakened and at last disappear altogether. But before the mind can be fit for this lofty meditation, it is necessary that it should be purged of ordinary impurities. Thus, the intending *yogin* should practice absolute non-injury to all living beings (*ahiṁsā*), absolute and strict truthfulness (*satya*), non-stealing (*asteya*), absolute sexual restraint (*brahmacarya*), and the acceptance of nothing but that which is absolutely necessary (*aparigraha*)" (Dasgupta, 1922/1991, p. 270). Dasgupta (1953/2006) has further stated these things in his Introduction to the third Volume of *the Cultural Heritage of India.* According to Haridas Bhattacharyya (1953/2006) "the *Yoga-Sūtra* agrees with Buddhism and Jainism that men's minds are constantly swayed by thoughts of expanding the self at the cost of others. Thoughts of injury, deceit, unlawful gain sex, and greed toss the soul from object to object and keep up the stream of thought and activity. It is very necessary for the *yogin* to control these wild propensities of the mind by cultivating the habits of non-injury (*ahiṁsā*), truthfulness (*satya*), non-stealing (*asteya*), continence (*brahmacarya*), and non-acceptance of gifts (*aparigraha)*" (p. 86).

1. Abstinence-from-injury (Ahiṁsā)

While explaining five *yamas*, Vyāsa has very categorically stated that "of these (five) abstinence from injury means the abstinence from malice towards all living creatures in all way and at all times. And the other abstinences and observances are rooted in it. In so far as their aim is the perfection of it, they are taught in order to teach it"[12]—Tr. Woods, (1914/2007), p. 178. The guiding word here is *anabhidrohah,* which is formed by adding prefix *abhi* to *drohah.* The word *droha* stands for hatred as well as malice and when it is added with prefix *abhi*, it is used to denote causing pain with a feeling of malice toward everyone. However, word *a* is added to it the meaning changes altogether and then it denotes complete absence of malice and pain towards all.

Vācaspati Miśra, while commenting on the gloss of Vyāsa, says: " 'rooted in it' would mean that, even if these are performed without observing abstinence from injury, they are as if they had not been performed, since they are quite fruitless." This is the meaning. The following up of them has nothing as its aim but the perfection of this [abstinence-from-killing]. 'If abstinence-from-killing has the others rooted in it, how can it be that they aim at the perfection of the abstinence-from-injury?' to this he replies, "in order to teach it"[13]—Tr. Woods, (1914/2007) p. 179. In the same manner Vijñāna Bhikṣu in his elaboration (*vṛtti*) of the gloss of Vyāsa on this aphorism says "this is to be qualified by the expression 'by not opposing the daily duties assigned to the *āśramas*' because it is not possible to avoid injury to tiny living things during the process of cleansing etc. (of oneself)"[14]—Tr. T.S. Rukmani, (2001), p. 189.

There is a deliberate order in the five *yamas*. *Ahiṁsā* (abstinence-from-injury or non-violence) comes first because one must remove one's brutal nature first. One must become non-violent and develop a cosmic love. Only and only then does one become fit for the practice of *yoga*. *Ahiṁsā* is abstention from injuring any living creature. On the spiritual path, the first step is to eliminate the beastly nature. The predominant trait in beasts is cruelty; therefore, the wise sages prescribed *ahiṁsā* as the first *yama*. *Ahiṁsā* is not merely non-killing. It is perfect harmlessness and positive love. It is to abstain from the slightest thought of harm to any living creature. The practitioner must abandon even unkind looks. There is no excuse or exception to this rule. Harsh words to beggars, servants or inferiors are also *hiṁsā* (cruelty). To fail to relieve pain or trouble in another is negative *hiṁsā*. To approve of another's harsh actions is also a kind of *hiṁsā.*

Absolute abstinence-from-injury is required in order to proceed ahead on the path of spiritual journey. In order to emphasise this point further, Patañjali says in the next aphorism (II.31) "when practiced without any exception on grounds of class, place, time or other obligations, they constitute the great vow (*mahā-vratam*)"[15]—Tr. K. Ramakrishna Rao (2011a, p. 606). It would be apparent that the *yamas* are universal and applicable to all and in all circumstances "notwithstanding the traditional context-driven exceptions that are taken for granted. For example, a fisherman is traditionally not causing injury when he is fishing or a soldier in battle killing the enemy. For the *yogin* taking the great vow, abstinence, however, is absolute, unqualified and unconditional" (Rao, 2011a, p. 606).

2. Truthfulness (Satya)

Truthfulness comes next in the list of self-restraints (*yamas*). Explaining this *yama*, Vyāsa states: "abstinence-from-falsehood (*satya*) means speech and mind such as correspond to the object-intended; and speech and mind corresponding to what is seen or inferred or heard. If speech is spoken in order that one's own knowledge may pass to some one else, it should not be deceitful or mistaken or barren of information; (then it would be abstinence from falsehood). It should be used for the service of all; not for the ruin of creatures. And even when used thus, should it be only for the ruin of creatures it would not be an abstinence from falsehood... Therefore, let (the *yogin*) consider (first) what is good for all creatures and (then) speak with abstinence-from-falsehood"[16]—Tr. Woods (1914/2007, p. 178). Vācaspati Miśra, in his commentary on the gloss of Vyāsa, says "The word such (*yathā*) raises an expectation which is fulfilled by the words 'corresponding to what is seen'. He brings this into connexion with the correlated word 'corresponding to (*tathā*)' in the expression 'speech and mind corresponding to'. (This should be,) whenever, there is a desire to say (something). (If spoken) otherwise (than as seen), it is not abstinence-from-falsehood...If it is not deceitful (or) the cause of deceit, (it is abstinence-from-falsehood)...An abstinence-from-falsehood even when it has these distinguishing characteristics, if it results in injury to another, would be a false kind of abstinence-from-falsehood, but would not be abstinence-from-falsehood, as he says in the words 'if it'"[17]—Tr. Woods (1914/2007, pp. 179-180).

It would thus appear that our thought must agree with word and so should word with action. This is truthfulness. How can something be considered as truth when there is no semblance in thought, word and action? To think of one thing, speak of something else and do something entirely different is nothing but crookedness. By telling lies we pollute our and others' mind and thus indulge in injury because the Self is truth. It can be realized only by speaking and observing truth in thought, word and deed. There are thirteen forms of truth: truthfulness, equal vision, self-control, absence of envious emulation, forgiveness, modesty, endurance, absence of jealousy, charity, thoughtfulness, disinterested philanthropy, self-possession, and unceasing and compassionate harmlessness. Truth means the strength to abide by the positive principles. We must speak truth and nothing but truth. Nevertheless, it must not be unpleasant because any unpleasant truth harms the other person. Any pleasing falsehood must also be avoided.

3. Abstinence-from-theft (Asteya)

When we want something and our means are insufficient to achieve it, we may indulge in acquiring it by stealing. Desire, thirst, and unceasing wish usually give rise to theft. Vyāsa explains thus this restraint: "Theft is the unauthorized (*aśāstrapūrvaka*) appropriation of things of value from another. While abstinence-from-theft, when free from coveting, is the refusal to do this"[18]—Tr. Woods (1914/2007, p. 178). Vācaspati Miśra, has thus explained the gloss of Vyāsa: "Since an (explanatory) negative idea depends on that of the positive he explains the distinguishing characteristic of theft by saying "theft is the unauthorized." Here, the generic idea is characterized by a qualification. This is the meaning. Since verbal and bodily operations are preceded by mental operations, it is the operation of mind, because it is dominant, that is mentioned in the words 'free from coveting'"[19]—Tr. Woods (1914/2007, p. 180).

Removing a thing without the knowledge of its owner and not wanting others to know about it is stealing. Taking pins, blotting paper, pencil, paper, etc. from the office is stealing. Similarly, hoarding too much money, eating too much, adding to one's craving all these are forms of stealing. Removal of cravings of all types is what is advocated in this *yama.*

4. Abstinence-from-incontinence (Brahmacarya)

The fourth self-restraint (*yama*) is practice of continence. When controlled the part of human energy expressed in sexual urge becomes transmuted into a higher spiritual energy called *ojas* in *Yoga*. Vyāsa has described this *yama* as follows "continence is control of the hidden organ of generation"[20]—Tr. Woods (1904/2007, p. 178). This has been explained by Vācaspati Miśra, in these words "He tells what continence is in the words 'hidden'. For even if his organ of generation is held in control, still if he becomes attached at the sight of a woman or upon (hearing) her talk or upon touching her limbs which are the seats of Kandarpa, he has no continence. So to exclude this case he says "the hidden organ. Other organs also that are very ardent for this (woman) are to be watched"[21]—Tr. Woods (1904/2007, p. 180). Celibacy not only frees a person from sex, it also sublimates his urge into something more creative. All great spiritual giants have practiced celibacy and have also spoke at length about this attribute. What is wanted is restraint and not suppression of sexual desire. Properly practiced and sublimated the sexual urge becomes a creative force that enables a spiritual aspirant to rise higher up on the ladder of spirituality.

5. Abstinence-from-acceptance-of-gifts (Aparigraha)

The fifth *yama* is abstinence-from-acceptance-of-gifts (*aparigraha*). This self-restraint is the opposite of acceptance of gifts from someone (*parigraha*); it is covetous or greedy nature of a practitioner. It is a mental state in which the sensual craving is dead. Vyāsa has thus enumerated these aspects in his gloss "Abstinence-from-acceptance-of-gifts is abstinence-from-appropriating objects, because one sees the disadvantages in acquiring them or keeping them or losing them or in being attached to them or in harming them"[22]—Tr. Woods (1914/2007, pp. 178-179).

Vācaspati Miśra while commenting on the gloss of Vyāsa has explained this point in these words: "He mentions the disadvantage due to attachment to these (objects) in the words (II. 15), 'since passions increase because of application to enjoyments and the skill of organs also increases.' The disadvantage which is characteristic of injury is also expressed by the words, 'Enjoyment is impossible unless one has harmed some living creatures.' Although obtained without effort, objects if unauthorized have disadvantages when one acquires them, since the acquisition of such things is censured. And even authorized objects, when acquired, are evidently disadvantageous, in that they must be kept and so on. Therefore, abstinence-from-acceptance-of-gifts is the refusal to appropriate them."[23]—Tr. Woods (1914/2007, p. 180).

Abstinence-from-acceptance-of-gifts (*aparigraha*) bestows peace and contentment by removing at one stroke fear, attachment, disappointment, anxiety, jealousy, anger and lust. It is indeed an aid to abstinence-from-injury (*ahiṁsā*) in that when the craving is not satiated one becomes angry, hates the person who stands in the way of gratification of that craving. He then tries to harm such an obstructer in different ways, starts speaking lies and begins to steal things to satisfy his desires. Therefore, this has been given the last position in the list of abstinences.

6. Abstinence-from-impatience (Kṣamā)

Patience requires one's biggest readiness to let go the offender even when punishing is within easiest reach. It requires forgiveness and reverence for the life of offender as explained in its definition in Raja Radhakant Deva's *Śabdakalpadruma* (vol. 2, p. 229), which thus defines *kṣamā*: "that which overlooks and bears even an offence on one's life is forgiveness"[24]—Author's translation. Its characteristics have been described in *Ekādaśītattva* in these words: "Forgiveness is that state in which any saddening event occurring either due to external or internal causes is neither retaliated in anger nor in physical hurt of the perpetrator"[25]—Author's translation. The 120th chapter of the *Matsya Purāṇa* has explained the characteristics of *kṣamā* in these words: "In the wake of a severe anger and physical assault when one neither loses composure nor retaliates and when his speech, mind and body is not vitiated and one who bears all untoward calmly such a state is knows as forgiveness"[26]—Author's translation. Thus forgiveness is exercising patience, releasing time and functioning in the here and now. It does not believe in retaliation, vengeance or retribution. It works on the principle of universal love, compassion and composure.

7. Abstinence-from-non-stead Forwardness (Ārjavam)

This self-restraint is concerned with following an attitude of straight-forwardness in all aspects of behaviour. There should be uniformity in thought, word and deed. Usually worldly people think one thing, speak the other and do still other one. All such dealings lack integrity of character. Why people indulge in such behavioural double-speak is not difficult to answer. Shaky convictions and lack of any scruple allure such men to change their stands time and again. This self-restraint requires that the *yogin* would renounce deception and wrongdoing in all walks of life. He would follow the straightforward path because a straightened approach along with honesty is always worth emulating to succeed on the path of Yoga.

8. Abstinence-from-cruelty (Ānṛśamsyam)

It is a restraining tendency towards cruelty and callous approach towards other living creatures. It calls for a compassionate attitude towards all living creatures without distinction. Usually, what one thinks about kindliness is included in it. However, it includes many other aspects also. Willfully and volitionally conquering callous, cruel and insensitive feelings and behaviour towards all beings is at the base of this self-restraint. It considers reverence for life as the ultimate goal so that universal love could be brought about in this world fraught with so much distinction, and caste, creed, and religion-based differences that have divided this world into so many fragments.

9. Abstinence-from-non-steadiness (Dhṛti)

This self-restraint aims at inculcating an unwavering and steadfast approach towards advancement in the chosen spiritual goal. It is overcoming non-perseverance, non-sincere and indecisive approach in spiritual practices. Any fear visualized on the path of spiritual journey or any indecision needs to be worked through and the help of Guru is most required when one has lost his path. It is a usual attitude that develops in any seeker of spiritual goal. It requires an attitude that calls for seeing each task through to its completion.

10. Abstinence-from-unwanted Desires (Damaḥ)

There are umpteen numbers of wish in every individual fulfilling of which can never be possible; they need to be properly managed and attenuated. This self-restraint calls for a proper dissection of those desires and then adequately managing them. Suppression is not proper because a suppressed desire raises its ugly head quite often and inasmuch as it is very powerful the chances of falling prey to tem cannot be ruled out. This self-restraint has been thus defined in the *Manusmṛti*: "That which removes flickering attitude by adequately appropriating them is *damaḥ*"[27]—Author's translation. It is concerned with adequate control of externally-oriented sense experiences.

Though the list of abstinences in the various *Purāṇas* show quite divergence, yet almost all sources agree on those described above. It is needless to point out that these self-restraints (*yamas*) are meant for inculcating the orderly and proper attributes as well as attitudinal, motivational, and affective orientation in a practitioner so that heis not waylaid on the path of spiritual progress.

Self-Observance (*Niyama*)

Self-observances (*niyama*) is obtained by adding prefix *ni* with *yama*. It has been defined by Monier Williams (1899) as "any act of voluntary penance or meritorious piety (esp. a lesser vow or minor observance) dependent on external conditions and not so obligatory as *yama*." These are the prescriptions for a *yogin* of good conduct. As against self-restraints they are to be observed. V.S. Apte (1890/1967) has explained it in these words: "any voluntary or self-imposed religious observance (dependent on external conditions); any minor observance or lesser vow; penance." Thus these methods aim at developing a positive approach towards everything in the world. A *yogin* must be attuned with his surrounding in such a manner that nothing disturbs his meditation. Positivity calls for certain do's as against don'ts. Each *yama* is basically 'don't' while a *niyama* is 'do' for *yogin.*

Techniques of Self-Observances (*Niyamas*)

In *Yoga-Sūtra* five self-observances have been described in aphorism 32 of book II. They are "*Niyama* is observance of cleanliness (*śauca*), contentment (*santoṣa*), austerity (*tapas*), self-study (*svādhyāya*), and devotion to God (*īśvarapraṇidhāna*)"[28]—Tr. K.R. Rao (2011a, p. 607). However, like self-restraints (*yamas*), the self-observances (*niyamas*) have been also described differently in various *Purāṇas* and yogic texts. The *Haṭhayoga Pradīṇikā* of *Yogi Svātmārāma* and *Skanda Purāṇa* mention ten such self-observances. The *Haṭhayoga Pradīpikā* enumerates them as "The ten *niyamas* mentioned by those proficient in the knowledge of *yogas* are: *tapa*, patience, belief in God, charity, adoration of God, hearing discourses on the principles of religion, shame, *japa* and *yajña*"[29]—Tr. Pancham Sinh, (1914, pp. 24-25). Similarly, the *Skanda Purāṇa* thus mentions ten *niyamas*: "Cleanliness, bathing, penance, charity, observing silence, sacrificing in the holy fire, study of religious texts, observance of various *vratas,* fasting, and controlling one's sensuous desires are the ten *niyamas*"[30]—Author's translation. Ten common *niyamas* found in most texts are described below.

1. Cleanliness (Śaucam)

This self-observance of cleanliness is important in the sense that it takes into account purity in word, deed and action. Vyāsa in his commentary has stated that "cleanliness is produced by earth or by water or the like, and by consumption and other (requirements) with regard to pure sacrificial food. This is outer. Inner (cleanliness) is the washing away of the blemishes of the mind-stuff"[31]—Tr. Woods (1914/2007, p. 181). Vācaspati Miśra while commenting on the *Vyāsabhāṣya* explains the (*cittamalam*) mind-stuff in these words "The 'stains of the mind-stuff' such as the arrogance and pride and jealousy; the removal of this is cleanliness of the central-organ"[32]—Tr. Woods (1914/2007, p. 182). In this connection it is imperative that external purity generates internal purity and *vice versa.* For example, when one takes a bath there occurs a change in his mind-set to accomplish finer aspects in his daily routine. It would thus be intuitively clear that yogic texts have stated in most unequivocal manner that both external cleanliness in our daily habits as well as keeping clean the mind-stuff with its various blemishes and taints are most important aspect of cleanliness and a *yogin* must be always on guard to stay clear of these stains. Purity also means being cleansed of bad habits and negative emotions. All negativity needs to be warded off with positivity in all aspects of life.

2. Contentment (Santoṣa)

Contentment cuts the root of all desires. It bestows peace and one-pointedness of mind. However, contentment should not be confused with satisfaction, complacency, carelessness, damn it, let go or similar other negativities. It is one's willingness to accept things as they are and to make the best possible use of them. Vyāsa has stated that "(To practise) contentment means not to covet more than the means at hand"[33]—Tr. Woods (1914/2007, p. 181). Explaining this self-observance, Vācaspati Miśra has stated that " 'Contentment' is the desire to take no more than is necessary for the general maintenance of life, because it follows the renunciation of what had been before one's own property. This is its distinction (from abstinence-from-acceptance-of-gifts)."[34]—Tr. Woods (1914/2007, p. 182). A contented practitioner of *Yoga* is always satisfied with his lot. He remains happy with whatever condition he is placed in, he never craves for those things that he does not have. Contentment is the mystic stream of joy that cools the unceasing cravings.

Our mind is always restless on account of irresistible stream of greed, lust, craving and desires. Greed is a type of internal fire that is difficult to extinguish and it consumes one slowly but steadily. Contentment is such a powerful antidote of such cravings. Contentment generates an unconditional positive regard in us and by inculcating it we start loving ourselves in such a way that life had never shown us before. It means allowing ourselves to seek happiness not from outside but from within and then one definitely comes to realize that the kingdom of God is within each one of us.

3. Austerity (Tapas)

Tapas means austerity or practice of penance. *Tapas* also means restraint of the senses and meditation. It leads to control of the mind. Austerities like occasional fasting or observing silence increase the power of endurance. Commenting on this type of self-observance, Vyāsa has stated "Austerity is the capacity to bear the opposites; and the opposites are hunger and thirst, cold and heat, standing and sitting, absence of all expressions and absence of speech. They also include vows such as the fasts of *kṛcchra, cāndrāyaṇa,* and *sāntāpana*"[35]—Tr. T.S. Rukmani (2001, *Yogavārttika* of *Vijñānabhikṣu*, Volume II, p. 196).

Mental austerity is more powerful than physical austerity. He who bears cold and heat does physical austerity and his power of endurance increases but he may not be able to bear insult. He will be easily upset by a harsh or unkind word for he has disciplined his body for bearing the physical extremes only. Mental austerity is keeping a balanced mind in all conditions of life to bear insult injury and persecutions, to remain serene, contented and peaceful and to remain cheerful in face of extremely adverse conditions. Such a *yogin* practices to have fortitude in meeting danger and develops patience and forbearance. In this manner this self-observance prepares a practitioner not to be upset on a trifle matter but to maintain his composure. It develops in a practitioner such a mental preparedness that he concentrates on practice only and waits for its fruition. This definitely does not happen through osmosis; we must do our work and let the benefits unfold in time.

4. Self-Study (Svādhyāya)

Self-study is not only the study of scriptures and books written by self-realized and wise persons but also an in depth inquiry into the nature of one's own self. It begins by asking the question, "who am I?" Vyāsa has very categorically stated that "Study is the recital of books that treat of release or the repetition of the syllable of adoration (*praṇava*)"[36]—Tr. Woods (1914/2007, pp. 181-182). Self-study is similar to sitting in the company of the wise men and listen from their mouth directly the discourses. When one is not able to seek the direct company of realized persons, he approaches the scriptures and the scriptures clears the doubts and also strengthens the flickering faith. It fills the mind with concerted resolve and refreshes inspirations by elevating the mind. It also helps in concentration and meditation, by cutting new positive grooves in mind and helps the mind to run in these grooves so as to hasten slowly the goal of self-realization.

5. Devotion to God (Īśvarapraṇidhāna)

It is celestial love and devotion to God. It consists of self-surrender by dedicating oneself for a higher cause or purpose in the name of God. This is the practice where the practitioner consecrates everything to the higher force. He no longer has any will of his own. He continuously goes on practicing "I am thine. All is thine. Thy will be done. I am merely an instrument in thine hands. Self-surrender is regarding every work as that of the Supreme Lord and renouncing all claims to its fruits. Vyāsa has thus described the value of such self-surrender, "Devotion to the Īśvara is the offering up of all actions to the Supreme Teacher. He who rests in himself, for whom the network of perverse-considerations (*vitarka*) has been destroyed, whether resting upon a bed or on a seat or wandering upon a road, would behold the destruction of the seed of the round-of-rebirths, would be permanently released, would participate in deathless delights." With regard to which it has been said, (i. 29), "Thereafter comes the right knowledge of him who thinks in an inverse way, and the removal of obstacles"[37]—Tr. Woods (1914/2007, p. 182). Vācaspati Miśra in his *Tattva Vaiśāradī* has explained *parikṣīṇavitarkajālaḥ* of Vyāsa in these words "In the phrase 'for whom the network of perverse-considerations has been destroyed' the words 'perverse-considerations' will be (later ii.33) described. And doubts and misconceptions should be added (as parts of the network). To this extent his intention is said to be pure"[38]—Tr. Woods (1914/2007, p. 182).

In surrendering the will to the divine a practitioner's will becomes one with the cosmic will. He becomes one with the Lord. There is no loss in surrendering one's will to God for in so doing the practitioner starts feeling continuously the reality of divine grace and the Lord's readiness to bestow help to him at all times. The divine flow streams into his being and moulds him in such a way as to make it a fit medium for the divine realization. In an important sense, it is an exercise in altruism for transcending the ego-compulsions.

6. Modesty (Hṛ)

It is an attribute that makes one free of any untoward pride. It develops an awareness of one's limitations that makes him humble in his approach. No matter how big an aspirant is, howsoever wise or high achiever one is, whatever progress one might have made in his spiritual journey, he or she must remember that there is more to be achieved. There is nothing like being complacent or feeling that one has reached the pinnacle and now he has become absolute. Modesty calls for remembering that limitless One is God only and each one of the living beings is limited in his capacity. It allows us to be meek and honour the Divine and surrender thereby one merges with the unlimited ocean of love and happiness. Modesty allows us to grow more and more in spirituality.

7. Self-Cognition (Mati)

Self-cognition involves acquisition of the spiritual knowledge. It pertains to the true knowledge of self. It is in that spirit that sir Monier Williams defined *mati* as "devotion, prayer, worship, hymn, sacred utterance." Any sacred utterance that develops self-cognition would be called as *mati*. In the *Devibhāgvata Purāṇa mati* has been defined in these words "There are two types of *mati* that are entirely accurate and entirely inaccurate"[39]— Author's translation. With entirely accurate knowledge one treads spiritual path that calls for tailoring one's life on the pattern of spiritual advices of his/her Guru. The other type is used by most of us in leading our daily life.

8. Oblation (Homa)

Sir Monier Williams has defined *homa* as "the act of making an oblation to the gods by casting clarified butter into the fire (*deva yajña*), oblation with fire, burnt-offering, any oblation or sacrifice." Any oblation that is offered in sacrificial fire is *homa*. It has been given such an important place that it has been described as one of five daily rituals (for the details of daily rituals *see* Husain, Beg and Dwivedi, 2013, pp. 197-233). It is considered as one of the most important *niyamas* inasmuch as sacrificial fire is symbolized as the mystic fire that carries our every act to the celestial.

9. Offering (Dānam)

It means offering everything for the welfare of someone. Vaman Shivaram Apte has defined it as "giving, granting, teaching, etc. (in general); giving in marriage; delivering, handing over, a gift, donation, present; liberality, charity, giving away as charity, munificence." It is sacrificing everything before the will of God. It is practiced by doing what we understand by charity. As a spiritual aspirant the approach needs to be of sacrificing our ego before the Almighty and small charities become the stepping stone to that goal. Unless one steps out of one's limited sense of ego, his/her spiritual progress remains a remote possibility. We need to cross our boundaries to become one with the Almighty. It is with that aim that this *niyama* has been included.

10. Incantation (Japam)

It involves reciting of the sacred *mantarm*. This is such an important aspect of spirituality that it has received considerable attention in spiritual literature. *Yoga-Sūtra* has described specifically about bit in book I. There it is said that "Repetition of it and reflection upon its meaning (should be made)"[40]—Tr. Woods (1914/2007, p. 61). Vyāsa in his commentary on this aphorism has explained that "As the Perfect Knowledge is eternal, the Vedic teachers assert that the relation between word and its meaning is eternal. In the case of the *Yogi* to whom the relation between the Connoted and the Connotative is known, its repetition and gradual development of its Truth, i.e. the repetition of *Praṇava* (*Aum*) and the Revelation of Īśvara connoted by *Praṇava*, are sure to follow. The mind of the *Yogi*, who repeats the *Praṇava* and reveals its truth, is made one-pointed. So, it has been said:—By study, *Yoga* is developed; by *Yoga* the study is confirmed; and the Highest-Self is revealed by the combined power of the study and Yoga"[41]—Tr. Bangali Baba (1976/2010, pp. 14-15). Woods (1914/2007, pp. 61-62) has explained this commentary on the said aphorism as follows "The repetition of the Mystic Syllable and reflection upon the Īśvara who is signified by the Mystic Syllable. Then in the case of this *yogin* who thus repeats the Mystic Syllable and reflects upon its meaning, mind-stuff attains to singleness-of-intent. And so it hath been said, "Through study let him practise *yoga*. Through *yoga* let him meditate on study, By perfectness in study and in *yoga*. Supreme Soul shines forth clearly."

Three types of *mantrajapam* have been described in the spiritual texts that are *vācika, upānśu* and *mānasika*. In the first type of *mantra japam* the practitioner's vocal organs are involved; in the second type only tongue moves while in the last only mental operations are involved. Each one is said to be superior to its predecessor.

The practice of self-restraints (*yamas*) and self-observances (*niyamas*) make it abundantly clear to us that true meaning of *yoga* or any other form of spiritual practice cannot dawn on us by merely mechanically undertaking various ritualistic practices but by embodying them in our lives. In becoming a person free of jealousy, dishonesty, discontent and destruction and in taking time to put our beliefs into action. By so doing we discover afresh its reral import and our true sense of being is revealed to us—one of pure love and utter joy. According to Sri Aurobindo (1972),

> "If there were nothing else to be said in favour of the spiritual genius of the Indian people or the claim of the Indian civilization to stand in the front rank as a spiritual culture, it would be sufficiently substantiated by this single fact that not only was this greatest and widest spiritual truth seen in India with the boldest largeness, felt and expressed with a unique intensity and approached from all possible sides, but it was made consciously the grand uplifting idea of life, the core of all thinking, the foundation of all religion, the secret sense and declared ultimate aim of human existence. The truth announced is not peculiar to Indian thinking; it has been seen and followed by the highest minds and souls everywhere. But elsewhere it has been the living guide only of a few thinkers or of some rare mystics or exceptionally gifted spiritual natures. The mass of men have had no understanding, no distinct perception, not even a reflected glimpse of this something Beyond; they have lived only in the lower sectarian side of religion, in inferior ideas of the Deity or in the outward mundane aspects of life. But the Indian culture did succeed by the strenuousness of its vision, the universality of its approach, the intensity of its seeking, in doing what has been done by no other culture. It succeeded in stamping religion with the essential ideal of a real spirituality; it brought some living reflection

of the very highest spiritual truth and some breath of its influence into every part of religious life" (pp. 127-128).

India's pride lies in the fact that almost in every generation and in every part of the country, from the time immemorial (more specifically from the time of her recorded history) she has produced spiritually enlightened holy men who embody for her all that the country holds most dear and sacred. Religion is a matter of personal experience; a transformation of one's entire being. It indeed is not an addition to one's intellectual fancy or theological furniture, but an exaltation of one's personality into the plane of the universal Spirit. In this regard, it worth noting what Radhakrishnan (1937/2001) has remarked "It is *Brahmadarśana*—insight into Reality, a direct awareness of the world of values.

"Religious experience is not to be confused with the pursuit of truth, beauty, or goodness. It is a life of adoring love transcending these. The Divine is not a mere sum of knowledge, love and beauty. The ultimate Reality which responds to our demands is more than rational...There is an element of mystery in all religion, an incomprehensible certainty which is not be explained by grammar or logic. Life is open only to life. Religious experience, when genuine, is characterized by vividness, directness, freshness, and joy. In it we feel the impact of Reality. It is spiritual discovery, not creation" (Radhakrishnan, 1937/2001, p. xiv).

In the right view all life is either subconsciously or consciously a *Yoga*, which is a methodized effort towards self-perfection by the expression of the potentialities latent in the being and a union of the human individual with the universal and transcendent existence. *Yoga* is practical psychology and the methods and techniques described in it are meant to resolve any problem that one may encounter in course of his or her progress towards self-realization.

Notes

1. *Yato'bhyudayaniḥśreyasa siddhiḥ sa dharmah. Vaiśeṣika Sūtra*
2. *Dhāraṇāt dharma ityāhuḥ dharmo dhārayate prajāh/*
   Yat syād dhāraṇasanyuktam sa dharma iti niścayah." Mahābhārata, Karṇa Parva (ch. 69/58).
3. *Yachhati niyachhati indriyagrāmamanena iti, Śabdakalpadruma*, Volume 4, p. 19.
4. *Viyāmo viyamo yāmo yamaḥ samyāmasamyamau, Amarakośa*, 3.9.18

5. *Atīndraḥ samagrahaḥ sargo dhṛtātmā niyamo yamaḥ. Mahābhārata*, 13.149.30.
6. *Antaryacchatīti yamah.* Śaṅkarācārya's commentary on *Mahābhārata*, 13.149.30.
7. *Yathākramameṣāmanuṣṭhānam Vyāsabhāṣya* on *Yoga-Sūtra*, II.29.
8. *Ahiṁsāsatyāsteyabrahmacaryāparigrhā yamāḥ. Yoga-Sūtra*, II.30.
9. *Ahiṁsā satyāsteyam brahmacaryam kṣamā dhṛtiḥ Dayārjavam mitāhārah śaucam caiva yamā daśa. Haṭhayoga Pradīpikā* 1. 17.
10. *Satyam kṣamārjavam dhyānam ānṛṇansyamahimsanam Damaḥ prasādomādhuryam mṛduteti yamā daśa. Skanda Purāṇa*, 5.91.
11. *Brahmacaryam dayā kṣāntirdhyānam satyamakalkatā Ahiṁsāsteyamādhuryam damañcaite yamāh smṛtāh. Garuḍa Purāṇa*, chapter 109.
12. *Tatrāhiṁsā sarvadā sarvabhūtānām anabhidrohah, uttare ca yamaniyamāstanmūlāstatsiddhipar-tayiava tatpratipāanāya pratipādyante, tadavadātarūpakaraṇāyaivopādīyante. Vyāsabhāṣya* on *Yoga-Sūtra*, II.30
13. *Tanmūlā iti. Ahiṁsāmaparipālyakṛtā apyakṛtakalpā, niṣphaltvādityarthaha. Tatsiddhiparataiayavānuṣthānam. Ahiṁsā cenmūlamuttareṣām katham te 'hiṁsāsiddhiparā ityat āha—tatpratipādanāyeti.* Vācaspati Miśra's *Tattva Vaiśāradī* on *Vyāsabhāṣya* II.30.
14. *Aśramavihitanityakarmāvirodheneti viśeṣaṇīyā śaucādiṣu kṣudrajantuhiṁsāyā aparihāryatvāt.* Vijñāna Bhikṣu's *Yoga Vārttika* on *Vyāsabhāṣya* II.30.
15. *Jātideśakālasamayānavachhinnāh sārvabhaumā mahāvratam. Yoga-Sūtra*, II.31.
16. *Satyam yathārthevāṁmanase. Yathā dṛṣtam yathānumitam yathā śrutam tathā vāṇmanaśceti. Paratra svabodhasaṁkrāntaye vāguktā sā yadi na vañcitā bhrantāvā pratipattibandhyā vā bhavediti. Eṣā sarvabhutopakārārtham pravṛttā na bhūtopaghātaya. Yadi caiavamapyabhidhūīyamānā bhūtopaghātaparaiva syānna satyam bhavet... tasmātparīkṣa sarvabhūtahitam satyam bruyāt. Vyāsabhāṣya* on *Yoga-Sūtra*, II.30
17. *Yathāśabdam sākāṁkṣam pūtrayati—yathādṛṣtamiti. Pratisambandhinam tathāśabdam pratikṣipati—tathāvāṁmanaśceti. Vivikṣāyāmkartavyāyāmiti. Anyathā tu na satyam...atah sā yadi na vañcitā vañcikā ...Evam lakṣaṇamapi satyam parapakāraphalam satyābhāsam na tu satyamityāḥ—eṣeti.* Vācaspati Miśra's *Tattva Vaiśāradī* on *Vyāsabhāṣya* II.30.
18. *Steyamaśāstrapūrvakam dravyāṇām paratah svīkaraṇam, tatpratiṣedhah punarasprihārūpamasteyamiti.—Vyāsabhāṣya* on *Yoga-Sūtra*, II.30.
19. *Abhāvasya bhāvādhīnanirūpaṇatayā steyalakṣaṇamāha—steyamaśāstrapūrvakamiti. Viśeṣeṇa sāmānyam lakṣyata ityarthah. Mānasa vyāpārapūrvakatvādvācanikakāyikavyāpārayoh prādhānyān-manovyāpāra ukto'spṛhārūpamiti*—Vācaspati Miśra's *Tattva Vaiśāradī* on *Vyāsabhāṣya* II.30.

20. *Brahmacaryam guptendriyasyaopasthasya samyamah—Vyāsabhāṣya* on *Yoga-Sūtra*, II.30.
21. *Brahmacaryasvarūpamāha—gupteti. Samyatopasthasyo'pi hi strīprekṣaṇatadālāpakandarpāyatana-tadaṅgasparśanasakto na brahmacaryavāniti tannirāsāyoktam guptendriyasyeti. Indriyāntarāṇyapi tatra lolupāni rakṣaṇīyānīti*—Vācaspati Miśra's *Tattva Vaiśāradī* on *Vyāsabhāṣya* II.30.
22. *Viṣayāṇāmarjanarakṣaṇakṣayasaṅgahimsādoṣadarśanādasvīkaraṇamaparigraha iti—Vyāsabhāṣya* on *Yoga-Sūtra*, II.30
23. *Aparigrahasvarūpamāha—viṣayāṇāmiti. Tatra saṅgadoṣa ukto bhogābhāsamanuvivardhante rāgāh kauśclāni cendriyāṇāiti (ii.15) himsālakṣaṇaśca doṣo nānupahṛtya bhutānyupabhogah sambhavatīti. Aśāstrīyāṇāmayatnopanatāmapi viṣayāṇāma ninditapratigrahādirū pārjanadoṣadarśanācchāstrīyāṇāma-pyupārjitānām ca rakṣaṇādido ṣadarśanādasvīkaraṇamaparigarhah.*—Vācaspati Miśra's *Tattva Vaiśāradī* on *Vyāsabhāṣya* II.30.
24. *Kṣamateātmoparsthitānām jīvānāmaparādham yā. Śabdakalpadruma*, Volume 2, p. 229.
25. *Bāhye cādhyātmike caiva duhkhe cotpādite kvacit/Na kupyati na vā hanta sā kṣamā parikīrtitā. Ekādaśītattva*
26. *Ākruṣto'bhihatoyattu nākrośenna hanedapi Aduṣtairvaṁmanahkāyaistitikṣuśca kṣamā smṛtā. Matsya Purāṇa*, chapter 120.
27. *Vikṣepasyāpahartāram tatsamam dāpayet damam. Manusmṛti* 8.192.
28. *Śauca santoṣa tapah svādhyāyeśvarapraṇidhānani niyamāh. Yoga-Sūtra*, II.32.
29. *Tapah santoṣa āstikyam dānamīśvarapūjanam*
Siddhāntavākyaśravaṇam hrīmatī ca japo hutam
Niyamā daśa samproktā yogaśāstraviśāradaih. Haṭhayoga Pradīpikā 1.18.
30. *Śaucam snānam tapo dānam maunejyādhyayanam vratam*
Upoṣaṇopadthadaṇdau daśaite niyamāh smṛtāh.Skanda Purāṇa 21.1.
31. *Śaucam mṛjjalādijanitam medhyābhyavaharaṇādi ca bāhyam. ābhyantaram cittamalānāmākṣālanam. Vyāsabhāṣya* II.32.
32. *Cittamalā madamānāsūyādayah. Tadapanayoh manah śaucam.*—Vācaspati Miśra's *Tattva Vaiúāradī* on *Vyāsabhāṣya* II.32
33. *Santoṣah sannihitasādhanādadhikasyānupāditsā—Vyāsabhāṣya* II.32.
34. *Prāṇayātrāmātrahetorabhyadhikasyānupāditsā santoṣah. Prāgeva svīkaraṇaparityāgaditi viśeṣah.*—Vācaspati Miśra's *Tattva Vaiśāradī* on *Vyāsabhāṣya* II.32.
35. *Tapo dvandvasahanam. Dvandvasca jighatsāpipāse śītoṣṇe sthānāsane kāṣthamaunākāramaune ca. Vratāni caiṣām yathāyogam kṛcchracāndrāyaṇasāmtāpanadīni.—Vyāsabhāṣya* II.32.
36. *Svādhyāyo mokṣaśāstrāṇāmadhyayanam praṇavajapovā.—Vyāsabhāṣya* II.32.

37. *Īśvarapraṇidhānam tasmin paramgurau sarvakarmārpaṇam. Śayyāsanstho'tha pathi vrajanvā svasthah parikṛīṇavitarkajālah/ Saṁsārbījakṣayamīkṣmāṇah syānnityamukto'mṛtabhogabhāgī// yatredamuktam—tatah pratyakcetanādhigamo'pyantarāyābhāvāsca iti.—Vyāsabhāṣya* II.32.
38. *Parikṣīṇavitarkajāla iti. Vitarko vakṣyamāṇah saṁśayaviparyayau ceti. Etāvatāśuddho'bhisandhi-ruktaḥ.*—Vācaspati Miśra's *Tattva Vaiśāradī* on *Vyāsabhāṣya* II.32.
39. *Matistu dvividhā loke yuktāyukteti sarvvathā. Devibhāgavata Purāṇa* 1.17.29.
40. *Tajjapastadarthabhāvanam.—Yoga-Sūtra*, I. 28.
41. *Sampratipattinityatayā nityaḥ śabdārthasambandhaḥ ityāgaminaḥ pratijānate. Vijñātavācya- vācakatvasya yoginaḥ tajjapastadarthabhāvanam. Praṇavasaya japaḥ praṇavābhidheyasya ceśarasya bhāvanam. Tadasya yoginah praṇavam japataḥ praṇavārtham ca bhāvayataścittamekāgram sampadyate. Tathā coktam—Svādhāyādyogamāsīta yogātsvādhyāyamānet. Svādhyāyayogasampatyā paramātmā prakāśate. Iti—Vyāsabhāṣya* I. 28.

References

Adler, A. (1929). *The Science of Living.* New York: Greenberg.

Apte, V.S. (1890/1966). *The Students Sanskrit-English Dictionary.* Delhi: Motilal Banrasidass.

Aurobindo, S. (1971). *Synthesis of Yoga.* Pondicherry: Sri Aurobindo Ashram Birth Centenary Library Edition.

Aurobindo, S. (1972). *The Foundations of Indian Culture.* Pondicherry: Sri Aurobindo Ashram Birth Centenary Library Edition.

Baba, B. (1976/2010). *The Yoga-Sūtra of Patañjali with the Commentary of Vyāsa.* Delhi: Motilal Banarasidass.

Bhattacharyya, H. (1953/2006). Yoga Psychology. In H. Bhattacharyya (Ed.) *The Cultural Heritage of India* (Volume III, pp. 53-90). Calcutta: The Ramakrishna Institute of Culture.

Bhawuk, D.P.S. (2011). *Spirituality and Indian Psychology: Lessons from the Bhagavad-Gita.* New York: Springer.

Dasgupta, S. (1922/1991). *A History of Indian Philosophy.* New Delhi: Motilal Banarasidass.

Dasgupta, S. (1953/2006). Introduction. In H. Bhattacharyya (Ed.) *The Cultural Heritage of India.* (Volume III, pp. 3-26). Calcutta: Ramakrishna Mission Institute of Culture.

Deva, R.R. (1857/1967). *Śabdakalpadruma.* Varanasi: Chowkhamba Sanskrit Series.

Dwivedi, C.B. (1967). Yogadarśana: A nucleus towards the synthesis of Indian Psychology. *Prabuddha Bharata, 72*(2), 69-74.

Hill, P.C. and Pargament, K.I. (2003). Advances in the conceptualization of religion and spirituality: Implications for physical mental health research. *American Psychologist, 58,* 64-74.

Husain, A. (2011). *Spirituality and Holistic Health: A Psychological Perspective.* New Delhi: Prasad Psycho Corporation.

Husain, A., Beg, M.A. and Dwivedi, C.B. (2013). *Psychology of Humanity and Spirituality.* New Delhi: Research India Press.

Koening, H.G., McCullough, M.E., and Larson, D.B. (2001). *Handbook of Religion and Health.* New York: Oxford University Press.

Miller, L.J. (2012). (Ed.) *The Oxford Handbook of Psychology and Spirituality.* Oxford: Oxford University Press.

Miller, W.R., and Thoresen, C.E. (1999). Spirituality and health. In W.R. Miller (Ed.), *Integrating Spirituality in Treatment.* Washington, D.C.: American Psychological Association.

Monier-Williams, M. (1899). *A Sanskrit-English Dictionary.* Oxford: Oxford University Press.

Pandey, R.K. (Ed.) (1997). *Kalpalatā. A Collection of Devotional Songs.* New Delhi: Sanskrit Sanskriti Pratisthanam.

Pargament, K.I. (2011). *Spiritually Integrated Psychotherapy: Understanding and Addressing the Sacred.* New York: Guilford Press.

Rao, K.R. (2011a). *Cognitive Anomalies, Consciousness and Yoga.* New Delhi: Matrix Publishers.

Rao, K.R. (2011b). Indian psychology: Implications and applications. In R. M.M. Cornelissen, G. Misra, and S. Varma (Eds.) *Foundations of Indian Psychology (Volume 1) Theories and Concepts.* Delhi: Pearson (pp. 7-26).

Rolland, R. (1960). *The Life of Ramakrishna.* Mayawati, Almora: Advaita Ashram.

Rukmani, T.S.(1981). *Yoga Vārttika of Vijñān Bhikṣu* (Volume I), New Delhi: Munshiram Manoharlal Publishers.

Rukmani, T.S. (1983). *Yoga Vārttika of Vijñān Bhikṣu* (Volume II), New Delhi: Munshiram Manoharlal Publishers.

Rukmani, T.S. (1987). *Yoga Vārttika of Vijñān Bhikṣu* (Volume III), New Delhi: Munshiram Manoharlal Publishers.

Rukmani, T.S. (1989). *Yoga Vārttika of Vijñān Bhikṣu* (Volume IV), New Delhi: Munshiram Manoharlal Publishers.

Sinh, P. (1914). (Tr.). *The Hathayoga Pradipika.* Allahabad: Panini.

Woods, J.H. (1914/2007). *The Yoga-system of Patañjali.* Delhi: Motilal Banarasi Dass.

4
Psychological Distress and Quality of Life in Women with Diabetes and Cancer

Anubhuti Dubey and *Kamini Mani Tripathi*

Chronic illnesses like cancer and diabetes have multiple causes ranging from heredity, life style factors, invasive environmental and psychological factors and these may contribute to onset, development and progression of illness. In most of the chronic illness conditions the long term effects may be difficult to predict. Chronic illnesses challenge every aspect of life. The more serious, the illness the greater the challenge it imposes. India is experiencing a rapid health transition, with large and rising burdens of chronic diseases, which are estimated to account for 53 per cent of all deaths and 44 per cent of disability-adjusted life-years (DALYs) lost in 2005 (Reddy *et al.*, 2005). Earlier estimates, from the Global Burden of Disease Study, projected that the number of deaths attributable to chronic diseases would rise from 3.78 million in 1990 (40.4% of all deaths) to 7.63 million in 2020 (66.7% of all deaths) (Murray and Lopez, 1996).

Data on cancer mortality are available from six centres across the country, which are part of the National Cancer Registry Programme of the Indian Council of Medical Research (ICMR). About 8,00,000 new cases of cancer are estimated to occur every year. The age-adjusted incidence rates in men vary from 44 per 1,00,000 in rural Maharashtra to 121 per 1,00,000 in Delhi (National Cancer Registry Programme, 2002). In women, the leading cancer sites include those related to tobacco (oral cavity, oesophagus, and lung), and cervix, breast, and ovary cancer. Sen and colleagues stated that the most frequently reported cancer sites in females in eastern India were breast (22.7% of total cases, ASR 25.1), followed by uterine cervix (17.5%, ASR 19.9), gallbladder (6.4%, ASR 8.1), ovary (ICD 56) (5.8%, ASR 6.3) and other female genital tract organs. Cancer of the uterine cervix, which is still the leading female cancer in India with an estimated 126,000 new cases every year, is now showing a slow decline in incidence in urban populations (Krishnamurthy, Yeole & Jussawall, 1997; Nandakumar, Anantha, and Venugopal, 1995). The change in the lifestyles and habits of urban women could be responsible for the decline. However, the disease remains common among women in rural areas. Case-control studies conducted in Kolkata and in other regions of India indicate early age at marriage, early age at first coitus, early age at first childbirth, sexual promiscuity (among both women and their spouses), sex with uncircumcised men, multiparity, low socio-economic status and poor genital hygiene as major risk factors for cervical cancer in India (Gawande, Wahab, Zodpey, and Vasudeo, 1998; Dutta *et al.*, 1990).

The number of people with diabetes mellitus in India is increasing across geographic, ethnic and administrative boundaries (Mohan, Sandeep, Deepa, Shah, and Varghere, 2007; Sadikot *et al.*, 2004). The ICMR estimates the prevalence of diabetes in adults to be 3.8 per cent in rural areas and 11.8 per cent in urban areas (Reddy *et al.*, 2005).

The biological causes of these diseases may be different but many of the symptoms they cause are similar, like fatigue, pain, loss of energy, loss of appetite, sleeplessness and restlessness, etc. These symptoms may interfere with everyday life and may require a change in existing pattern of life. The common psychological and mental health problems emerges with are depression, anxiety, fear and concern for the future, physical limitation and decreased work ability can lead to financial difficulties.

Cancer and Distress

Cancer may be life-threatening, treatment can be physically disabling, and cancer survivors live with the possibility of recurrence. A number of medical, personal, and socio-cultural factors have been shown to affect psychosocial adaptation to cancer, including extent of symptoms, relationship with the medical team, and history of psychiatric problems, coping skills, social support and socio-economic status (Zabora *et al.*, 2001; Rowland, 1999). Some level of psychosocial distress is normal after a diagnosis of cancer, given the nature of the disease, however, for the majority of individuals diagnosed with cancer the cancer-related depression and anxiety can be expected to squander with time, but for others, psychosocial distress may considerably intervene with comfort, quality of life, and the ability to make appropriate treatment decisions and adhere to treatment (Massie and Holland, 1989; Rowland, 1999). In situation of cancer, distress is defined as continuing along a continuum ranging from common normal feeling of vulnerability, sadness and fear to problems that can become disabling such as depression, anxiety and panic, social isolation and spiritual crisis (National Comprehensive Cancer Network, 2007). Among these, anxiety is the most frequently seen in cancer patients. It can occur in four forms, i.e. situational anxiety, disease related anxiety, treatment related anxiety and as an exacerbation of pre-treatment anxiety disorder (Sarita, 2004). On account of cancer diagnosis, treatment or impending complications, the cancer related depression is a pathological affective response to loss of normality and one's personal world. Depression is suspected when symptoms of sadness persist and are accompanied by increasing dysfunction, feeling of worthlessness, lowered self-esteem, suicidal preoccupation or inability to anticipate anything with pleasure (Miranda, de Resende, Melo, Costa Al Jr, and Friedman, 2002).

Sexual dysfunction is common following radical pelvic surgery and tends to remain a chronic problem. Along with organic causes there is a strong psychogenie element brought about by loss of fertility, disfigurement, depression and anxiety about one's desirability as a sexual partner (Corney *et al.*, 1993).

Breast cancer is a serious, stressful and life-threatening disease. It is assumed that the diagnosis of cancer evokes far greater distress than many other diseases, regardless of prognosis (Stechlin and Beach, 1966; Thomas, Pandey, Ramdas, and Nair, 2002). Several studies have documented the significant disruptions in the patient's Quality of Life (QOL) during the initial phases of the breast cancer diagnosis and its subsequent treatment (Vinokur, Threatt, Caplan, and Zimmerman, 1989; Levy *et al.*, 1992). Patients undergoing a mastectomy have been observed to experience significant QOL changes at various levels: physical, functional, emotional domains of QOL and well-being (Vinokur, Threatt, Caplan, and Zimmerman, 1989; Arora *et al.*, 2001). Studies have also identified the relationship between mastectomy and poor sexual adjustment and body image (Arora *et al.*, 2001; Stanton, Krishnan, and Collins, 2001).

Diabetes and Distress

Diabetes may produce central nervous system impairment than interferes with memory (Taylor and Rachman, 1988) especially among the elderly (Mooradian, Perryman, Fitten, Kavonian and Marley, 1998). Diabetes may also intensify the difficulties in psychosocial functioning, contributing to eating disorders and sexual dysfunction in men and women, as well as depression (Talbot, Nouwen, Gingras, Balanger and Audet, 1999) among other problems. In large New York City study, serious psychological distress (depression, anxiety and other disorders) was reported by 10.4 per cent of persons with diabetes (80/857) (McVeigh, Mostashari and Thorpe, 2004). Self-care behaviour in diabetes was adversely affected by the occurrence of natural calamities (Ramachandran, 2005). Lesser degree of psychological distress not amounting to psychiatric morbidity is more common (Sridhar and Madhu, 2002). Women with type 2 diabetes mellitus reported poorer quality of life compared to men (Sridhar, Madhu and Veena, 2000). Diabetes doubled the odds of depression (Anderson, Freedland, Clouse and Listman, 2001); *i.e.* persons with diabetes were twice as likely to have depression compared to those without diabetes. The odds of depression occurring in women were higher than in men. Depression may be related to complexities in management of diabetes, or to neurohormonal abnormalities (Sridhar and Madhu, 2002).

Objective

Psychological problems in cancer patients often go unrecognized until they are specifically sought (Pandey *et al.,* 2007). The diagnosis of breast or cervix cancer and its subsequent treatment has significant impact on the woman's physical functioning, mental health and her well-being, and thereby causes substantial disruption to quality of life (QOL). The main objective of present research is to find out the differences in psychological distress in women having diabetes and cancer and role of psychological distress in quality of life and sexual and physical adjustment with the disease.

Hypothesis

It was hypothesized that two chronic illnesses, i.e. diabetics and cancer will produce the same level of psychological distress in women patients.

Method

Sample

The sample consisted of 80 women participants having one of the chronic diseases, i.e. diabetes (N = 40) or cancer (N = 40) for at least more than two years. All the females were married. All of them were residing at Gorakhpur city area.

Materials

The detailed description of the tools used in the present study is given below.

Depression, Anxiety, Stress Scale (DASS): DASS is a quantitative measure of distress. It is 42 items questionnaire developed by Loviband and Loviband (1995). It includes three self-report scales designed to measure the negative emotional states of depression, anxiety and stress. Each of the three subscales contains 14 items. The depression scale assesses dyspohoria, hopelessness, devaluation of life, self-deprecation, lack of interest/involvement, anhedonia and inertia. The anxiety scale assesses autonomic arousal, skeletal muscle effects, situational anxiety, and subjective experience of anxious affect. The stress scale is sensitive to the levels chronic non-specific arousal. It assess difficulty relaxing, nervous arousal, being easily upset, irritable and impatient. The respondents are asked to use four point severity/frequency scales to rate the extent to which they have experienced each state over the past week. The factor structure, reliability, and validity of the Depression Anxiety Stress Scales (DASS; S.H. Lovibond and P.F. Lovibond, 1995) and the 21-item short form of these measures (DASS–21) were examined in nonclinical volunteers ($n = 49$) and patients with Diagnostic and Statistical Manual of Mental Disorders (4th ed.; American Psychiatric Association, 1994) diagnoses of panic disorder ($n = 67$), obsessive-compulsive disorder ($n = 54$), social phobia ($n = 74$), specific phobia ($n = 17$), and major depressive disorder ($n = 46$). This study replicates previous findings indicating that the DASS distinguishes well between features of depression, physical arousal, and psychological tension and agitation and extends these observations to the DASS–21. In addition, the internal consistency and concurrent validity of the DASS and DASS–21 were in the acceptable to excellent ranges (Antony *et al.*, 1998).

Quality of Life: The scale is based on the tool of WHO Quality of Life (1998). The items related to physical appearance and sexual quality of life was selected from this questionnaire. In this scale there were 20 items related to different aspects of quality of life, 5 items related to sexual aspects of life and 4 items were related to physical appearance. The responses were made on five-point scale ranging from (5) very much to (1) not at all. In this scale high scores lead to high evaluation of quality of life and *vice versa*.

Procedure: The respondents having diabetes were contacted at their homes and the cancer patients were contacted at the OPDs of Hanuman

Prasad Cancer Hospital, Gorakhpur. Some cancer patients were indoor patients and some were outdoor patients. Rapport was established with participants and the purpose of the study was disclosed to them and requested them to participant in the study. The set of scales were given to them. The instructions for each tool had been read to the participants and sufficient probing was made. The data was collected individually.

Results

The obtained data was subjected to statistical analysis related to descriptive and one way Analysis of Variance, correlational analysis and stepwise Multiple Regression Analysis.

Table 4.1: Mean, S.D. and F ratio of Depression, Anxiety and Stress in two groups

Distress Variables	*Cancer Patients*		*Diabetic Patients*		*F*
	Mean	*S.D.*	*Mean*	*S.D.*	
Depression	24.50	10.36	18.15	8.07	10.14**
Anxiety	19.15	4.02	15.25	3.86	13.00**
Stress	35.10	7.60	29.40	10.13	5.26**

Note: P < .01** P < .05*

Table 4.1 presented the mean, S.D and one way ANOVA for three distress related variable, i.e. depression, anxiety and stress in two groups of chronically illness patients. There were significant difference found for depression, anxiety and stress in cancer and diabetic patient groups and the mean scores showed that cancer patients were more distressed than diabetic patients on all the three variables, i.e. depression, anxiety and stress.

Table 4.2: Mean, S.D. and F ratio of QOL, Physical Appearance and Sexual Functioning in two groups

QOL Domains	*Cancer Patients*		*Diabetic Patients*		*F*
	Mean	*S.D.*	*Mean*	*S.D.*	
QOL	58.25	6.62	64.55	8.24	7.09**
Physical Appearance	8.95	2.48	9.90	1.61	2.05
Sexual Functioning	13.55	1.23	16.30	6.13	3.85*

Note: P < .01** P < .05*

Table 4.2 showed the mean, S.D. and one way ANOVA for Quality of Life (QOL) related variable, i.e. QOL in general, physical appearance and sexual functioning in two groups of chronically illness patients. There were significant difference found for QOL general and sexual functioning in cancer and diabetic patient groups and the mean scores showed that cancer patients were evaluating their QOL and sexual functioning less well than diabetic patients. However, for physical appearance both groups were no showing significant differences.

Table 4.3: Coefficient of correlation in distress related variables and quality of life domains

Variables	*Distress related variables*			*Quality of life domains*		
	Stress	*Depression*	*Anxiety*	*Sexual functioning*	*Physical appearance*	*Quality of life*
Stress	—	.58**	.49**	–0.1	–.11	–.63**
Depression		—	66**	.08	–.13	–.42**
Anxiety			—	–.13	–.25	–.35**
Sexual functioning				—	.19	.16
Physical appearance					—	.37**
Quality of life						—

Correlation was computed to find out the relationship in distress related variable and quality of life in whole patients group, i.e. diabetic patients and cancer patients in Table 4.3. This table showed that distress related variables, i.e. were positively and significantly correlated to each other. Stress and Anxiety were found to be significantly and negatively correlated with quality of life, physical appearance and sexual functioning. Physical appearance was also found to be positively correlated with sexual functioning.

Stepwise multiple regression analysis was done to find out the predictive power distress related variables in predicting quality of life for patients with cancer and diabetes.

Table 4.4: Quality of life domains as predicted by distress related variables

Predictors	*Criterion = Quality of Life*					
	R	*R²*	*R² Change*	*Beta*	*t*	*F*
Depression	.42	.17	.17	–.42	–2.82	7.96**

Table 4.4 presented that quality of life was significantly predicted by depression [F = 7.96 (*df* = 1, 79) P <0.01]. Depression explained 17 per cent variance in the criterion variable Quality of Life. The beta value showed that depression had negative contribution in criterion variable. It suggested that the higher the depression in patients the poor she evaluates her quality of life.

Discussion

The main purpose of this study was to examine the psychological distress in women having diabetes and cancer of breast and cervix. It was hypothesized that two chronic illnesses, i.e. diabetics and cancer will produce the same level of psychological distress in women patients.

Distress in Cancer and Diabetes

The present findings showed significant differences in distress in cancer and diabetic patients. The cancer patients are more distressed than diabetic patients. Breast cancer is the leading cause of cancer death among women around the world. In India there is mix incidence pattern with breast cancer being second to cancer of the cervix in rural areas (Parkin *et al.,* 1997; National Cancer Registry Programme, 1992; Holland, and Gooen-Piels, 2000), however, in metropolitan cities like Mumbai, New Delhi and Trivandrum, the incidence of breast cancer has crossed that of cervix. Initial diagnosis has been shown to evoke a state of shock, fear and disbelief (Holland, and Gooen-Piels, 2000) thus creating not only a psychological crisis but an existential one as well (Thomas, Pandey, Ramdas, and Nair, 2002).

Keller and Henrich (1999) found that women are more likely than man to absorb in illness related behaviour including perceiving and reporting symptoms, utilizing informal and health care services. It is reported that doctors take symptoms reported by man more seriously while symptoms reported by women are often interpreted as psychological ensuing higher frequency of prescriptions for psychotropic drugs. Despite female patients reporting symptoms and higher overall distress due to illness compared to male patients, general satisfaction with life, however, did not differ significantly between genders.

Distress related finding of this present research showed that all the three distress related variables, i.e. stress, anxiety and depression were significantly more in cancer patients. The women who develop breast cancer or cervical cancer found that it affects their femininity specially the breast cancer be considered as important factor in determining feminine identity and the women with cancer are in the present study are younger in age than the women with diabetes. This may be one reason that they are more distressful in comparison to diabetic women. Many medical journals have reported the psychological trauma produced by diagnosis and treatment of breast cancer actually the cancer in women of sex related sited produce the psychiatric morbidity and sexual dysfunction (Corney *et al.,* 1993). The incidence of anxiety, depression and sexual dysfunction in women who underwent either breast conservation surgery or breast removal surgery (Fallowfield, Hall, Maguine and Baum, 1990) and women who are awaiting a biopsy because of suspected breast cancer are psychologically distress (Dekeyser *et al.*, 1998).

In present investigation majority of the cancer patients don't have a family history of cancer. However, they were exhibiting the symptoms of stress, anxiety and depression. The researches (Hyland *et al.*, 2001) suggested that if there remains a family history of cancer leads to more distress in other family members. In the present study the diabetic patients are less distressed as the disease of cancer in general is perceived in India as more life threatening than diabetes. One more reason may be that the treatment of cancer is more painful and have a lot of emotional, social, financial side effects. Basically dealing with the side effects of cancer treatment like fatigue, hair loss, weight changes, distracted life all are stressful (Carver *et al.*, 1998; Frierson, Thiel, and Anderson, 2006).

Physical Appearance

Here in the present study physical appearance is conceptualized in terms of physical attractiveness, physical activity and energy before the diagnosis of the disease and the present status. In researches the body change stress refers to subjective psychological stress that accompanies women's negative and distressing thoughts, emotions, and behaviours resultant from breast cancer and breast surgeries. However, in the present investigation there are no significant differences emerged in relation to perception of physical appearance in women patients with cancer and diabetes. Both of these diseases produces physical changes, as well as, the process of aging although the negative side effect of cancer such as hair loss, weight changes are profound in cancer group as this is appeared in the lower mean of physical appearance in cancer group. Several researches have highlighted the importance of the body image concerns of women with chronic physical illness (Chrisler and Parrett, 1995; DeVellis, Revenson and Blalock, 1997).

In the present research we incorporated the physical appearance items in the quality of life scale as this is an important concern for chronically ill patients. Quality of Life batteries usually do not include measures of body image (e.g. SF-36, Ware, Snow and Kosinski, 2000), although some do (e.g. EORTC QLQ-C30, Aaronson, 1993). Some investigators devise their own measures, with items including satisfaction with the scar (Wimberly *et al.*, 2005) or concerns about body integrity (Carver *et al.*, 1998).

Sexual Functioning

Sexual problems may be the result of physical changes, medication and the chronic illness (DeVellis, Revenson and Blalock, 1997; Krukofsky, 1988). Disease severity age and relationship quality have all been shown to impact sexual functioning (Curry *et al.*, 1993, 1994). In addition high levels of depression may result in decreased libido, and feelings of unattractiveness due to illness-related changes in the body (e.g. hair loss, weight again) also may negatively affect women's sexuality (Petri, 2000). The present findings showed significant differences in diabetes and cancer patients with reference to their sexual functioning. The sexual functioning of cancer patients was more affected by the disease than the diabetic patients. Sexual functioning is a problem for patients with certain kinds of cancers like cervix or breast but depression is a more common problem for patients with all kinds of cancer.

Quality of Life

Quality of life among the chronically ill patients is now assessed with emphasis especially placed on how much the disease and its treatment interfere with the activities of daily living, such as sleeping, eating, going to the working, and engaging in recreational activities a cancer treatment has disappointing survival rates and produces adverse side effect, the treatment may be more harmful than the disease itself (Aaronson *et al.*, 1993). Moreover, the quality of life researches have made it possible to assess the impact of unpleasant therapies.

In the present investigation there is significant difference found in cancer and diabetic patients in evaluating quality of life. The cancer patients have assessed their quality of life better than the diabetic patients.

Cancer produce many different symptoms which affect the quality of life, the intensity of disease and psychological distress also aggravate the problem of cancer patients in the areas of social, emotional support, health habit, spiritual philosophical view of life and body image concerns (Taplin *et al.*, 1995; Arora *et al.*, 2001; Ganz *et al.*, 2002).

Conclusion

The need for psychosocial intervention amongst cancer patients cannot be understated. The goals of planning a psychosocial intervention in the Indian breast/uterus cancer context would be to support the patient's ability to cope with the stress of treatment, helping them to tolerate short-term loss for long-term gain, and to assist in symptom management (Jacobsen *et al.,* 1995; Payne, Sullivan and Massie, 1996). Counselling for psychological distress and treatment of depressive disorder would improve the well-being and/or metabolic control in diabetes mellitus (Katon, *et al.*, 2005).

References

Aaronson, N.K., Ahmedzai, S., Bergman, B., *et al.* (1993). The European organization for research and treatment of cancer QLQ-C30: A quality-of-life instrument for use in international clinical trials in oncology. *Journal of the National Cancer Institute*, 85, 365-76.

Anderson, R.J., Freedland, K.E., Clouse, R.E., and Listman, P.J. (2001). The prevalence of comorbid depression in adults with diabetes. *Diabetes Care,* 24, 1069-78.

Antony, M M., Bieling, P.J., Cox, B.J., Enns, M.W., Swinson, R.P. (1998). Psychometric properties of 42-item and 21-item versions of the Depression Anxiety Stress Scales in clinical groups and community sample. *Psychological Assessment*, Vol. 10(2), 176-181.

Arora, N.K., Gustafson, D.H., Hawkins, R.P., McTavish, F., Cella, D.F., Pingree, S., *et al.* (2001). Impact of surgery and chemotherapy on the quality of life of younger women with breast carcinoma: a prospective study. *Cancer,* 92, 1288-98.

Carver, C.S., Pozo-Kaderman, C., Prince, A.A., *et al.* (1998). Concerns about aspects of body image and adjustment to early stage breast cancer. *Psychosomatic Medicine*. 8, 60, 168-174.

Chrisler, J., and Parrett, K. (1995). Women and autoimmune disorders. In A. Stanton and S. Gallant (Eds.), *The Psychology of Women's Health Progress and Challenges in Research and Application* (pp. 171-195). Washington, DC: American Psychological Association.

Corney, R.H., Crowther, M.E., Everett, H., Howells, A. and Shepherd, J.H. (1993), Psychosexual dysfunction in women with gynaecological cancer following radical pelvic surgery. *BJOG: An International Journal of Obstetrics and Gynaecology*, 100, 73-78.

Curry, S., Levine, S., Corty, E., Jones, P., and Kurit, D. (1994). The impact of systemic lupus erythematosus on women's sexual functioning. *Journal of Rheumatology*, 21, 2254-2260.

Curry, S., Levine, S., Jones, P., and Kurit, D. (1993). Medical and psychosocial predictors of sexual outcome among women with systemic lupus erythematosus. *Arthritis Care and Research*, 6, 23-30.

DeKeyser, F.G., Wainstock, J.M., Rose, L., Converse, P.J., and Dooley, W. (1998). Distress, symptom distress, and immune function in women with suspected breast cancer. *Oncology Nursing Forum*, 25, 1415-1422.

DeVellis, B., Revenson, T., and Blalock, S.J. (1997). Rheumatic disease and women's health. In S. Gallant, G.P. Keita, and R. Royak-Schaler (Eds.), *Health care for Women: Psychological, Social and Behavioural Influences* (pp. 333-347). Washington, DC: American Psychological Association.

Dutta, P.K., Upadhyay, A., Dutta, M., Urmil, A.C., Thergaonkar, M.P., and Ganguly, S.S. (1990). A case control study of cancer cervix patients attending Command Hospital, Pune. *India Journal of Cancer*, 27, 101-8.

Fallowfield, L.J., Hall, A., Maguire, G.P. and Baum, M. (1990). Psychological outcomes of different treatment policies in women with early breast cancer outside a clinical trial. *British Medical Journal*, 22; 301 (6752): 575-580.

Frierson, G.M., Thiel, D.L., and Anderson, B.L. (2006). Body Change Stress for Women with Breast Cancer: The Breast-Impact of Treatment Scale. *Annals of Behavioural Medicine*, 32(1), 77-81.

Ganz, P.A., Desmond, K.A., Leedham, B., Rowland, J.H., Meyerowitz, B.E., Belin, T.R. (2002). Quality of life in long-term, disease-free survivors of breast cancer: a follow-up study. *Journal of National Cancer Institute*, 94, 39-49.

Gawande, V., Wahab, S.N., Zodpey, S.P., and Vasudeo, N.D. (1998). Parity as a risk factor for cancer cervix. *Indian Journal of Medical Science*, 52, 147 50.

Haig, R.A. (1992). Management of depression in patients with advanced cancer. *Medical Journal of Australia*, 156, 499-503.

Holland, J.C., and Gooen-Piels, J. (2000). Principles of Psycho-Oncology. In *Cancer Medicine*. 5th edition. Edited by Bast R.C., Kufe, D.W., Pollock, R.E., Weichselbaum, R.R., Holland, J.F., Frei, E. and B.C. Decker, Ontario.

Hyland, F., Kinmonth, A.L., Marteau, T.M., Griffin, S., Murrell, P., Spiegelhalter, D. *et al.* (2001) Raising concerns about family history of breast cancer in primary care consultations: Prospective, population based study. Women's Concerns Study Group. *British Medical Journal*, 322, 27-28.

Jacobsen, P.B., Bovbjerg, D.H., Schwartz, M.D., Hudis, C.A., Gilewski, T.A., Norton, L. (1995). Conditioned emotional distress in women receiving chemotherapy for breast cancer. *Journal of Consulting Clinical Psychology,* 63, 108-114.

Katon, W., Cantrell, C.R., Sokol, M.C., Chiao, E., and Gdovin, J.M. (2005). Impact of antidepressant drug adherence on comorbid medication use and resource utilization. *Archives of Internal Medicine*, 165, 2497-503.

Krishnamurthy, S, Yeole, B.B., and Jussawalla, D.J. (1995). Uterine cervical adenocarcinomas and squamous carcinomas in Bombay: 1965-1990. *Journal of Obstetrics and Gynecology Research,* 23, 521-7.

Krukofsky, B. (1988). Sexuality counselling of people with chronic illness. In W. Weinstein and E. Rosen (Eds.), *Sexuality Counselling: Issues and Implications* (pp. 259-273). Belmont, CA: Brooks/Cole.

Levy, S.M., Haynes, L.T., Herberman, R.B., Lee, J., McFeeley, S., and Kirkwood, J. (1992). Mastectomy versus breast conservation surgery: mental health effects at long-term follow-up. *Health Psychology*, 11, 349-54.

Lovibond, S.H. and Lovibond, P.F. (1995). *Manual for the Depression Anxiety Stress Scales*. (2nd. Ed.) Sydney: Psychology Foundation. ISBN 7334-1423-0.

Massie, M.J. and Holland, J.C. (1989). Overview of normal reactions and prevalence of psychiatric disorders. In Holland J.C., and Rowland, J.H. (eds): *Handbook of Psycho Oncology: Psychological Care of the Patient With Cancer* (pp 273-282.) New York, NY, Oxford University Press.

McVeigh, K.H., Mostashari, F., and Thorpe, L.E. (2003). Serious psychological distress among persons with diabetes – New York City, 2003. *MMWR Morbidity Mortality Weekly Report,* 53, 1089-92.

Miranda, C.R., de Resende, C.N., Melo, C.F., Costa, Al Jr, and Friedman, H. (2002). Depression before and after uterine cervix and breast cancer neoadjuvant chemotherapy. *International Journal of Gynecological Cancer,* 12, 773-776.

Mohan, V., Sandeep, S., Deepa, R., Shah, B., Varghere C. (2007). Epidemiology of type 2 diabetes: Indian scenario. *Indian Journal of Medical Research,* 125, 217-30.

Murray, C.J.L., and Lopez, A.D. (1996). *Global Health Statistics. Global Burden of Disease and Injury Series*. Boston MA: Harvard School of Public Health.

Nandakumar, A., Anantha, N., and Venugopal, T.C. (1995). Incidence, mortality and survival in cancer of the cervix in Bangalore, India. *British Journal of Cancer,* 71, 1348-52.

National Cancer Registery Programme (1992). *Biennial Report (1988–89): An epidemilogical study*. Indian Council of Medical Research, New Delhi.

National Cancer Registery Programme (2002). Two year report of the population-based cancer registries 1997-98. Incidence and distribution of cancer. New Delhi: Indian Council of Medical Research.

National Comprehensive Cancer Network (NCCN) (2007). *Standards of care and management of distress penal.* Distress management management version [http://www.nccn.org/professionals/physician_gls/PDF/distress.pdf].

Pandey, M., Devi, N., Thomas, B.C., Vinod Kumar, S., Krishnan, R. and Ramdas, K. (2007), Distress overlaps with anxiety and depression in patients with head and neck cancer. *Psycho-Oncology*, 16: 582–586.

Parkin, D.M., Whelan, S.L., Ferlay, J., Raymond, L., and Young, J., (eds) (1997). *Cancer incidence in five continents. Volume VII.* International agency for research on cancer, Lyon, France. IARC Science Publication No. 143.

Payne, D.K., Sullivan, M.D., and Massie, M.J. (1996). Women's psychological reactions to breast cancer. *Seminal Oncology*, 23, 89-97.

Petri, M. (2000). Systemic lupus erythematosus: Women's health issues. *Bulletin on the Rheumatic Diseases,* 49, 1-3.

Ramachandran, A. (2005). Experiences of the WHO Collaborating Centre for Diabetes in India in managing tsunami victims with diabetes. *Practical Diabetes International,* 22, 98-99.

Reddy, K.S., Shah, B., Varghese, C. and Ramadoss, A. (2005). *Responding to the threat of chronic diseases in India.* Published Online. DOI 10.1016/S0140-6736(05).

Rowland, J.H. (1999). Anxiety and the blues after breast cancer: How common are they? *CNS Spectrums*, 4, 40-54.

Sadikot, S.M., Nigam, A., Das, S., Bajaj, S., Zargar, A.H., Prasannakumar, K.M., *et al.* (2004). The burden of diabetes and impaired glucose tolerance in India using the WHO 1999 criteria: prevalence of diabetes in India study (PODIS). *Diabetes Research Clinical Practice,* 66, 301-7.

Sarita, G.P. (2004). Impact of chemotherapy on distress and quality of life of cancer patients. *Dissertation submitted* to University of Kerala, Trivandrum, India.

Sen, S., Sankaranarayanan, R., Mandal, S., Ramkumar, A.V., Parkin, D.M. and Siddiqui, M. (2002). Cancer patterns in eastern India: The first report of Kolkata cancer registry. *International Journal of Cancer*, Vol. 100(1), 86 91.

Sridhar, G.R., and Madhu, K. (2002). Depression and psychosocial stress in diabetes mellitus. In: Kapur, A, Joshi, J.K., editors. *Novonordisk diabetes update proc*. Mumbai: Business Network Inc., pp. 87-92.

Sridhar, G.R., and Madhu, K. (2002). Psychosocial and cultural issues in diabetes mellitus. *Current Science,* 83, 1556-64.

Sridhar, G.R., Madhu, K., and Veena, S. (2000). Gender differences in well-being among persons with diabetes in India. *Diabetes Research Clinical Practice*, 50: 981.

Stanton, A.L., Krishnan, L., and Collins, C.A. (2001). Form or function? Part 1. Subjective cosmetic and functional correlates of quality of life in women treated with breast-conserving surgical procedures and radiotherapy. *Cancer*, 91, 2273-81.

Stechlin, J.S., and Beach, K.H. (1966). Psychological aspects of cancer therapy. A surgeon's viewpoint. *JAMA,* 197, 100-104.

Taplin, S.H., Barlow, W., Urban, N., Mandelson, M.T., Timlin, D.J., Ichikawa, L., and Nefcy, P., (1995). Stage, age or comorbidity and the direct costs of colon, prostrate, and breast cancer care. *Journal of National Cancer Institute,* 87, 417-26.

Thomas, B.C., Pandey, M., Ramdas, K., and Nair, M.K. (2002). Psychological distress in cancer patients: Hypothesis of a distress model. *European Journal Cancer Prevention*, 11, 179-85.

Vinokur, A.D., Threatt, B.A., Caplan, R.D., and Zimmerman, B.L. (1989). Physical and psychosocial functioning and adjustment to breast cancer: long-term follow-up of a screening population. *Cancer*, 63, 394-405.

Ware, J.E., Snow, K.K., and Kosinski, M. (2000). *SF-36 Health Survey: Manual and Interpretation Guide.* Lincoln, RI: Quality Metric Incorporated.

Wimberly, S.R., Carver, C.S., Laurenceau, J., Harris, S.D., and Antoni, M.H. (2005). Perceived partner reactions to diagnosis and treatment of breast cancer: Impact on psychosocial and psychosexual adjustment. *Journal of Consulting and Clinical Psychology*, 73, 300-311.

Zabora, J., Brintzenhofeszoc, K., Curbow, B., *et al.* (2001). The prevalence of psychological distress by cancer site. *Psycho-Oncology,* 10, 19-28.

5

An Ecological Model of the Impact of Sexual Assault on Women's Mental Health

Laxmi Vajpeyi

The impact of sexual assault on women's mental health has been extensively studied and has been the subject of multiple prior reviews (Briere and Jordan, 2004; Chivers-Wilson, 2006; Ellis, 1983; Goodman, Koss, and Russo, 1993; Koss, 1993; Koss, Bailey, Yuan, Herrera, and Lichter, 2003; Koss *et al.*, 1994; Kilpatrick and Acierno, 2003; Kilpatrick, Amstadter, Resnick, and Ruggiero, 2007; Resick, 1993; Rogers and Gruener, 1997). The reviews from the early 1990s are remarkably consistent with more recent syntheses of the literature: rape is one of the most severe of all traumas, causing multiple, long-term negative outcomes. Between 17 per cent and 65 per cent of women with a lifetime history of sexual assault develop Post-traumatic Stress Disorder (PTSD; Clum, Calhoun, and Kimerling, 2000; Kilpatrick *et al.*, 1989; Kilpatrick and Resnick, 1993; Kilpatrick, Saunders, Veronen, Best, and Von, 1987; Rothbaum, Foa, Riggs, Murdock, and Walsh, 1992). Many (13%-51%) meet diagnostic criteria for depression (Acierno *et al.*, 2002; Becker, Skinner, Abel, Axelrod, and Treacy, 1984; Burnam *et al.*, 1988; Clum *et al.*, 2000; Dickinson, deGruy, Dickinson, and Candib, 1999; Frank and Anderson, 1987; Golding, 1996; Kilpatrick *et al.*, 1987; Winfield, George, Swartz, and Blazer, 1990). Most sexual assault victims develop fear and/ or anxiety (73%-82%; Frank and Anderson, 1987; Ullman and Siegel, 1993), and 12 per cent to 40 per cent experience generalized anxiety (Siegel, Golding, Stein, Burnam, and Sorenson, 1990; Winfield *et al.*, 1990). Approximately 13 per cent to 49 per cent of survivors become dependent on alcohol, whereas 28 per cent to 61 per cent may use other illicit substances (Frank and Anderson, 1987; Ullman, 2007; Ullman and Brecklin, 2002a). It is not uncommon for victims to experience suicidal ideation (23%-44%; Frank and Stewart, 1984; Frank, Turner, Stewart, Jacob, and West, 1981; Kilpatrick *et al.*, 1985; Petrak, Doyle, Williams, Buchan, and Forster, 1997), and 2 per cent to 19 per cent may attempt suicide (Davidson, Hughes, George, and Blazer, 1996; Frank *et al.*, 1981; Kilpatrick *et al.*, 1985).

Though there is little disagreement that sexual assault is highly detrimental to women's mental health, how to conceptualize that harm has been the subject of debate. A trauma response theoretical model has been proposed as a useful conceptual framework for guiding research and intervention (Goodman *et al.*, 1993; Herman, 1992), though concerns have been raised that the clinical diagnosis of PTSD risks pathologizing victims (Berg, 2002; Gilfus, 1999) as well as perpetuating ethnocultural biases (Marsella, Friedman, and Spain, 1999; Wasco, 2003). Framing the impact of sexual assault solely within a PTSD framework would indeed be limiting, and hence, violence against women scholars have advocated for ecologically informed trauma models of rape recovery (Koss and Harvey, 1991; Neville and Heppner, 1999). Sexual assault does not occur in social and cultural isolation: we live in a rape-prone culture that propagates messages that victims are to blame for the assault, that they caused it and, indeed, deserve it (Buchwald, Fletcher, and Roth, 1993; Burt, 1998; Lonsway and Fitzgerald, 1994; Sandy, 1998). Victims are faced with negotiating postassault help seeking and, ultimately, their pathway to recovery within multiple hostile environments. If survivors turn to their family and friends for social support, how will they react, as they, too, have been inundated with these cultural messages? If victims turn to formal systems, such as the legal, medical, and mental health systems, they may face disbelief, blame, and refusals of help instead of assistance. The trauma of rape extends far beyond the actual assault, and society's response to this crime can also affect women's well-being.

The purpose of this review is to examine the psychological impact of adult sexual assault through an ecological theoretical perspective to understand how factors at multiple levels of the social ecology contribute to the deleterious mental health effects that have been so consistently reported in the literature. The utility of an ecological framework is that it can suggest multiple strategies, at multiple levels of analysis, for alleviating the psychological harm caused by sexual assault. We will begin with a brief discussion of the different ecological theories that have been utilized in violence against women research. Since Koss and Harvey (1991) and Neville and Heppner (1999) first called for more ecologically informed research on psychological sequel and recovery, numerous studies have been conducted on the relationships between extra individual level factors and mental health outcomes. Our review will synthesize this developing literature to identify positive, negative, and still inconclusive findings regarding the relationships between individual, assault, and ecological factors and survivors' psychological distress.

> **Key Points of the Research Review**
>
> - The negative mental health squeal of sexual assault stems from multiple factors, not just characteristics of the victim. Aspects of the assault itself, post-assault disclosures and help seeking, and socio-cultural norms help shape the way in which this trauma affects women's psychological well-being.
> - Women's victimization is cumulative, and the response from the social world is cumulative, both of which affect how any one incident of sexual violence will affect women's mental health?
> - Self-blame has been studied from both individual-level and extra-individual perspectives, and we conceptualize it as a meta-construct that develops from and is shaped by multiple levels in the ecological system.

Ecological Theories in Violence against Women Research

There are multiple ecological theories evolving in the social sciences, and it is beyond the scope of this article to explore each one (*see* McLaren and Hawe, 2005 for a review). In violence against women scholarship, two specific approaches have been drawn on to inform research, prevention, and treatment. First, from community psychology, Kelly's (1966, 1968, 1971) ecological theory posits that the functions of individuals and community organizations are interdependent and that individuals have differential patterns of experiences given different ecological settings. Ecological settings consist of person constructs, which are individual characteristics such as race/ethnicity, gender, and beliefs and attitudes; events, which refer to the specific problem(s) that prompts an individual to need assistance and/or seek help and instigates a community help-system network to respond; and environments, which include structural features of a community (e.g. resources), functional features (e.g. service delivery processes), as well as the attitudes and values of the community as a whole (Kelly, Ryan, Altman, and Stelzner, 2000). Koss and Harvey (1991) and Harvey (1996) adapted these ideas to propose an ecological model of rape recovery, and Campbell and colleagues have used this model in empirical research to evaluate how the legal, medical, and mental health systems respond to victims' needs and how those system experiences affect victims' psychological, physical, and sexual health outcomes (Campbell, 1998; Campbell *et al.*, 1999; Campbell *et al.*, 2001; Campbell, Sefl, and Ahrens, 2004). Second, from developmental psychology, Bronfenbrenner's (1979, 1986, 1995) ecological theory of human development has similar conceptual foundations in its premise that human development occurs through constantly evolving interactions between individuals and their multiple, interconnected environmental contexts. Bronfenbrenner's model subdivides environmental influences into multiple levels reflecting the relative size, immediacy of interaction, and degree of formality/informality of the environmental setting. The individual level comprises bio-psycho-social characteristics of the person; the microsystem focuses on direct interpersonal interactions between individuals and members of their immediate environment such as families, friends, and peers; the mesosystem reflects interconnections and linkages between individuals and between individuals and systems; the exosystem includes organizations and social systems (e.g., legal, medical, and mental health); the macro system includes societal norms, expectations, and beliefs that form the broader social environment; and the chronosystem encompasses the changes that occur over time between persons and their multiple environments. Bronfenbrenner's conceptualization shaped the theoretical models created by Heise (1998) and White and Kowalski (1998) to explain the underlying causes of violence against women and risk factors for perpetration. Similarly, Grauerholz's (2000) model of sexual revictimization examines how personal, interpersonal, and socio-cultural factors contribute to child sexual abuse survivors' increased risk for subsequent sexual victimization later in life. Both the Centres for Disease Control and Prevention (CDC; 2004) and the World Health Organization (WHO; Jewkes, Sen, and Garcia-Moreno, 2002; Krug, Mercy, Dahlberg, and Zwi, 2002) have adapted this approach to develop multilevel models for the prevention of gender-based violence.

As noted previously, Neville and Heppner (1999) also extended Bronfenbrenner's model to explain how sexual assault affects women's well-being and recovery processes, which they termed CIEMSAR: culturally inclusive ecological model of sexual assault recovery. The fundamental premise of their model is that sexual assault survivors' mental health is shaped by many factors, not just the assault itself or pre-existing individual characteristics. With each disclosure and interaction with the social world, victims are given explicit and implicit messages about how they are to make sense of this crime and apportion blame.

First, at the individual level of analysis, characteristics of the victim could certainly influence the recovery process. Neville and Heppner's (1999) model examined age, race/ethnicity, and social class as socio-demographic correlates of post-assault psychological distress; to that base, our model includes additional demographic features recently examined in the literature such as education, marital status, employment status, and income. Neville and Heppner noted race/ethnicity can be conceptualized at multiple levels of the social ecology, but that most research on post-assault sequel has not conceptualized race/ethnicity from a socio-cultural perspective. In other words, racial differences have been examined without a full exploration of cultural identity. We concur with this analysis and followed the convention established by Neville and Heppner to discuss race/ethnicity at both the individual level of analysis and the macro level of analysis, depending on the way in which this construct was conceptualized in the particular study. Also at the individual level, our model considers the role of personality characteristics, pre-existing mental health conditions, and biological/genetic factors in victims' post-assault distress, which were not examined in Neville and Heppner's model.

Finally, victims' coping processes are also influential in recovery, although it is unclear at which level of analysis this construct best fits (e.g., coping by mobilizing social support reflects an interaction of individual and microsystem processes). We follow Neville and Heppner's precedent and place this construct at the individual level, as it reflects the choices and propensities of the survivors, but explore it "last" in the individual processes as a way of symbolizing its interconnections to the higher levels in the model (i.e. microsystems).

Second, characteristics of the assault itself affect women's psychological well-being. Neville and Heppner (1999) examined how the victim-offender relationship and the severity of injury differentially affect victims' distress. In addition to those factors, our model explores the roles of threats to kill the victim, weapon use, assault force or violence, and substance use at the time of the assault in relation to victims' post-assault psychological sequel, which has been a growing area of inquiry in recent years.

Third, at the micro system level, our model explores the impact of disclosures to informal sources of support (e.g. family and friends) on victims' post-assault psychological distress. Neville and Heppner (1999) conceptualized social support as the meso system level, but we have elected to reframe this construct as a micro system process (when that support is specifically from family, friends, or peers). Bronfenbrenner

(1979) defined the micro system as the face-to-face interactions and interrelations between individuals and others in their immediate setting; because the provision of (or denial of) social support occurs through direct interactions with family, friends, or peers, we conceptualized this as a microsystem process. Since, Neville and Heppner's model was developed, research on social support has flourished, and we can now refine the model in light of this new empirical knowledge base.

Fourth, although Bronfenbrenner's original model separates mesosystems (i.e. processes that contribute to linkages between systems and/or other individuals in the ecological environment) from exo systems (i.e. formal systems with which individuals may or may not have contact), our analysis of the extant literature on post-assault sequel suggests that empirically based distinctions between these levels are not yet warranted, which is consistent with Neville and Heppner's (1999) model. For example, victims may seek assistance from a Rape Crisis Center (RCC), which could be conceptualized as a formal help resource (i.e. exosystem) and in the process of helping the survivors, RCC staff may help establish connections with other formal systems (such as the legal or medical systems) and/or work with survivors to help them access more informal supports in their lives (i.e. mesosystems). Therefore, we distinguish our combined meso/exosystem level from the prior microsystem level by whether the interactions take place between informal supports (microsystem) versus formalized supports (meso/exosystem).

Fifth, as noted previously, race/ethnicity can be conceptualized at the macrolevel of analysis when explored from a socio-cultural perspective to understand the cultural identity and its role in rape recovery. Victims' post-assault distress is also influenced by the rape-prone culture in which we live, which remains highly acceptant of rape myths and stereotypes that woman, are to blame for their own victimization (Rozee and Koss, 2001).

Sixth, the chronosystem was not included in Neville and Heppner's (1999) original model, but we have incorporated it to reflect Bronfenbrenner's idea that person-environment interactions are reciprocal and change over time. There are normative transitional events (e.g. school changes) and non-normative events (e.g. sexual assault) that shape how individuals interact with their environments and how their environments respond to them. The chronosystem examines the cumulative effects of multiple sequences of developmental transitions over the life course. Therefore, a history of sexual assault and other victimizations across the lifespan would influence the recovery process at each victimization (if more than one is experienced). Neville and Heppner conceptualized sexual revictimization as an individual-level variable, but we view it as an historical lifespan factor that shapes how other levels in the model affect a recent victimization.

Finally, Neville and Heppner (1999) conceptualized self-blame as a macrolevel phenomenon, informed by Ward's (1995) analysis that women internalize societal rape myths, which leads to negative self-appraisals. We concur that societal rape myths contribute to internalized self-blame, but since the development of Neville and Heppner's original model, multiple empirical studies have established that survivors encounter a great deal of victim blaming in their interactions with both formal and informal systems (e.g., Filipas and Ullman, 2006). In addition, some victims, particularly racial/ethnic minorities, are more likely to be subjected to victim-blaming treatment (e.g. Campbell *et al.*, 2001). Survivors of certain types of assault, such as acquaintance/date rape and those who have been sexually revictimized, are also more susceptible to being blamed for the assault (e.g., Arata, 1999; Filipas and Ullman, 2006). In view of these findings, we argue that self-blame transcends anyone level of the model, as it stems from individual, assault, micro-, meso/exo-, macro-, and chronosystem-level processes. Therefore, we conceptualize self-blame as a meta-construct that results from interactions across all levels of the social ecology.

In the review, people focused on empirical studies of adult sexual assault, which is often operationalized in research as assaults that occurred at age 14 or older (Koss, Gidycz, and Wisneiwski, 1987). Age 14 is also the developmental demarcation identified by Burnam *et al.* (1988) for significantly different post-assault mental health outcomes. As such, our review does not include studies of childhood sexual abuse (only), but would include studies of victims who were sexually victimized multiple times in their lives, provided that one of the assaults clearly occurred in adulthood (as defined above). Studies that assessed lifetime sexual victimization but did not distinguish whether there was an assault sustained during adulthood (as defined above) were not included in this review (though we note that the substantive findings from these studies do not differ from those that met our inclusion criteria). Similarly, studies of criminal victimization were not reviewed unless subgroup analyses were available that separated victims of sexual assault from victims of other types of crimes. Because sexual assault is one form of intimate partner violence (Campbell and Soeken, 1999; Cole, Logan, and Shannon, 2005; Eby, Campbell, Sullivan, and Davidson, 1995), we searched the domestic violence/intimate partner violence literature as well to ensure that studies of intimate partner sexual assault were also included. Because our goal was to develop a model of mental health impact (not physical or sexual health impact), to be included in this review, a study must have empirically examined a link between at least one of the factors in the ecological model described above and a psychological health outcome such as PTSD, depression, fear/anxiety, general psychological distress, sociality, and/or substance use (*see* Table 5.1).

Individual-Level Factors

1. Socio-Demographic Variables

Several socio-demographic variables have been studied in relation to post-assault sequel. Most studies have not found racial/ethnic differences in post-assault distress; specifically, no difference has been found for PTSD (e.g. Campbell *et al.*, 1999; Elliott, Mok, and Briere, 2004; Ullman and Brecklin, 2002a; Ullman, Filipas, Townsend, and Starzynski, 2006), depression (Elliott *et al.*, 2004; Frank and Stewart, 1984; McFarlane *et al.*, 2005; Wyatt, 1992), fear/anxiety (McFarlane *et al.*, 2005; Wyatt, 1992), or general distress (Kilpatrick, Veronen, and Best, 1984). Studies of lifetime victimization have reported that Hispanic and non-Hispanic women do not differ in depression, substance use/dependence, phobia, panic, or obsessive-compulsive disorder (Burnam *et al.*, 1988), and White and non-White women do not differ in suicidal ideation/attempts (Ullman and Brecklin, 2002b). However, one study with a small number of African-American participants found that African-American women were more likely than White women to be anxious after sexual assault (Burge, 1988), and a second study of intimate partner sexual assault victims identified that Hispanic women had significantly higher levels of PTSD than African-American and White women (McFarlane *et al.*, 2005). Ruch and Chandler (1983) defined trauma as the general effect of the assault on victims' lives, and under that definition, they found that White women were more traumatized than racial/ethnic minority survivors. With respect to victims' age, several studies have found that older survivors experience increased depression and general trauma (Frank and Stewart, 1984; Ruch and Chandler, 1983; Ruch and Leon, 1983); however, younger age has been found to predict PTSD and depression (Elliott *et al.*, 2004) and older victims have been found to have fewer PTSD symptoms when assaulted by relatives (Ullman *et al.*, 2006). Several studies found no effect of age

Table 5.1: The Impact of Multilevel Ecological Factors on Sexual Assault Victims' Psychological Sequel.

Ecological Level	*Major Findings*
Individual level factors (victim and assault characteristics)	Mixed findings on the impact of socio-demographic variables (i.e., age, race, income, education, employment), assault characteristics (i.e., victim-offender relationship, injury, alcohol use), and biological factors (i.e., cortisol levels) on post-assault well-being.
	Personality traits such as neuroticism predict PTSD among sexual assault survivors.
	Poorer pre-assault mental health predicts multiple negative outcomes, such as depression and anxiety.
	Avoidance coping strategies predict multiple negative outcomes, such as longer recovery time, depression, and PTSD.
	Perceived life threat during assault and perceived dangerousness of assailant predict negative outcomes, such as depression, anxiety, and PTSD symptomatology.
Microsystem factors	Positive social reactions and support from informal providers (e.g., family, friends, significant others) predicts less mental distress post assault.
	Negative social reactions from informal support providers predict multiple negative outcomes such as depression, anxiety, and post-traumatic stress.
Meso/exosystem factors	Legal System: secondary victimization (i.e. victim blaming, minimal help) predicts higher symptomatology such as PTSD and depression.
	SANEs, rape crisis centres, and other community mental health programmes help mitigate the negative effects of other medical systems (e.g. E.R.) and predict less mental health distress post assault.
Macro-system factors	The rape-prone culture, institutionalized racism, cultural differences in responding to rape, and acceptance of rape myths create a difficult socio-cultural context for sexual assault survivors to recover.
Chronosystem factors	Cumulative trauma and revictimization over the lifetime predicts negative outcomes such as depression, anxiety, and PTSD.
Self-blame: Multilevel meta-construct	Self-blame is associated with PTSD and depression at the individual level. At the micro and meso/exo levels, receiving blame exacerbates self-blame and is associated with PTSD symptomatology. At the macro level, internalized socio-cultural beliefs affect victims' self-blame. At the chronosystem level, victims of cumulative trauma have been found to have greater self-blame and higher levels of trauma.

on distress (Bownes, O'Gorman, and Sayers, 1991; Campbell *et al.*, 1999; Kilpatrick *et al.*, 1984; Kramer and Green, 1991; Ullman and Filipas, 2001b).

In the examination of income level, marital status, and employment status with post-rape distress, most studies that attempted to relate these variables with specific post-rape diagnoses have not found an association (e.g., Bownes *et al.*, 1991; Campbell *et al.*, 1999; Mackey *et al.*, 1992; Ullman and Brecklin, 2002a; Ullman and Filipas, 2001b). However, when these variables are studied in relation to more general indices of trauma or stress, associations have been found. One study found that victims who were "economically stressed" were less likely to report that they were "recovered" from the assault months or years afterward (Burgess and Holmstrom, 1978), a single study found that being married was related to increased trauma (Ruch and Chandler, 1983), and a similar study identified that being unemployed was related to post-assault trauma two weeks after assault (Ruch and Leon, 1983). Furthermore, Ullman and Brecklin's (2002b) study of lifetime victimization indicated that those who were employed or married experienced less suicidal ideation, but no difference was found for suicide attempts.

The relationship between education and post-assault distress is also unclear. Two studies reported that less education is related to PTSD (Burge, 1988; Ullman and Brecklin, 2002a): one identified that higher education predicted lowered levels of PTSD (Ullman and Filipas, 2001b), and one found that a lack of a college education was related to suicide attempts (Ullman and Brecklin, 2002b). However, an equivalent number of studies have found no effect of education on post-traumatic stress (Campbell *et al.*, 1999; Ullman *et al.*, 2006) or depression (Frank and Stewart, 1984). Studies of lifetime victimization have found that depression, substance abuse, phobia, panic disorder, obsessive-compulsive disorder, and suicidal ideation do not differ based on level of educational attainment (Burnam *et al.*, 1988; Ullman and Brecklin, 2002b).

2. *Personality Factors*

Few studies have been conducted on the relationship between personality factors and post-assault psychological distress. Researchers commonly conceptualize personality using the Five-Factor Model, which consists of five dimensions: openness, conscientiousness, extraversion, agreeableness, and neuroticism. Cox, MacPherson, Enns, and McWilliams

(2004) reported that neuroticism (including traits such as anxiety, impulsiveness, hostility, and depression; John and Srivastava, 1999) was found to predict PTSD, and that the self-criticism, an additional personality variable, also predicted PTSD.

3. Preexisting Mental Health Conditions

Several studies have identified that preexisting mental health conditions are positively related to post-assault mental health sequel. Victims who had attempted suicide pre assault experienced significantly more post-assault depression and anxiety (Frank *et al.*, 1981), and pre-existing mental health diagnosis and substance abuse problems were positively associated with post-assault trauma (Frank and Anderson, 1987; Ruch and Chandler, 1983; Ruch and Leon, 1983). Pre-assault depression and suicidal history significantly predicted depression levels 4 months post-assault (Atkeson *et al.*, 1982). Anxiety attacks and obsessive-compulsive symptoms also predicted depression at 8 and 12 months. Psychiatric treatment history before the sexual assault predicted depression at a year post-assault (Atkeson *et al.*, 1982). Conversely, several studies have not found that pre-rape psychopathology predicts post-rape distress (Bownes *et al.*, 1991; Frank *et al.*, 1981; Frank and Stewart, 1984; Kilpatrick *et al.*, 1984). However, these studies examined psychiatric history generally (e.g., visits to psychiatrist, psychiatric hospitalization), suggesting that although pre-rape psychiatric history overall may not be associated with post-rape symptomatology, more specific mental health variables (e.g., diagnoses) may be associated with post-assault distress.

4. Genetic and Biological Factors

To date, no studies have examined genetic factors as predictors of post-rape distress, but several biological factors have been examined in a limited body of work. Normally, in reaction to stress, the body reacts by releasing hormones such as cortical (Chivers-Wilson, 2006). However, traumatic events such as sexual assault seem to alter cortical response, possibly contributing to PTSD (Yehuda, 2006). Among adult rape victims, cortisol levels immediately after the assault have been alternately identified as a positive correlate of PTSD (Resnick, Yehuda, and Acierno, 1997) and unrelated to PTSD (Resnick, Yehuda, Pitman, and Foy, 1995). Some have theorized that sexual assault survivors who develop PTSD may have abnormally low cortisol levels due to a history of sexual victimization

(Resnick *et al.*, 1997), which may function to maintain the stress response, contributing to PTSD (Shalev and Sahar, 1998). MHPG (3-Methoxy-4-Hydroxyphenylglycol), a metabolite of norepinephrine (a stress hormone), has also been found to contribute to PTSD (Yehuda, Resnick, Schmeidler, Yang, and Pitman, 1998). Survivors of sexual assault without PTSD showed associations between MHPG and cortisol, suggesting that these responses are coordinated in an adaptive response to trauma (Yehuda *et al.*, 1998).

5. Coping Responses

Finally, victims' coping responses affect their postassault psychological health. As noted previously, coping is a "transitional" construct that includes both individual-level and situational factors (Roth and Cohen, 1986). Survivors may use approach strategies (i.e., emotional or cognitive activity oriented towards the threat) and/or avoidance strategies (i.e. emotional or cognitive activity oriented away from the threat) for any given situation and at any given point in time during their recovery process. Survivors may use a consistent coping orientation over time to deal with stress, but this orientation may change depending on the availability of resources (e.g., personal resources and/or support in the environment). For example, Ullman and colleagues have found that rape survivors who receive negative social support are more likely to use avoidance coping and have increased PTSD symptomatology (Ullman, 1996c; Ullman, Townsend, Filipas, and Starzynski, 2007). Therefore, coping can be explained as an underlying orientation towards stress that can be influenced by time, situation/context, and environmental support.

The empirical research on sexual assault survivors' coping distinguishes between maladaptive or adaptive recovery strategies. Maladaptive approaches involve some level of avoidance, such as staying at home, withdrawal, disengagement, and substance abuse, which are associated with longer recovery time and higher levels of depression, anxiety, fear, and PTSD (Burgess and Holmstrom, 1979; Gutner, Rizvi, Monson, and Resick, 2006; Frazier and Burnett, 1994; Frazier, Mortensen, and Steward, 2005; Meyer and Taylor, 1986; Santello and Leitenberg, 1993; Ullman *et al.*, 2007). Adaptive strategies, such as expressing emotions, seeking social support, and reducing stress, have been found to be related to faster recovery and less depression, anxiety, fear, and PTSD (Burgess and Holmstrom, 1979; Frazier and Burnett, 1994; Frazier *et al.*, 2005; Gutner *et al.*, 2006; Meyer and Taylor, 1986; Valentiner,

Foa, Riggs, and Gershuny, 1996). However, several studies have found mixed findings regarding coping and post-assault distress. For example, Valentiner *et al.* (1996) reported that seeking social support was not associated with PTSD severity, and instead, the actual type of support received by survivors predicted adjustment. Furthermore, Ullman (1996a, 1996b, 1996c) found that approach strategies such as joining a support group and going to a therapist were actually related to more distress. It has also been suggested that avoidance can be beneficial for recovery. Frazier and Burnett (1994) found that avoidance strategies such as keeping busy and suppressing negative thoughts were related to less distress. This finding is also consistent with Roth and Cohen's (1986) theory that the use of avoidance immediately after a stressful life event may be helpful to adjustment. These mixed findings suggest that perhaps coping strategies should be examined in relation to the context in which they are used (i.e., microsystem influences).

Assault-Related Factors

Numerous studies have investigated how characteristics of the assault itself affect victims' post-assault distress. With respect to victim-offender relationship, most studies have found that experiencing rape perpetrated by a stranger is not associated with differential levels of post-rape symptomatology (e.g. Arata and Burkhart, 1996; Campbell *et al.*, 1999; Frank, Turner, and Stewart, 1980; Kilpatrick *et al.*, 1984; Kramer and Green, 1991; Mackey *et al.*, 1992; Riggs, Kilpatrick, and Resnick, 1992; Ullman and Filipas, 2001b), but some studies have reported that surviving stranger rape was associated with increased PTSD (Bownes *et al.*, 1991; Ullman *et al.*, 2006), depression (Ellis, Atkeson, and Calhoun, 1981) and general trauma (Ruch and Chandler, 1983). Ellis and colleagues (1981) reported that stranger rapes tended to be more violent and invasive than non-stranger rapes and suggested that this may contribute to findings of increased post-rape symptomatology. Sexual assault by a partner has been found to be a significant predictor of PTSD (Temple, Weston, Rodriguez, and Marshall, 2007; Ullman *et al.*, 2006), although when compared to other types of assailants, there was no difference in depression (Koss, Dinero, Seibel, and Cox, 1988; Riggs *et al.*, 1992) or anxiety (Koss *et al.*, 1988). Some have suggested that the perceived dangerousness of the assailant (rather than simpler stranger/non-stranger distinction) may be related to the severity of PTSD symptoms (Cascardi, Riggs, Hearst-Ikeda, and Foa, 1996).

Many studies report that injury incurred as a result of sexual assault is related to post-assault PTSD, depression, and anxiety (e.g., Bownes *et al.*, 1991; Sales, Baum, and Shore, 1984), but many have not found a relationship between psychological distress and injury (Campbell *et al.*, 1999; Kilpatrick *et al.*, 1984; Ullman and Filipas, 2001b). One study identified that threats to kill the victim did not affect post-rape depression or anxiety (Frank *et al.*, 1980), but Sales *et al.* (1984) reported that threats to kill predicted depression and anxiety immediately after the assault. Most examinations of post-rape distress have not found an effect for weapon use (Campbell *et al.*, 1999; Frank *et al.*, 1980; Kilpatrick *et al.*, 1984; Sales *et al.*, 1984), although one study identified that victims with PTSD had experienced more weapon use than those without PTSD (Bownes *et al.*, 1991). However, this sample differed from those that found no weapon effect, in that all victims had reported the rape to the police. Although most attempts to associate assault force or violence with post-assault distress have found that these variables are positively related (Bownes *et al.*, 1991; Sales *et al.*, 1984; Ullman and Siegel, 1993), others have found that violence/force does not predict post-assault depression and anxiety (Atkeson *et al.*, 1982) or general post-assault distress (Kilpatrick *et al.*, 1984).

A limited number of studies have assessed the relationship of victim substance use before or during sexual assault to post-assault distress. These studies have not found an association between substance abuse and post-traumatic symptoms (Arata and Burkhart, 1996; Campbell *et al.*, 1999; Resnick *et al.*, 1997; Schwartz and Leggett, 1999). The relatively high level of perpetrator violence and relatively low level of victim resistance that are common among substance-facilitated rapes (Ullman, Karabatsos, and Koss, 1999) could contribute to post-assault symptomatology; therefore, the mental health outcomes of substance-facilitated rapes should be further examined.

Micro System Factors

Although several studies have investigated sexual assault survivors' disclosure processes (Ahrens, 2006; Ahrens, Campbell, Ternier-Thames, Wasco, and Sefl, 2007; Fisher, Daigle, Cullen, and Turner, 2003; Golding, Siegel, Sorenson, Burnam, and Stein, 1989; Ullman and Brecklin, 2003) and the positive and negative social reactions they receive from both formal and informal support providers (Ahrens *et al.*, 2007; Golding *et al.*, 1989; Sudderth, 1998; Ullman, 2000), fewer studies have actually examined how these social reactions affect mental health outcomes such as depression and PTSD. Overall, this literature suggests that social support from family, friends, and intimate partners facilitates sexual assault survivors' recovery. The availability of family and friends, living with family, and feeling close to family members are related to better adjustment (Burgess and Holmstrom, 1979; Kramer and Green, 1991; Ruch and Chandler, 1983; Ruch and Leon, 1983; Sales *et al.*, 1984). Positive social reactions from family and friends are related to less psychological distress (Campbell, Ahrens, Sefl, Wasco, and Barnes, 2001; Coker *et al.*, 2002), and similarly, in studies that did not differentiate between informal and formal sources of support, positive social support was also related to lower symptomatology (Atkeson *et al.*, 1982; Thompson *et al.*, 2000). Negative social reactions from family, friends, and peers have consistently been found to be related to increased anxiety, depression, and PTSD (Borja, Callahan, and Long, 2006; Campbell *et al.*, 2001; Davis, Brickman, and Baker, 1991; Moss, Frank, and Anderson, 1990). Studies that have measured both informal and formal sources of support together substantiate this effect (Ullman, 1996a, 1996b, 1996c; Ullman and Filipas, 2001a; Ullman, Townsend, Filipas, and Starzynski, 2007).

Interestingly, it appears that negative social reactions have a stronger detrimental effect on survivors' mental health than positive social reactions have for bolstering well-being (Borja *et al.*, 2006; Campbell *et al.*, 2001; Fowler and Hill, 2004; Ruch and Leon, 1983). It may be that negative social reactions are more salient for survivors' recovery because survivors are more likely to first disclose to family and friends (Ahrens *et al.*, 2007; Filipas and Ullman, 2001; Starzynski, Ullman, Filipas, and Townsend, 2005), and they likely expect sympathetic reactions from these people. If survivors receive unexpected negative reactions from family and friends, it may be particularly upsetting. However, the direction of causality between psychological distress and social support is unresolved. For example, Starzynski *et al.* (2005) found that increased levels of distress symptoms predicted seeking social support from both informal and formal support providers. In addition, what happens in one instance of seeking support has implications for further help seeking and distress. Ahrens *et al.* (2007) revealed that when initial disclosures were negative, victims refrained from further disclosures and were less likely to seek further help, which was associated with higher self-reported distress. These findings emphasize the need for longitudinal studies of victims' recovery process to examine the temporal relationships between social support and post-assault psychological sequel.

Meso/Exosystem Factors

Sexual assault victims have extensive post-assault needs and may turn to multiple formal social systems for assistance: approximately 26 per cent to 40 per cent of victims report the assault to the police and pursue prosecution through the criminal justice system, 27 per cent to 40 per cent seek medical care and medical forensic examinations, and 16 per cent to 60 per cent obtain mental health services (Campbell *et al.*, 2001; Ullman, 1996a, 1996b, 2007; Ullman and Filipas, 2001a). If victims are able to receive the services they need and are treated in an empathic, supportive manner, then social systems can help facilitate recovery. Conversely, if victims do not receive needed services and are treated insensitively, then these systems can magnify victims' feelings of powerlessness, shame, and guilt. Post-assault help-seeking from formal social systems can become a "second rape," that is, a secondary victimization to the initial trauma. These experiences of secondary victimization can have a negative impact on victims' psychological well-being (Campbell *et al.*, 1999; Campbell *et al.*, 2001; Campbell and Raja, 1999, 2005).

The Legal System

Throughout their contact with legal system, victims are asked to recount the assault many times. During this questioning, they are often asked victim-blaming questions about what they were wearing, their prior sexual history, and whether they responded sexually to the assault (Campbell, 2005, 2006; Campbell and Raja, 2005). In self-report characterizations of their psychological health, rape survivors indicate that as a result of their contact with legal system personnel, they felt bad about themselves (87%), guilty/self-blaming (73%), depressed (71%), violated (89%), distrustful of others (53%), and reluctant to seek further help (80%; Campbell, 2005; Campbell and Raja, 2005). The harm of secondary victimization is also evident on objective measures of PTSD symptomatology. In a series of studies on victim/police contact, Campbell and colleagues found that low legal action (i.e., case did not progress/was dropped) and high secondary victimization were associated with increased PTSD symptomatology (Campbell *et al.*, 2001; Campbell and Raja, 2005). In tests of complex interactions, Campbell *et al.* (1999) identified that the victims of non-stranger rape whose cases were not prosecuted and who were subjected to high levels of secondary victimization had the highest PTSD of all—worse than those who chose not to report to the legal system at all.

The Medical System

Sexual assault victims may also seek help from the medical system for injury detection and care, medical forensic examination, screening and treatment for Sexually Transmitted Infections (STIs), pregnancy testing, and emergency contraception. Although most victims are not physically injured to the point of needing emergency care (Ledray, 1996), traditionally, police, rape crisis centres, and social service agencies have advised victims to seek treatment in hospital emergency departments (EDs) for a medical forensic examination (Martin, 2005). During this medical care, doctors and nurses ask victims similar questions as do legal personnel regarding their prior sexual history, sexual response during the assault, manner of dress, and what they did to "cause" the assault. Medical professionals may view these questions as necessary and appropriate, but rape survivors find them upsetting (Campbell and Raja, 2005). Comparative studies suggest that victims encounter significantly fewer victim-blaming questions and statements from medical system personnel relative to legal professionals (Campbell, 2005, 2006; Campbell *et al.*, 1999; Campbell *et al.*, 2001; Campbell and Raja, 2005), but this still has a demonstrable negative impact on victims' mental health. Campbell (2005) found that as a result of their contact with ED doctors and nurses, most rape survivors stated that they felt bad about themselves (81%), guilty (74%), depressed (88%), violated (94%), distrustful of others (74%), and reluctant to seek further help (80%; see also Campbell and Raja, 2005). Victims who do not receive basic medical services rate their experiences with the medical system as more hurtful, which has been associated with higher PTSD levels (Campbell *et al.*, 2001; Campbell and Raja, 2005). Specifically, non-stranger rape victims who received minimal medical services but encountered high secondary victimization had significantly higher levels of PTSD symptoms than victims who did not seek medical services at all (Campbell *et al.*, 1999).

The Mental Health System

Few studies have examined if and how sexual assault victims benefit from community-based mental health system services (Acierno, Brady, Grey, Kilpatrick, Resnick, and Best, 2002). In general, victims tend to rate their experiences with mental health professionals positively and characterize their help as useful and supportive (Campbell *et al.*, 2001; Ullman, 1996a, 1996b). Whether positive satisfaction results in demonstrable mental health benefit is largely unknown although Campbell *et al.* (1999) found that community-based mental health services were particularly helpful for victims who had had negative experiences with the legal and/or medical systems. Victims who encountered substantial difficulty obtaining needed services and experienced high secondary victimization from the legal and medical systems had high PTSD symptomatology; but among this high-risk group of survivors, those who had been able to obtain mental health services had significantly lower PTSD, suggesting that there may have been some benefit from receiving such services. In this same sample, however, 25 per cent of women who received post-assault mental health services rated this contact as hurtful and 19 per cent characterized it as severely hurtful (Campbell *et al.*, 2001).

The Advocacy Community

Sexual assault victims may also seek help from Rape Crisis Centres (RCCs) or domestic violence shelter programmes. One of the key roles RCC staff fulfil is to help victims negotiate their contact with the legal and medical systems (i.e. mesosystemic processes). Sexual assault survivors who have the assistance of an RCC advocate during their contact with the legal and medical systems are significantly less likely to experience secondary victimization and also report significant less emotional distress after their system contact (Campbell, 2006). RCCs also provide direct services (i.e. exosystemic processes) to survivors, such as individual and group counselling (Campbell and Martin, 2001). Wasco *et al.* (2004) and Howard *et al.* (2003) compared self-reported PTSD symptoms pre- and post-counselling among victims receiving RCC counselling services and found significant reductions in distress levels and self-blame over time and increases in social support, self-efficacy, and sense of control. Because these studies did not examine the content of services or include comparison groups, it is unclear whether these observed improvements are attributable to the services provided.

Macrosystem Factors

Although there has been extensive research on how individual level, micro-system, and meso-system factors impact rape survivors' well-being, the research on macro-system factors is very limited. As noted previously, race/ethnicity can be conceptualized at multiple levels of analysis. Whereas, many studies have examined racial/ethnic differences in rape recovery, fewer have examined socio-cultural identity in post-rape recovery. For example, Neville, Heppner, Oh, Spanierman, and Clark (2004) examined the self-esteem of African American and White college rape survivors, and although they did not find any differences in the post-rape symptoms, self-blame and coping experienced by these survivors, they did find differences in their cultural attributions. African American women were more likely to internalize the "Jezebel" image as to why they were sexually assaulted. Engaging in these cultural blame attributions (e.g. "African-American women are not valued in this society") was related to greater self-blame attributions and, in turn, related to lower self-esteem among African-American women. These findings are reminiscent of Wyatt's (1992) findings that African-American rape survivors were more likely to feel that they are at risk for being victimized and sexually assaulted than their White counterparts. Similarly, Lefley, Scott, Llabre, and Hicks (1993) found that among Hispanic, White, and African American rape survivors, Hispanics were more likely to be blaming and punitive towards themselves and other victims, whereas, the White rape survivors were least punitive (*see* also Williams and Holmes, 1982). Not surprisingly, Hispanic rape survivors had the highest psychological distress and White rape survivors the least. Luo (2000) explored cultural-specific beliefs about rape among Chinese marital rape survivors and found that Chinese rape survivors had similar symptoms to those reported in the Western literature (e.g., fear, anxiety, self-blame, depression, loss of self-esteem), but her qualitative findings suggest that specific Chinese cultural beliefs such as collectivism, a strong emphasis of family honour, and a focus on female virginity have a strong negative impact on recovery.

Research on sexual assault has yet to take into account fully how the rape-prone culture in which we live not only condones male violence against women but also negatively affects the recovery of sexual assault survivors (Rozee and Koss, 2001). To date, most research on social factors, such as rape myth acceptance, has been primarily conducted with participants who have not been sexually assaulted (*see* Lonsway and Fitzgerald, 1994 for a review). Harned's (2005) qualitative study found that victims of date/partner rape blamed themselves because their experiences did not fit the typical rape stereotype (i.e. violent stranger rape). Likewise, women often reported that they cared about the perpetrator and thus did not believe he had meant to cause them harm.

Harned (2005) argued that these beliefs signify the impact of rape myths on female victims and teaches them to blame themselves for the assault while taking away the responsibility from the perpetrator's actions. Similarly, Peterson and Muehlenhard (2004) reported that sexual assault survivors who were high in rape myth acceptance were less likely to acknowledge that what had happened to them was, indeed, sexual assault. High rape myth acceptance appears to decrease the likelihood that victims will disclose the assault and seek support (Botta and Pingree, 1997; Moor, 2007).

Chrono System Factors

The primary chrono system factor that may affect victims' recovery outcomes is their prior history of victimization throughout the lifespan. *Revictimization* is generally defined as the experience of sexual victimization in both childhood and adulthood (Messman-Moore and Long, 2003). A recent review of the literature identified that two of every three women who reported sexual victimization had been assaulted more than once (Classen, Palesh, and Aggarwal, 2005). Many studies have found that revictimization is more strongly associated with negative psychological outcomes (e.g. depression, suicide attempts, PTSD, anxiety) than a single sexual assault alone (Arata, 2002; Classen *et al.*, 2005; Follette, Polusny, Bechtle, and Naugle, 1996; Messman-Moore, Long, and Siegfried, 2000; Miner, Flitter, and Robinson, 2006). Multiple sexual assaults may have a cumulative effect, increasing the severity of psychological sequelae with each assault (Nishith, Mechanic, and Resick, 2000). These distress outcomes may increase an individual's vulnerability to additional assaults, which may in turn exacerbate the existing psychological distress (Grauerholz, 2000; Messman-Moore and Long, 2003).

In addition, sexual assault is not the only form of violence women experience in their lifetimes, as physical and emotional abuse in childhood and in adult intimate partner relationships are highly prevalent (Pimlott-Kubiak and Cortina, 2003). Even though the focus of this review is the impact of sexual assault on women's mental health, we cannot define the scope of inquiry so narrowly that it bears little resemblance to the lived experiences of survivors. Other victimizations (prior or concurrent) undoubtedly affect how survivors respond to a subsequent sexual victimization. For example, in a sample of battered women, Campbell and Soeken (1999) summed how many sexual assaults women had endured in their lifetimes (childhood sexual assault, non-intimate partner adult sexual assault, and intimate partner adult sexual assault) and found that more assaults were associated with increased levels of depression. Other researchers have substantiated that sexual assault within intimate partner violence is associated with increased depression, PTSD, and anxiety, above that explained by physical violence alone (Bennice *et al.*, 2003; Cole *et al.*, 2005). Campbell, Greeson, Bybee, and Raja (2008) examined the cumulative impact of experiencing childhood sexual abuse, adult sexual assault, intimate partner violence, and sexual harassment on women's levels of PTSD symptomatology, and indeed, the women who experienced all four forms of violence at the highest levels were significantly higher on self-report distress than those who endured fewer forms at lower levels.

Although revictimization and/or other victimization experiences are often conceptualized as individual-level factors that affect survivors' mental health, Grauerholz (2000) convincingly argued that revictimization itself is an ecological phenomenon (*see* also Heise, 1998; Jewkes *et al.*, 2002; White and Kowalski, 1998). For example, for victims of childhood sexual abuse, their post-assault distress would be determined by aspects of the child, the assault sustained, informal support, formal systems, and socio cultural factors. If victims of childhood sexual abuse are then revictimized in adolescence, the post-assault sequel from that victimization would include the experiential vestiges of the prior victimization (and multilevel factors that contributed to post-assault distress at that time, i.e. a chronosystem effect). In addition, the model would "repeat" itself in the context of the new victimization—new interactions in the ecology would shape the distress experience from the most recent assault (also a chronosystem effect). Women's victimization is cumulative and the response from social world is cumulative, and so it is little wonder then that the mental health consequences of revictimization are so severe.

Self-Blame as a Multilevel Meta-Construct

Self-blame has been studied as from both individual-level and extra individual perspective, and therefore, we conceptualize self-blame as a meta-construct that develops from and is shaped by multiple levels in the ecological system. At the individual level, Janoff-Bulman (1979) identified two types of self-blame: characterological self-blame, which she theorized would be maladaptive because it involves blaming ones own character for the negative event; and behavioural self-blame, which involves blaming one's actions for the event. This latter type of self-blame may actually be adaptive because it enhances perceived control and the belief that future rapes can be avoided. Empirical support for Janoff-Bulman's model has been mixed. General self-blame has been found to be associated with PTSD and depression (Boeschen, Koss, Figueredo, and Coan, 2001; Filipas and Ullman, 2006; Frazier, 1990; Frazier and Schauben, 1994; Meyer and Taylor, 1986; Ullman, Townsend, Filipas, and Starzynski, 2007; Wyatt, Newcomb, and Notgrass, 1991). Some studies have found that characterological self-blame is indeed more harmful and behavioural self-blame can protect against distress (Hill and Zuarta, 1989; Koss and Figueredo, 2004; Koss, Figuerdo, and Prince, 2002), but others suggest that behavioural self-blame is more detrimental (Frazier, 2003; Frazier *et al.*, 2005). Maladaptive coping strategies have also been linked with higher levels of self-blame and PTSD symptomatology (Filipas and Ullman, 2006; Frazier *et al.*, 2005).

Yet, survivors' self-blame comes both from internal and external forces, as multiple ecological factors directly contribute to victims' negative attributions. For example, certain assault characteristics (e.g., greater severity of the assault, using alcohol/drugs) contribute to increase self-blame and thereby more post-assault distress (Koss *et al.*, 2002; Wyatt *et al.*, 1991). Starzynski *et al.* (2005) reported that survivors with higher behavioural self-blame were less likely to reach out to both informal and formal support providers, perhaps out of concern that they would receive more criticism of their behaviour or choices. Such apprehension may be warranted, as negative social reactions from informal supports have consistently been found to be associated with increased self-blame (Ahrens, 2006; Littleton and Breitkopf, 2006; i.e. a micro-system effect). Ullman and colleagues have documented univariate relationships between negative social reactions, self-blame, and PTSD symptoms, but in multivariate analyses, self-blame did not mediate the effect of negative social reactions on symptoms.

At the meso/exosystem level, Campbell *et al.* have documented in multiple studies that survivors often encounter victim-blaming treatment from legal and medical system personnel, and not surprisingly, survivors state that they do start to blame themselves more for the assault (Campbell, 2005, 2006; Campbell *et al.*, 2001). In recent years, the emergence of community interventions, such as Sexual Assault Nurse Examiner (SANE) programmes, have made a positive systemic effort to curb victim blaming and provide empowering post-assault care to survivors (Campbell,

Patterson, and Lichty, 2005). Interestingly, rape victims who received postassault care in a SANE programme did not indicate that this model of care exacerbated their self-blame (Campbell, Patterson, Adams, Diegel, and Coats, 2008). At the macrosystem level, Long, Ullman, Starzynski, Long, and Mason (2007) reported that less educated and older African American women tended to blame themselves more for the rape than younger, more educated African American women. The authors suggest that less educated African-American women may have fewer resources to help counter the negative views about themselves (e.g. rape myth education) compared to college-educated women. The finding that older women blamed their behaviour more than younger women may be because of their lack of exposure to sexual assault education and the nature of culture in which they were raised, which was more accepting of violence against African-American women. A chronosystem effect has also been supported such that victims of repeated sexual assault have more self-blame, societal blame, and higher levels of trauma symptoms (Arata, 1999; Filipas and Ullman, 2006). Although we suspect it would be challenging to disentangle empirically the sources, levels, and relative impact of victims' self-blame, the extant literature clearly indicates that self-blame is fed and nurtured along an often destructive path by multiple people, settings, and cultures over time.

Conclusions and Future Directions

In this review, we extended the work of Neville and Heppner (1999) to examine how multilevel ecological factors affect sexual assault victims' psychological sequelae. Our analysis indicates that the mental health consequences of rape are caused by multiple factors beyond characteristics of the victim or the assault. Indeed, many studies found no relationship between socio-demographic variables and post-assault distress. Survivors' preassault mental health may affect the recovery process, but because prior research has not assessed prior victimizations in relation to preexisting mental health, it is difficult to know what these findings actually reflect. An emerging field of study suggests biological processes are important in recovery, but why women have different cortisol levels (and thereby different degrees of post-traumatic symptomatology), and whether cortisol levels vary by victimization history, is not yet understood. The degree of violence and threat in the assault itself affects women's mental health outcomes to some extent, but whether the offender is a stranger or known person is not consistently predictive of victims' psychological outcomes.

Overall, it would be difficult to predict fully women's post-assault sequelae only from individual or assault characteristics.

Research findings are more consistent at the micro-, meso/exo-, macro-, and chronosystem levels. Receiving social support from family, friends, and peers is helpful, but these positive reactions may not be as powerful as unexpected negative reactions. This is not to say that positive social support is unimportant; rather, the findings suggest that negative reactions are more central to the prediction of depression and PTSD severity. If victims seek help from the legal system, it is probable that their cases will not be prosecuted, and the treatment they receive from legal system personnel will likely leave them feeling blamed, doubted, and judged, which, not surprisingly, is associated with increased PTSD symptomatology. If survivors seek medical care for a forensic examination and evaluation and management of sexually transmitted infections and pregnancy, they will typically encounter fewer difficulties obtaining needed assistance (relative to legal system contact) but may still be treated in ways that exacerbate their post-assault distress. By contrast, community mental health services and rape crisis centre advocacy can buffer these negative effects. Although empirical research on macro system factors is limited, institutionalized racism and pervasive rape myths contribute to societal acceptance of sexual assault, which creates a more difficult social context for victims to negotiate their recoveries. Cumulative trauma, a manifestation of the chronosystem, is highly detrimental to women's well-being.

A critical next step in the development of an ecological model of rape recovery is to examine interactions across different levels of the social ecology. For example, what individual or assault characteristics, in conjunction with what kinds of coping strategies, are associated with more positive or negative psychological outcomes? Then, adding the next layer of conceptual complexity, how do these individual-level features play out in different post-assault help-seeking experiences? It may be that some survivors are more likely to have negative experiences with formal social systems, such as the legal and medical systems, and this contact may be more or less detrimental to some survivors than others— although such findings would not excuse any victim-blaming treatment from social system personnel. Similarly, how these individual and extra individual factors co-occur for women who have been repeatedly sexually victimized throughout the lifespan is essential to examine. It is not difficult to imagine that negative informal or formal help-seeking experiences in an earlier assault would curb later help seeking for a subsequent assault and compound victims' psychological distress. We suspect that the mixed findings in the literature regarding individual and assault characteristics may be due not only to methodological differences across studies, but may also reflect unexamined cross-level interactions.

Although the literature on post-assault recovery has advanced rapidly since Neville and Heppner's review, sexual assault survivors are a heterogeneous population and we still know very little about the recovery processes of many sub-groups of survivors. Prevalence research suggests that women with disabilities (e.g. mobility/visual/hearing impairments, mental/emotional disabilities, cognitive/developmental disabilities, and/or chemical dependency) are at disproportionately high risk for being sexually assaulted (e.g. as many as 85% of women with disabilities have been raped; Elman, 2005), but how their recovery process unfolds is largely unknown. Similarly, the experiences of lesbian, bisexual, and transgendered survivors, elderly women, and immigrant women are largely missing in the literature. For this review, we made concerted effort to find research on sexual assault within Intimate Partner Violence (IPV), and this work indicates that the combined effect of IPV and sexual assault is highly detrimental to women's mental health, but these survivors are understudied in both the IPV and sexual violence literatures. There is also a pressing need to examine specific cultural factors to understand how women from different racial/ethnic backgrounds are affected by mainstream and culture-specific beliefs and norms.

A key advantage of an ecological model of mental health impact is that it can suggest multiple strategies for intervention. Although individual and assault characteristics are difficult, if not impossible, to modify in their own right, it is possible to address myths and stereotypes about sexual assault and its victims, which could have positive effects on victims' recoveries. Public education efforts must emphasize that women's experiences of rape are usually not "stereotypical rapes" (i.e. violent stranger assaults). There is no universal experience of rape: all kinds of women may be victimized, and women may exhibit markedly diverse responses to this traumatic crime. At the micro system level, rape awareness programmes need to provide information for informal support providers about the varied reactions survivors may exhibit. In addition, such programmes should emphasize to informal support providers that positive reactions such as emotional support and tangible aid are helpful for recovery, and negative reactions, such as egocentrism and blame, may overshadow any positive efforts. At the meso/exosystem level, there are many promising intervention models for improving the community response to rape. Emerging data suggest that Sexual Assault Nurse Examiner (SANE) programmes and Sexual Assault Response Teams (SARTs) significantly improve the provision of consistent, victim-centred medical and crisis intervention services, and simultaneously increase rates of successful prosecution (*see* Campbell, Patterson, and Lichty, 2005 for a review). In addition, restorative justice programmes for sexual assault provide a mechanism outside of the traditional criminal justice system to address victims' needs (*see* Koss, 2006; Koss and Achilles, 2008 for reviews). Rape crisis center services are beneficial to victims, and increasing the availability and accessibility of these programmes to more survivors may also contribute to more consistently positive post-assault help-seeking experiences (Campbell, 2006). Intervening at the macro system level may be the most difficult, but the comprehensive models developed by the CDC (2004) and WHO (Jewkes, Sen, and Garcia-Moreno, 2002) outline strategies for working with multiple systems and settings; specifically, they suggest using a wide variety of tactics, such as policy change, organizational change, systems advocacy, media campaigns, and rape awareness/prevention education, to create broad-based systemic change. Similarly, efforts that focus on the prevention of sexual assault reduce the likelihood of multiple victimizations in women's lifetimes, thereby curbing negative chronosystem effects. Both Kelly's and Bronfenbrenner's ecological theories emphasize that changes at anyone level of the social ecology can have extended effects at other levels. As a result, there are many feasible approaches to improving the societal response to rape victims and addressing their post-assault recovery needs.

References

Acierno, R., Brady, K., Gray, M., Kilpatrick, D.G., Resnick, H., and Best, C.L. (2002). Psychopathology following interpersonal violence: A comparison of risk factors in older and younger adults. *Journal of Clinical Geropsychology*, 8, 13-23.

Ahrens, C. (2006). Being silenced: The impact of negative social reactions on the disclosure of rape. *American Journal of Community Psychology*, 38, 263-274.

Ahrens, C., Campbell, R., Ternier-Thames, K., Wasco, S., and Sefl, T. (2007). Deciding whom to tell: Expectations and outcomes of rape survivors' first disclosures. *Psychology of Women Quarterly*, 31, 38-49.

Arata, C.M. (1999). Coping with rape: The roles of prior sexual abuse and attributions of blame. *Journal of Interpersonal Violence,* 14, 62-78.

Arata, C.M. (2002). Child sexual abuse and sexual revictimization. *Clinical Psychology: Science and Practice,* 9, 135-164.

Arata, C.M. and Burkhart, B.R. (1996). Post-traumatic stress disorder among college student victims of acquaintance assault. *Journal of Psychology and Human Sexuality,* 8, 22, 79-92.

Becker, J.V., Skinner, L.J., Abel, G.G., Axelrod, R., and Treacy, E.C. (1984). Depressive symptoms associated with sexual assault. *Journal of Sex and Marital Therapy,* 10, 185-192.

Bennice, J.A., Resick, P.A., Mechanic, M., and Astin, M. (2003). The relative effects of intimate partner physical and sexual violence on post-traumatic stress disorder symptomatology. *Violence and Victims,* 18, 87-94.

Berg, S.H. (2002). The PTSD diagnosis: Is it good for women? *Affilia,* 17, 55-68.

Boeschen, L.E., Koss, M.P., Figueredo, A.J., and Coan, J.A. (2001). Experiential avoidance and posttraumatic stress disorder: A cognitive mediational model of rape recovery. *Journal of Aggression, Maltreatment and Trauma,* 4, 211-245.

Borja, S.E., Callahan, J.L., and Long, P.J. (2006). Positive and negative adjustment and social support of sexual assault survivors. *Journal of Traumatic Stress,* 19, 905-914.

Botta, R.A., and Pingree, S. (1997). Interpersonal communication and rape: Women acknowledge their assaults. *Journal of Health Communication,* 2, 197-212.

Bownes, I.T., O'Gorman, E.C., and Sayers, A. (1991). Assault characteristics and post-traumatic stress disorder in rape victims. *Acta Psychiatrica Scandinavia,* 83, 27-30.

Briere, J., and Jordan, C.E. (2004). Violence against women: Outcome complexity and implications for assessment and treatment. *Journal of Interpersonal Violence,* 19, 1252-1276.

Bronfenbrenner, U. (1979). *The Ecology of Human Development: Experiments by Nature and Design.* Cambridge, MA: Harvard University Press.

Bronfenbrenner, U. (1986). Ecology of the family as a context for human development: Research perspectives. *Developmental Psychology,* 22, 723-742.

Bronfenbrenner, U. (1995). Developmental ecology through space and time: A future perspective. In P. Moen, G.H. Elder, Jr., and K. Luscher (Eds.), *Examining Lives in Context: Perspectives on the Ecology of Human Development* (pp. 619-647). Washington, DC: APA Books.

Buchwald, E., Fletcher, P., and Roth, M. (Eds.). (1993). *Transforming a rape culture.* Minneapolis, MN: Milkweed.

Burge, S.K. (1988). Post-traumatic stress disorder in victims of rape. *Journal of Traumatic Stress,* 1, 193-210.

Burgess, A.W., and Holmstrom, L.L. (1978). Recovery from rape and prior life stress. *Research in Nursing and Health,* 1, 165-174.

Burgess, A.W., and Holmstrom, L.L. (1979). Adaptive strategies and recovery from rape. *American Journal of Psychiatry,* 136, 1278-1282.

Burnam, M.A., Stein, J.A., Golding, J.M., Siegel, J.M., Sorenson, S.B., Forsythe, A.B., *et al.* (1988). Sexual assault and mental disorders in a community population. *Journal of Consulting and Clinical Psychology*, 56, 843-850.

Burt, M.R. (1998). Rape myths. In M.E. Odem and J. Clay-Warner (Eds.), *Confronting Rape and Sexual Assault* (pp. 129-144). Lanham, MD: Rowman and Littlefield.

Campbell, J.C., and Soeken, K.L. (1999). Forced sex and intimate partner violence: Effects on women's risk and women's health. *Violence Against Women,* 5, 1017-1035.

Campbell, R. (1998). The community response to rape: Victims' experiences with the legal, medical, and mental health systems. *American Journal of Community Psychology,* 26, 355-379.

Campbell, R. (2005). What really happened? A validation study of rape survivors' help-seeking experiences with the legal and medical systems. *Violence and Victims,* 20, 55-68.

Campbell, R. (2006). Rape survivors' experiences with the legal and medical systems: Do rape victim advocates make a difference? *Violence Against Women,* 12, 1-16.

Campbell, R., Ahrens, C., Sefl, T., Wasco, S.M., and Barnes, H.E. (2001). Social reactions to rape victims: Healing and hurtful effects on psychological and physical health outcomes. *Violence and Victims,* 16, 287-302.

Campbell, R., Greeson, M.R., Bybee, D., and Raja, S. (2008). The Co-occurrence of childhood sexual abuse, adult sexual assault, intimate partner violence, and sexual harassment: A mediational model of PTSD and physical health outcomes. *Journal of Consulting and Clinical Psychology,* 76, 194-207.

Campbell, R., and Martin, P.Y. (2001). Services for sexual assault survivors: The role of rape crisis centers. In C. Renzetti, J. Edleson, and R. Bergen (Eds.), *Sourcebook on Violence Against Women* (pp. 227-241). Thousand Oaks, CA: Sage.

Campbell, R., Patterson, D., Adams, A.E., Diegel, R., and Coats, S. (2008). A participatory evaluation project to measure SANE nursing practice and adult sexual assault patients' psychological well-being. *Journal of Forensic Nursing,* 4, 19-28.

Campbell, R., Patterson, D., and Lichty, L.F. (2005). The effectiveness of sexual assault nurse examiner (SANE) programme: A review of psychological, medical, legal, and community outcomes. *Trauma, Violence, and Abuse: A Review Journal,* 6, 313-329.

Campbell, R., and Raja, S. (1999). The secondary victimization of rape victims: Insights from mental health professionals who treat survivors of violence. *Violence and Victims,* 14, 261-275.

Campbell, R., and Raja, S. (2005). The sexual assault and secondary victimization of female veterans: Help-seeking experiences in military and civilian social systems. *Psychology of Women Quarterly,* 29, 97-106.

Campbell, R., Sefl, T., and Ahrens, C.E. (2004). The impact of rape on women's sexual health risk behaviours. *Health Psychology,* 23, 67-74.

Campbell, R., Sefl, T., Barnes, H.E., Ahrens, C.E., Wasco, S.M., and Zaragoza-Diesfeld, Y. (1999). Community services for rape survivors: Enhancing psychological well-being or increasing trauma? *Journal of Consulting and Clinical Psychology,* 67, 847-858.

Campbell, R., Wasco, S.M., Ahrens, C.E., Sefl, T., and Barnes, H.E. (2001). Preventing the "second rape": Rape survivórs' experiences with community service providers. *Journal of Interpersonal Violence,* 16, 1239-1259.

Cascardi, M., Riggs, D.S., Hearst-Ikeda, D., and Foa, E.B. (1996). Objective ratings of assault safety as predictors of PTSD. *Journal of Interpersonal Violence,* 11(1), 65-78.

Centres for Disease Control and Prevention. (2004). *Sexual Violence Prevention: Beginning the dialogue*. Atlanta, GA: Author.

Chivers-Wilson, K.A. (2006). Sexual assault and post-traumatic stress disorder: A review of the biological, psychological, and sociological factors and treatments. *McGill Journal of Medicine,* 9, 111-118.

Classen, C.C., Palesh, O.G., and Aggarwal, R. (2005). Sexual revictimization: A review of the empirical literature. *Trauma, Violence, and Abuse,* 6, 103-129.

Clum, G.A., Calhoun, K.S., and Kimerling, R. (2000). Associations among symptoms of depression and post-traumatic stress disorder and self-reported heath in sexually assaulted women. *Journal of Nervous and Mental Disease,* 188, 671-678.

Coker, A.L., Smith, P.H., Thompson, M.P., McKeown, R.E., Bethea, L., and Davis, K.E. (2002). Social support protects against the negative effects of partner violence on mental health. *Journal of Women's Health and Gender-Based Medicine,* 11, 465-476.

Cole, J., Logan, T., and Shannon, L. (2005). Intimate sexual victimization among women with protective orders: Types and associations of physical and mental health problems. *Violence and Victims,* 2, 695-715.

Cox, B.J., MacPherson, P.S.R., Enns, M.W., and McWilliams, L.A. (2004). Neuroticism and self-criticism associated with posttraumatic stress disorder in a nationally representative sample. *Behaviour Research and Therapy,* 42, 105-114.

Davidson, J.R., Hughes, D.C., George, L.K., and Blazer, D.G. (1996). The association of sexual assault and attempted suicide within the community. *Archives of General Psychiatry,* 53, 550-555.

Davis, R.C., Brickman, E., and Baker, T. (1991). Supportive and unsupportive responses of others to rape victims: Effects on concurrent victim adjustment. *American Journal of Community Psychology,* 19, 443-451.

Dickinson, L.M., deGruy, F.V., Dickinson, W.P., and Candib, L.M. (1999). Health-related quality of life and symptom profiles of female survivors of sexual abuse in primary care. *Archives of Family Medicine,* 8, 35-43.

Eby, K.K., Campbell, J.C., Sullivan, C.M., and Davidson, W.S., II. (1995). Health effects of experiences of sexual violence for women with abusive partners. *Health Care for Women International,* 16, 563-576.

Elliott, D.M., Mok, D.S., and Briere, J. (2004). Adult sexual assault: Prevalence, symptomatology, and sex differences in the general population. *Journal of Traumatic Stress,* 17, 203-211.

Ellis, E.M. (1983). A review of empirical rape research: Victim reactions and response to treatment. *Clinical Psychology Review,* 3, 473-490.

Ellis, E.M., Atkenson, B.M., and Calhoun, K.S. (1981). An assessment of long-term reaction to rape. *Journal of Abnormal Psychology,* 90, 263-266.

Elman, R.A. (2005). *Confronting the sexual abuse of women with disabilities.* VAWNet Document, National Online Resource Centre on Violence against Women, Minneapolis: University of Minnesota. Retrieved from http://www.vawnet.org/SexualViolence/Research/VAWnetDocument

Filipas, H.H., and Ullman, S.E. (2001). Social reactions to sexual assault victims from various support sources. *Violence and Victims,* 16, 673-692.

Filipas, H.H., and Ullman, S.E. (2006). Child sexual abuse, coping responses, self-blame, PTSD, and adult sexual revictimization. *Journal of Interpersonal Violence,* 21, 652-672.

Fisher, B.S., Daigle, L.E., Cullen, F.T., and Turner, M.G. (2003). Reporting sexual victimization to the police and others. *Criminal Justice and Behaviour,* 30, 6-38.

Foa, E.B., Rothbaum, B.O., Riggs, D.S., and Murdock, T.B. (1991). Treatment of post-traumatic stress disorder in rape victims: A comparison between cognitive-behavioural procedures and counselling. *Journal of Consulting and Clinical Psychology,* 59, 715-723.

Follette, V.M., Polusny, M.A., Bechtle, A.E., and Naugle, A.E. (1996). Cumulative trauma: The impact of child sexual abuse, adult sexual assault, and spouse abuse. *Journal of Traumatic Stress,* 9, 25-35.

Fowler, D.N., and Hill, H.M. (2004). Social support and spirituality as culturally relevant factors in coping among African-American women survivors of partner abuse. *Violence Against Women,* 10, 1267-1282.

Frank, E., and Anderson, B.P. (1987). Psychiatric disorders in rape victims: Past psychiatric history and current symptomatology. *Comprehensive Psychiatry,* 28, 77-82.

Frank, E., and Stewart, B.D. (1984). Depressive symptoms in rape victims: A revisit. *Journal of Affective Disorders,* 7, 77-85.

Frank, E., Turner, S.M., and Stewart, B.D. (1980). Initial response to rape: The impact of factors within the rape situation. *Journal of Behavioural Assessment,* 2, 39-53.

Frank, E., Turner, S.M., Stewart, B.D., Jacob, M., and West, D. (1981). Past psychiatric symptoms and the response to sexual assault. *Comprehensive Psychiatry,* 22, 479-487.

Frazier, P. (2003). Perceived control and distress following sexual assault: A longitudinal test of a new model. *Journal of Personality and Social Psychology,* 84, 1257-1269.

Frazier, P.A. (1990). Victim attributions and post-rape trauma. *Journal of Personality and Social Psychology,* 59, 298-304.

Frazier, P.A. (1991). Self-blame as a mediator of post-rape depressive symptoms. *Journal of Social and Clinical Psychology,* 10, 47-57.

Frazier, P.A., and Burnett, J.W. (1994). Immediate coping strategies among rape victims. *Journal of Counselling and Development,* 72, 633-639.

Frazier, P.A., Mortensen, H., and Steward, J. (2005). Coping strategies as mediators of the relations among perceived control and distress in sexual assault survivors. *Journal of Counselling Psychology,* 52, 267-278.

Frazier, P.A., and Schauben, L.J. (1994). Causal attributions and recovery from rape and other stressful life events. *Journal of Social and Clinical Psychology,* 13, 1-14.

Gilfus, M.E. (1999). The price of the ticket: A survivor-centered appraisal of trauma theory. *Violence Against Women,* 5, 1238-1257.

Golding, J.M. (1996). Sexual assault history and limitations in physical functioning in two general population samples. *Research in Nursing and Health,* 19, 33-44.

Golding, J.M., Siegel, J.M., Sorenson, S.B., Burnam, M.A., and Stein, J.A. (1989). Social support sources following sexual assault. *Journal of Community Psychology,* 17, 92-107.

Goodman, L.A., Koss, M.P., and Russo, N.F. (1993). Violence against women: Physical and mental health effects. Part I: Research findings. *Applied and Preventative Psychology,* 2, 79-89.

Grauerholz, L. (2000). An ecological approach to understanding sexual revictimization: Linking personal, interpersonal, and socio-cultural factors and processes. *Child Maltreatment,* 5, 5-17.

Gutner, C.A., Rizvi, S.L., Monson, C.M., and Resick, P.A. (2006). Changes in coping strategies, relationship to perpetrator, and post-traumatic distress in female crime victims. *Journal of Traumatic Stress,* 19, 813-823.

Harned, M. (2005). Understanding women's labelling of unwanted sexual experiences with dating partners, *Violence Against Women,* 11, 374-413.

Harvey, M.R. (1996). An ecological view of psychological trauma and trauma recovery. *Journal of Traumatic Stress,* 9, 3-23.

Heise, L.L. (1998). Violence against women: An integrated, ecological framework. *Violence Against Women,* 4, 262-290.

Herman, J.L. (1992). Complex PTSD: A syndrome in survivors of prolonged and repeated trauma. *Journal of Traumatic Stress,* 5, 377-391.

Hill, J.L., and Zuarta, A.J. (1989). Self-blame attributions and unique vulnerability. *Journal of Social and Clinical Psychology,* 8, 368-375.

Howard, A., Riger, S., Campbell, R., and Wasco, S.M. (2003). Counselling services for battered women: A comparison of outcomes for physical and sexual abuse survivors. *Journal of Interpersonal Violence,* 18, 717-734.

Janoff-Bulman, R. (1992). *Shattered Assumptions: Towards a New Psychology of Trauma.* New York: The Free Press.

Jewkes, R., Sen, P., and Garcia-Moreno, C. (2002). Sexual violence. In E.G. Krug, L.L. Dahlberg, J.A. Mercy, A.B. Zwi, and R. Lozano (Eds.), *World report on violence and health* (pp. 147-181). Geneva: World Health Organization.

John, O.P., and Srivastava, S. (1999). The Big Five trait taxonomy: History, measurement, and theoretical perspectives. in L.A. Pervin and O.P. John (Eds.), *Handbook of Personality: Theory and Research* (pp. 102–138). New York: Guilford Press.

Kelly, J.G. (1966). Ecological constraints on mental health services. *American Psychologist,* 21, 535-539.

Kelly, J.G. (1968). Towards an ecological conception of preventive interventions. In J.W. Carter, Jr. (Ed.), *Research Contributions from Psychology to Community Mental Health* (pp. 75-99). New York: Behavioural Publications.

Kelly, J.G. (1971). Qualities for the community psychologist. *American Psychologist,* 26, 897-903.

Kelly, J.G., Ryan, A.M., Altman, B.E., and Stelzner, S.R. (2000). Understanding and changing social systems: An ecological view. In J. Rappaport and E. Seidman (Eds.), *Handbook of Community Psychology* (pp. 133-160). New York: Plenum Press.

Kilpatrick, D.G., and Acierno, R. (2003). Mental health needs of crime victims: Epidemiology and outcomes. *Journal of Traumatic Stress*, 16, 119-132.

Kilpatrick, D.G., Amstadter, A.B., Resnick, H.S., and Ruggiero, K.J. (2007). Rape-related PTSD: Issues and interventions. *Psychiatric Times*, 24, 50-58.

Kilpatrick, D.G., Best, C.L., Veronen, L.J., Amick, A.E., Villeponteaux, L.A., and Ruff, G.A. (1985). Mental health correlates of criminal victimization: A random community survey. *Journal of Consulting and Clinical Psychology,* 53, 866-873.

Kilpatrick, D.G., and Resnick, H.S. (1993). PTSD associated with exposure to criminal victimization in clinical and community populations. In J.R.T. Davidson and E.B. Foa (Eds.), *PTSD in review: Recent research and future directions* (pp. 113-143). Washington, DC: American Psychiatric Press.

Kilpatrick, D.G., Saunders, B.E., Amick-McMullan, A., Best, C.L., Veronen, L.J., and Resnick, H.S. (1989). Victim and crime factors associated with the development of crime-related post-traumatic stress disorder. *Behaviour Therapy,* 20, 199-214.

Kilpatrick, D.G., Saunders, B.E., Veronen, L.J., Best, C.L., and Von, J.M. (1987). Criminal victimization: Lifetime prevalence, reporting to police, and psychological impact. *Crime and Delinquency,* 33, 479-489.

Kilpatrick, D.G., Veronen, L.J., and Best, C.L. (1984). Factors predicting psychological distress among rape victims. In C.R. Figley (Ed.), *Trauma and its Wake* (pp. 113-141). Bristol, PA: Brunner/Mazel.

Koss, M.P. (1993). Rape: Scope, impact, interventions, and public policy responses. *American Psychologist,* 48, 1062-1069.

Koss, M.P. (2006). Restoring rape survivors: Justice, advocacy, and a call to action. *Annals of the New York Academy of Sciences,* 1087, 206-234.

Koss, M., and Achilles, M. (2008). *Restorative Justice Responses to Sexual Assault.* Retrieved March 3, 2008, from http://www.vawnet.org

Koss, M.P., Bailey, J.A., Yuan, N.P., Herrera, V.M., and Lichter, E.L. (2003). Depression and PTSD in survivors of male violence: Research and training initiatives to facilitate recovery. *Psychology of Women Quarterly,* 27, 130-142.

Koss, M.P., Dinero, T.E., Seibel, C.A., and Cox, S.L. (1988). Stranger and acquaintance rape: Are there differences in the victim's experience? *Psychology of Women Quarterly,* 12, 1-24.

Koss, M.P., and Figueredo, A.J. (2004). Cognitive mediation of rape's mental health impact: Constructive replication of a cross-sectional model in longitudinal data. *Psychology of Women Quarterly,* 28, 273-286.

Koss, M.P., Figueredo, A.J., and Prince, R.J. (2002). A cognitive mediational model of rape recovery: Preliminary specification and testing in cross-sectional data. *Journal of Consulting and Clinical Psychology,* 70, 926-941.

Koss, M.P., Gidycz, C.A., and Wisniewski, N. (1987). The scope of rape: Incidence and prevalence of sexual aggression and victimization in a national sample of higher education students. *Journal of Consulting and Clinical Psychology,* 55, 162-170.

Koss, M.P., Goodman, L.A., Browne, A., Fitzgerald, L.F., Keita, G.P., and Russo, N.F. (1994). *No Safe Haven: Male Violence Against Women at Home, at Work, and in the Community.* Washington, DC: American Psychological Association.

Koss, M.P., and Harvey, M.R. (1991). *The Rape Victim: Clinical and Community Interventions.* Thousand Oaks, CA: Sage.

Krakow, B., Hollifield, M., Johnston, L., Koss, M., Schrader, R., Warner, T.D., *et al.* (2001). Imagery rehearsal therapy for chronic nightmares in sexual assault survivors with post-traumatic stress disorder: A randomized control trial. *Journal of the American Medical Association,* 296, 537-545.

Kramer, T.L., and Green, B.L. (1991). Post-traumatic stress disorder as an early response to sexual assault. *Journal of Interpersonal Violence,* 6, 160-173.

Krug, E.G., Mercy, J.A., Dahlberg, L.L., and Zwi, A.B. (Eds.). (2002). *World Report on Violence and Health.* Geneva: World Health Organization.

Ledray, L. (1996). The sexual assault resource service: A new model of care. *Minnesota Medicine,* 79, 43-45.

Lefley, H.P., Scott, C.S., Llabre, M. and Hicks, D. (1993). Cultural beliefs about rape and victim's responses in three ethnic groups. *American Journal of Orthopsychiatry,* 63, 623-632.

Littleton, H., and Breitkopf, C.R. (2006). Coping with the experience of rape. *Psychology of Women Quarterly,* 30, 106-116.

Long, L.M., Ullman, S.E., Starzynski, L.L., Long, S.M., and Mason, G.E. (2007). Age and educational differences in African-American women's sexual assault experiences. *Feminist Criminology,* 2, 117-136.

Lonsway, K.A., and Fitzgerald, L.F. (1994). Rape myths: In review. *Psychology of Women Quarterly,* 18, 133-164.

Luo, T. (2000). "Marrying my rapist?" The cultural trauma among Chinese rape survivors. *Gender and Society,* 14, 581-597.

Mackey, T., Sereika, S.M., Weissfeld, L.A., Hacker, S.S., Zender, J.F., and Heard, S.L. (1992). Factors associated with long-term depressive symptoms of sexual assault victims. *Archives of Psychiatric Nursing,* 6, 10-25.

Marsella, A.J., Friedman, M.J., and Spain, E.H (1999). Ethnocultural aspects of post-traumatic stress disorder: An overview of issues and research directions. In A.J. Marsella, M.J. Friedman, E.T. Gerrity, and R.M. Scurfield (Eds.), *Ethnocultural Aspects of Post-traumatic Stress Disorder: Issues, Research, and Clinical Applications.* Washington, DC: American Psychological Association.

Martin, P.Y. (2005). *Rape work: Victims, Gender, and Emotions in organization and community context.* New York: Routledge.

McFarlane, J., Malecha, A., Watson, K., Gist, J., Batten, E., Hall, I. *et al.* (2005). Intimate partner sexual assault against women: Frequency, health consequences, and treatment outcomes. *Obstetrics and Gynecology,* 105, 99-108.

McLaren, L., and Hawe, P. (2005). Ecological perspectives in health research. *Journal of Epidemiology and Community Health,* 59, 6-14.

Messman-Moore, T.L., and Long, P.J. (2003). The role of childhood sexual abuse sequelae in the sexual revictimization of women: An empirical review and theoretical reformulation. *Clinical Psychology Review,* 23, 537-571.

Messman-Moore, T.L., Long, P.J., and Siegfried, N.J. (2000). The revictimization of child sexual abuse survivors: An examination of the adjustment of college women with child sexual abuse, adult sexual assault, and adult physical abuse. *Child Maltreatment,* 5, 18-27.

Meyer, C.B., and Taylor, S.E. (1986). Adjustment to rape. *Journal of Personality and Social Psychology,* 50, 1226-1234.

Miner, M.H., Flitter, J.M.K., and Robinson, B.E. (2006). Association of sexual revictimization with sexuality and psychological function. *Journal of Interpersonal Violence,* 21, 503-524.

Moor, A. (2007). When recounting the traumatic memories is not enough: Treating persistent self-devaluation associated with rape and victim-blaming myths. *Women and Therapy,* 30, 19-33.

Moss, M., Frank, E., and Anderson, B. (1990). The effects of marital status and partner support on rape trauma. *American Journal of Orthopsychiatry,* 60, 379-391.

Neville, H.A., and Heppner, M.J. (1999). Contextualizing rape: Reviewing sequelae and proposing a culturally inclusive ecological model of sexual assault recovery. *Applied and Preventative Psychology,* 8, 41-62. Culturally inclusive ecological model of sexual assault recovery. *Applied* and *Preventative Psychology,* 8, 41-62.

Neville, H.A., Heppner, M.J., Oh, E., Spanierman, L.B., and Clark, M. (2004). General and culturally specific factors influencing black and white rape survivors' self-esteem. *Psychology of Women Quarterly,* 28, 83-94.

Nishith, P., Mechanic, M.B., and Resick, P.A. (2000). Prior interpersonal trauma: The contribution to current PTSD symptoms in female rape victims. *Journal of Abnormal Psychology*, 109, 20-25.

Peterson, Z.D., and Muehlenhard, C.L. (2004). Was it rape? The function of women's rape myth acceptance and definitions of sex in labelling their own experiences. *Sex Roles,* 51, 129-144.

Petrak, J., Doyle, A., Williams, L., Buchan, L., and Forster, G. (1997). The psychological impact of sexual assault: A study of female attenders of a sexual health psychology service. *Sexual and Marital Therapy,* 12, 339-345.

Pimlott-Kubiak, S., and Cortina, L.M. (2003). Gender, victimization, and outcomes: Reconceptualizing risk. *Journal of Consulting and Clinical Psychology,* 71, 528-539.

Resick, P.A. (1993). The psychological impact of rape. *Journal of Interpersonal Violence,* 8, 223-255.

Resick, P.A., Galovski, T.E., Uhlmansiek, M., Scher, C.D., Clum, G.A., and Young-Xu, Y. (2008). A randomized control trial to dismantle components of cognitive processing therapy for posttraumatic stress disorder in female victims of interpersonal violence. *Journal of Consulting and Clinical Psychology,* 76, 243-258.

Resick, P.A., Nishith, P., Weaver, T.L., Astin, M.C., and Feuer, C.A. (2002). A comparison of cognitive-processing therapy with prolonged exposure and a waiting condition for the treatment of chronic post-traumatic stress disorder in female rape victims. *Journal of Consulting and Clinical Psychology,* 70, 867-879.

Resnick, H.S., Yehuda, R., and Acierno, R. (1997). Acute post-rape plasma cortisol, alcohol use, and PTSD symptom profile among recent rape victims. *Annals New York Academy of Sciences,* 821, 433-436.

Resnick, H.S., Yehuda, R., Pitman, R.K., and Foy, D.W. (1995). Effect of previous trauma on acute plasma cortisol level following rape. *American Journal of Psychiatry,* 152, 1675-1677.

Riggs, D.S., Kilpatrick, D.G., and Resnick, H.S. (1992). Long-term psychological distress associated with marital rape and aggravated assault: A comparison to other crime victims. *Journal of Family Violence,* 7, 283-296.

Rogers, C., and Gruener, D. (1997). Sequelae of sexual assault. *Primary Care Update for OB/GYNs,* 4, 143-146.

Roth, S., and Cohen, L.J. (1986). Approach, avoidance and coping with stress. *American Psychologist,* 41, 340-347.

Rothbaum, B.O., Foa, E.B., Riggs, D.S., Murdock, T., and Walsh, W. (1992). A prospective examination of posttraumatic stress disorder in rape victims. *Journal of Traumatic Stress,* 5, 455-475.

Rozee, P.D., and Koss, M.P. (2001). Rape: A century of resistance. *Psychology of Women Quarterly,* 25, 295-311.

Ruch, L.O., and Chandler, S.M. (1983). Sexual assault trauma during the acute phase: An exploratory model and multivariate analysis. *Journal of Health and Social Behaviour,* 24, 174-185.

Ruch, L.O., and Leon, J.J. (1983). Sexual assault trauma and trauma change. *Women & Health,* 8, 5-21.

Starzynski, L.L., Ullman, S.E., Filipas, H.H., and Townsend, S.M. (2005). Correlates of women's sexual assault disclosure to informal and formal support sources. *Violence and Victims,* 20, 417-432.

Sudderth, L.K. (1998). "It'll come right back at me": The interactional context of discussing rape with others. *Violence Against Women,* 4, 572-594.

Temple, J.R., Weston, R., Rodriguez, B.F., and Marshall, L.L. (2007). Differing effects of partner and nonpartner sexual assault on women's mental health. *Violence Against Women,* 13, 285-297.

Thompson, M.P., Kaslow, N.J., Kingree, J.B., Rashid, A., Puett, R., Jacobs, D., *et al.* (2000). Partner violence, social support, and distress among inner-city African American women. *American Journal of Community Psychology,* 28, 127-143.

Ullman, S.E. (1996a). Do social reactions to sexual assault victims vary by support provider? *Violence and Victims,* 11, 143-156.

Ullman, S.E. (1996b). Correlates and consequences of adult sexual assault disclosure. *Journal of Interpersonal Violence,* 11, 554-571.

Ullman, S.E. (1996c). Social reactions, coping strategies, and self-blame attributions in adjustment to sexual assault. *Psychology of Women Quarterly,* 20, 505-526.

Ullman, S.E. (2000). Psychometric characteristics of the social reactions questionnaire: A measure of reactions to sexual assault victims. *Psychology of Women Quarterly,* 24, 169-183.

Ullman, S.E. (2007). Mental health services seeking in sexual assault victims. *Women and Therapy,* 30, 61-84.

Ullman, S.E., and Brecklin, L.R. (2002a). Sexual assault history, PTSD, and mental health service seeking in a national sample of women. *Journal of Community Psychology,* 30, 261-279.

Ullman, S.E., and Brecklin, L.R. (2002b). Sexual assault history and suicidal behaviour in a national sample of women. *Suicide and Life-Threatening Behaviour,* 32, 117-130.

Ullman S.E., and Brecklin, L.R. (2003). Sexual assault history and health-related outcomes in a national sample of women. *Psychology of Women Quarterly,* 27, 46-57.

Ullman, S., and Filipas, H.H. (2001a). Correlates of formal and informal support seeking in sexual assault victims. *Journal of Interpersonal Violence,* 16, 1028-1047.

Ullman, S.E., and Filipas, H.H. (2001b). Predictors of PTSD symptom severity and social reactions in sexual assault victims. *Journal of Traumatic Stress,* 14, 369-389.

Ullman, S.E., Filipas, H.H., Townsend, S.M., and Starzynski, L.L. (2006). The role of victim-offender relationships in women's sexual assault experiences. *Journal of Interpersonal Violence,* 21, 798-819.

Ullman, S.E., Karabatsos, G, and Koss, M.P. (1999). Alcohol and sexual assault in a national sample of college women. *Journal of Interpersonal Violence,* 14, 603-625.

Ullman, S.E., and Siegal J.M. (1993). Victim-offender relationship and sexual assault. *Violence and Victims,* 8, 121-134.

Ullman, S.E., Townsend, S.M., Filipas, H.H., and Starzynski, L.L. (2007). Structural models of the relations of assault severity, social support, avoidance coping, self-blame, and PTSD among sexual assault survivors. *Psychology of Women Quarterly,* 31, 23-37.

Valentiner, D.P., Foa, E.B., Riggs, D.S., and Gershuny, B.S. (1996). Coping strategies and posttraumatic stress disorder in female victims of sexual and nonsexual assault. *Journal of Abnormal Psychology,* 105, 455-458.

Ward, C.A. (1995). *Attitudes toward rape: Feminist and social psychological perspectives*. London: Sage.

Wasco, S.M. (2003). Conceptualizing the harm done by rape: Applications of trauma theory to experiences of sexual assault. *Trauma, Violence, and Abuse,* 4, 309-322.

Wasco, S.M., Campbell, R., Howard, A., Mason, G., Schewe, P., Staggs, S., *et al.* (2004). A statewide evaluation of services provided to rape survivors. *Journal of Interpersonal Violence,* 19, 252-263.

White, J.W., and Kowalski, R.M. (1998). Male violence toward women: An integrated perspective. In R.G. Green and E. Donnerstein (Eds.), *Human Aggression: Theories, Research, and Implications for Social Policy* (pp. 203-228). San Diego, CA: Academic Press.

Williams, J.E., and Holmes, K.A. (1982). In judgment of victims: The social context of rape. *Journal of Sociology and Social Welfare, 9,* 154–169.

Winfield, I., George, L.K., Swartz, M., and Blazer, D.G. (1990). Sexual Assault and Psychiatric Disorders.

6

Parenting Type and Perceived Problem Behaviour of Children

Ruchi Kakkar and *Aradhana Shukla*

Adult depressive symptoms insecurity in close relationships and disrupted family relationships each have important implications for the quality of the family life and for children's psychological well-being of the interpersonal (Downey and Coyne, 1990; Miller, Cowan, Cowan, Hetherington, and Clingempeel, 1993; Cowan, Cohn, Cowan, and Pearson, 1996). The mediating role of the interpersonal and parent-child relationships in the link between (a) parent depressive symptoms and (b) adult relationship insecurity and children's psychological well-being has received support in several previous studies (e.g., Miller *et al.*, 1993; Cowan *et al.*, 1996). Few studies, however, have considered the role of parent's psychological health and relationships functioning at the adult, interpersonal and parent-child levels in explaining variation in children's emotional and behavioural well-being. In the present study, we considered the effects of parent depressive symptoms and adult relationship insecurity in accounting for long term variations in children's internalizing symptoms and externalizing problems *via* disruption in the quality of the interpersonal and parent-child relationships.

Individuals with high levels of depressive symptoms are more likely to attribute hostility to other family members as well as to withdraw from social interaction (Conger and Elder, 1994), and depressive symptoms in one or both spouses are related to marital exchanges characterized by heightened hostility, tension and discord (Cummings and Davies, 1994; Downey and Coyne, 1990). Previous research has also identified links between symptoms of psychological distress, including depression and attachment insecurity (e.g., Roberts, Gotlib,

Kassel, 1996) and insecurity in close relationships is associated with increased levels of couple conflict (e.g., Crowell *et al.*, 2002; Cowan *et al.*, 1996). Depression, therefore, may indirectly affect the marital relationship by influencing individuals' expectations about a spouse or partners' support and emotional availability (Cummings and Cicchetti, 1990). A recent cross-sectional study found associations between parent dysphoria, marital attachments, marital conflict and young children's adjustment (Cummings, Keller, and Davies, 2005). Although the associations have been documented, few studies have tested hypotheses regarding the relation between depression, security in close relationships, and interpersonal conflict in the context of a prospective, longitudinal research design.

Parental depression is considered a significant risk factor for the development of a range of psychological adjustment problems of children, including a negative attribution style, social and academic difficulties, internalizing symptoms, and externalizing problems (Cummings and Davies, 1994; Downey and Coyne, 1990). Marital and parent-child relationships are regarded as possible mechanisms through which the effects of parent distress are communicated to other family members, including partners and children's (Cummings and Davies, 1994). The effects of parent depression on children's adjustment have been found to be mediated by both marital distress (e.g., Davies, Dumenci, and Windle, 1999; Du Rocher Schudlich and Cummings, 2003) and hostile and rejecting parenting (e.g., Kane and Garber, 2004; Oyserman, Bybee, and Mowbray, 2002).

Parental depression may also indirectly affect the parent-child relationship by increasing marital conflict (Conger *et al.*, 1992; Low and Stocker, 2005). According to Belsky (1984), parenting behaviour can be determined as a functional of individual parent factors, child characteristics, and the social context in which the parent-child relationship exists, with emphasis on the marital relationship as a primary emotional context in which parent-child functioning occurs. Tests of the family stress model found support for a process perspective whereby parental depression predicted increased marital conflict, which in turn influenced adolescent adjustment problems *via* the impact on parent-child relations (Conger *et al.*, 1992, 1993). Against a backdrop of interparental conflict, children appear to experience the parent-child relationship as more hostile and insecure (e.g., Harold, Fincham, Osborne, and Conger, 1997; Harold, Shelton, Goeke Morey, and Cummings, 2004). The level of parent acceptance in the context of marital conflict has also been identified as a particularly salient dimension of the parent-child relationship for young adolescents (Fauber, Forehand, Thomas, and Wierson, 1990). In one of the few studies to consider the effect of parent depression on multiple dyadic relationships in the family, present depression was related to children's externalizing problems indirectly through effects on the quality of the marital relationship and parenting style (Miller *et al.*, 1993; Leinonen, Solantaus, and Punamaki, 2003; Cummings *et al.*, 2005).

Similar relations has been found between adult security in close relationships and family functioning. Adult insecurity has been related to higher levels of energy and intrusive parenting and lower levels of positive effect (Adams, Gunnar, and Tanaka, 2004). Paralleling the parent depression literature, Cowan *et al.* (1996) found the mothers' and fathers' attachment histories indirectly affected young children's adjustment by influencing marital quality and parenting behaviour. Documented links between adult attachments and parenting behaviour have relied almost exclusively on mothers and pre-school children. Less well understood is how male and female insecurity in close relationships and the parenting of adolescents are related.

Keeping these views in consideration this study was planned and it was aimed to find out the pattern of disruptive behaviour of the participants as affected by type of parenting, parental age and gender of child. The objectives and hypotheses of this study are as follows:

1. The first objective of this study was to find out the pattern of parenting on disruptive behaviour of the child. It was formulated that single parent children, double parent children and separated parent children would be different in relation to the scores of disruptive behaviour scale.
2. The second objective of this study was to explore the pattern of parental gender on disruptive behaviour of their child. It was assumed that the gender of the parent would lay its impact on their children's disruptive behaviour.
3. The third objective of this study was to find out the impact of child's gender on disruptive behaviour. It was contended that the gender of the child would lay its impact on disruptive behaviour.

Keeping these objectives and hypotheses in consideration this study was planned in factorial perspective.

Method

Sample: Three hundred sixty participants arranging between 10-18 years served as participants and they were arranged according to the requirements of three way factorial design with three types of parenting (single parenting, double parenting and separated parenting), parental gender (male, female) and gender of the child (boy, girl). 30 participants in each cell. The schematic presentation of experimental design is given in Table 6.1.

Table 6.1: Schematic presentation of Experimental Design

	A					
	A1		A2		A3	
	B		B		B	
	B1	B2	B1	B2	B1	B2
C1	30	30	30	30	30	30
C1	30	30	30	30	30	30

Legends:

A *Parenting type*	B *Gender of parent*	C *Gender of child*
A1 Double parent	B1 Male	C1 Boy
A2 Single parent	B2 Female	C2 Girl
A3 Separated parent		

Tools

In this scale only one tool was used and it is mentioned below:

Problem behaviour Check List: Parent rating from Achenbac, (1991). In this one tool was used and this is described below: This scale consists of 113 five point items representing behaviour problem of child as experienced by parents. The scale provided score on two broad bound dimensions of child behaviour problems—externalizing problems (aggressive, disruptive and antisocial behaviour) and internalizing problems (anxiety, depression and social with drawal). Prior to the conduction the Ss were instructed as follows:

> मैं आपके सामने कुछ शारीरिक मानसिक प्रकारों के लक्षण प्रस्तुत कर रही हूँ। आप इसे ध्यानपूर्वक देखें और अपने बच्चों/विद्यार्थियों में इनकी उपस्थिति देखकर सामने लिखे पाँच बिन्दुओं, बहुत अधिक, अधिक सामान्य, कम, बहुत कम, में किसी एक पर चिह्न लगाकर व्यक्त करें। समय की सीमा नहीं है। फिर भी कार्य शीघ्रता से करें।

Results

Data were analyzed by three way analysis of variance and they are given below:

Impact of type of parenting, parental gender and gender of the child on disruptive behaviour: Data were analyzed by three way ANOVA and interpreted in terms of type parenting, parental gender and gender of the child on disruptive behaviour. Findings were presented in Table 6.2.

Table 6.2: Summary table of ANOVA showing the impact of type of parenting, parental gender and gender of the child on disruptive behaviour

Sources of Variation	*Ss*	*Df*	*Ms*	*F*
A	8.99	2	4.49	5.69
B	.10	1	.10	8.86
C	4.39	1	4.39	5.56
AB	13.73	2	6.86	8.69
AC	15.23	2	7.61	8.64
BC	.99	1	.99	.84
ABC	16.74	2	8.37	10.60
Error (within)	274.92	348	0.79	359

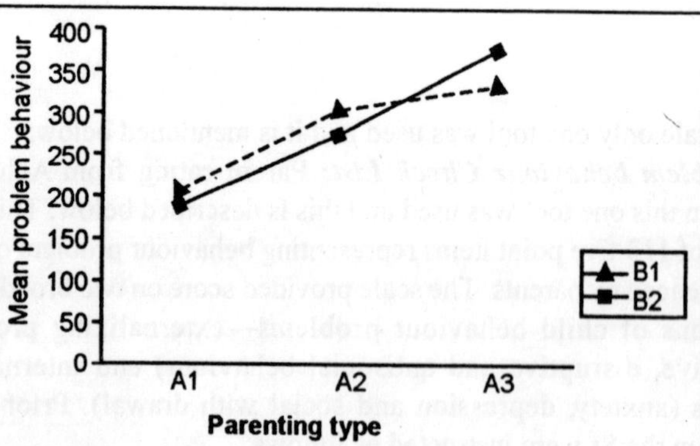

Legends

A Parenting type
A1 Double Parent
A2 Single Parent
A3 Separated Parent

B Gender of Parent
B1 Male
B2 Female

Fig. 6.1: Mean value showing the impact of type of parenting and parental gender the experience of problem behaviour of children

The main effect of type of parenting was significant (F2, 348 = 5.69 $p < .01$). Mean values pooled parental gender and gender of child were 198.83, 290.03 and 355.84 (Fig. 6.1). It was noted that the experience of problem behaviour was highest in separated parents followed by single parents and double parents, respectively. Moreover, discrepancy was higher between double and single parents. The next main effect of parental gender was also insignificant (F1, 348 = 8.86 $p > .05$). It was noted that males (fathers) were highly disruptive behaviour (X = 280.71) than females (mothers) but the different was nominal (X = 282.68). The third main effect of gender of the child was also significant (F1, 348 = 5.56 $p < .01$). It was that boys were experienced less in disruptive behaviour (X = 277.80) as compared to girls (X = 28).

Of problem behaviour was high in fathers than mothers. Moreover, it was also noted that the discrepancy related with parental gender was absolutely high in separated parents. The type of parenting and gender of the child interaction was also significant (F, 2.359 = 8.69 P < .01) and it is appeared in Fig. 6.2. Figure reveals that the magnitude of children's gender 5.34).

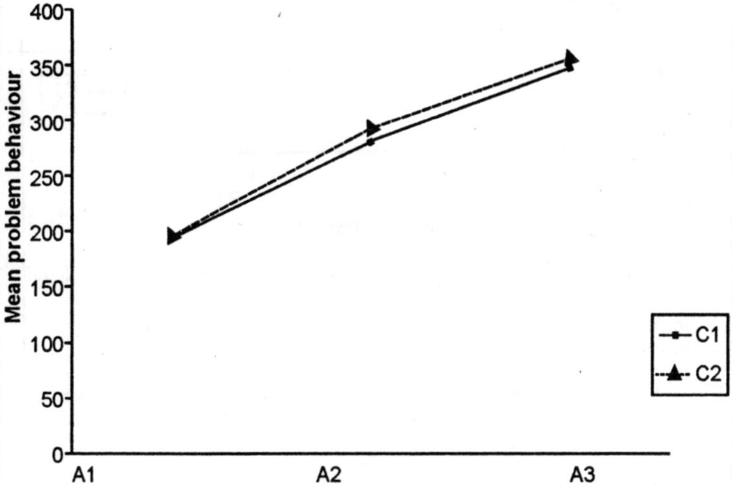

Legends

A Parenting type
A1 Double Parent
A2 Single Parent
A3 Separated Parent

C Gender of child
C1 Boys
C2 Girl

Fig. 6.2: Mean values showing the impact of type of parenting and child gender on problem behaviour

The two way interaction of type of parenting X parental gender was also significant (F, 2.359 = 8.69 $p < .01$) and it is appeared in Fig. 6.1. Figure reveals that the experience related discrepancy was commonly shared by all parenting type. However, the magnitude of discrepancy was more pronounced at middle group, namely double parenting. The parental gender X children's gender was non-significant (F, 1.332 = .69 $p < .05$). It showed that both variable were not able to yield their impact.

The three way interaction of parenting type X parental gender X children's gender was significant (F, 2.359 = 10.60 $p < .01$) and it is mentioned in Fig. 6.3. Figure reveals that all variables laid their impact on the experience of problem behaviour.

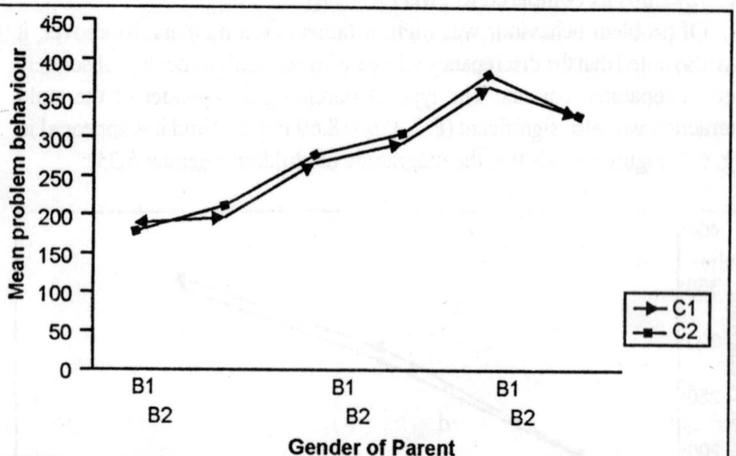

Legends

A = Parenting type	B = Gender of the parent	C = Gender of child
A1 = Double Parent	B1 = Male	C1 = Boys
A2 = Single Parent	B2 = Female	C2 = Girl
A3 = Separated Parent		

Fig. 6.3: Mean values showing the impact of type of parenting, parental gender and child gender on problem behaviour of children

Discussion

Obtained data were analyzed by three way ANOVA and interpreted in terms of parenting type, parental gender and the gender of child as affecters of the problematic behaviour of children. Prior to the inscription of this work some hypotheses were formulated and the findings will be discussed accordingly.

1. Differentials in parenting type would evince the difference in problem behaviour: Our first and foremost notion was concerned with the impact of parenting type on problem behaviour. It was contended the variation parenting type would cause variation in problem behaviour. It was found that the children of separated parents enabled their parent to show more problem behaviour of their parents because divorced parents are at greater risk for symptoms of depression than the married parents (Amato, 2000; Simons and Johnson, 1996; Forhand *et al.*, 1990). In addition, it is also noted that single parents who are not divorcee and live alone/alone with their children due to death of spouse or dive to job condition are not so depressed as compared to separated parents who live alone due to divorce. Parental depressive symptoms may be one factor in divorced homes that increases children's risk for adjustment problems (Whiteside and Becker, 2000). For example, depressed parents may model negative affect and poor coping strategies (Hammen, 1997). A study by Larson and Gillman, 1999 suggests that children and adolescents are susceptible to "emotional transmission" from single mothers, that is, children's momentary mood states are likely to change to match the mood states experienced by their single mothers when they are together. Thus, when divorced single mothers are sad or irritable, their children may also experience these mood states.

The heightened depressive symptoms experienced by divorced mothers may have a specific effect on their parenting, namely, withdrawal and disengagement from interactions with their children, as Field and her colleague have demonstrated (Hart, Aaron and Field, 2003). Mothers experiencing depressive symptoms may be more self-focused, have less motivation for social interaction, and be less socially involved than mothers who are not experiencing symptoms of depression (Hammen, 1997). Parental withdrawal may be one manifestation of these depressive symptoms. Indeed, some studies suggest that mothers are less involved with their children in divorced families then in 2-parent families. In the Verginia Longitudinal Study, divorced mothers of pre-adolescent children reported spending less time with their sons (but not their daughters) then did non-divorced mothers, although this finding was not replicated in a second study of early adolescents (Hetherington and Clingempeel, 1992; Hart, Aaron and Field, 2003). In a study of 953 adolescents, divorce was associated with memories of lowered for by family SES or interpersonal conflict (Woodward, Fergusson and Belsky, 2000). These findings suggests that divorced mothers are more withdrawn and disengaged from their children than the married mothers. This withdrawal may represent an extension of maternal depressive symptoms into the parenting domain. In the present study, we examine depressive symptoms and maternal withdrawal as a sing le construct: "depressive/withdrawn parenting". We use this term to describe a parent who is experiencing symptoms of depression, and is less sociable and less engaged on both an emotional and a behavioural level, in the child's daily life.

No research to date has examined depressive/withdrawn parenting as a mediator of the effects of divorce on children's adjustment. In addition, there are no studies that have tested parental withdrawal (independent of depressive symptoms) as a mediator. We are aware of one study that has examined the mediational role of maternal depressive symptoms, but there was no evidence that this variable accounted for the higher levels of conduct problems and depression reported by adolescents from divorced families as compared to non-divorced families (Simons *et al.*, 1999). Given the evidence that both depressive symptoms and parental withdrawal are more common in divorced families, it is surprising that these variables have received so little attention as mediators of divorce effects.

2. Gender of the parent would lay its impact on their children disruptive behaviour: Our second notion was concerned with the gender difference of parents as affecters of children disruptive behaviour. It was found that fathers experienced more problem than mothers. It may be due to the fact that sense father usually go out from home due to job so whenever they come to home they used to experience their children's disruptive comparatively high then mothers.

Neki (1976) has analyzed the child rearing practices in the development of dependency by comparing the Indian and the Western cultures. He found that the Western culture encourages independence whereas the Indian child rearing fosters dependence. Srivastava, Banerjee and Tripathi (1995) studied parental views regarding the perceived values and costs in having a child. He identified two main value types—psychological and economic. The urban parents considered children to be more of psychological value such as children make life more meaningful and are a source of love and provide company. In contrast rural parents value children for their economic values, i.e. performance of domestic chores, followed by psychological value of children. Child rearing values also reflected family relations and changes in them. Regarding the costs of children the parental responses indicated the impact of urbanization and industrialization. Majority of the parents were worried about their children's future and wished their children to be successful in life. Parents' response indicated the change in the Indian setting from a collectivistic orientation in which greater emphasis was on societal functioning and family was the social unit to a personalized orientation due to the contemporary setup in the urban areas.

The context of childhood in the traditional Indians families involves a complex structure in which an interplay of personal and contextual factors take place a dynamic fashion. Attention to balance the influences beyond one's control is always evident. It is believed that placement of the stars at the time of birth of the child determines her fate. The horoscope or *Janampatri* is often made and consulted on critical occasions (e.g. marriage, illness, job, etc.) All this indicates a belief in some form of pre-determinism in parents (Misra, Srivastava and Gupta, 1999).

The traditional Indian view holds that each and every individual is endowed with certain competencies and ordered life course. Many people subscribe to the view that parents transfer merits and demerits to their children. A child is considered as an extension of her parents. The similarities between parents and children identified and emphasized during conversations in the family. Fathers and mothers also consider their children as self objects, through which they are defined. As a result, for many Indian parents socialization happens to be an occasion for their own self-articulation. The locus of this articulation is often perceived to be lying within the psyche of parents themselves.

Thus, it is very surely fair to say that gender of the parent may influence the perception of disruptive behaviour in their children.

***3. Gender of the child would lay its impact on disruptive behaviour*:** Last but not least was the hypothesis in which an attempt was made to find out the pattern of disruptive behaviour in children as affected by their gender. It was found that the disruptive behaviour of boys was perceived more than the problem of girls.

Previous studies did not explicitly test for gender differences in early-starter patterns of antisocial behaviour. As noted, although girls and boys have been shown to have analogous pattern of aggression over time (Broidly *et al.*, 2003), the absolute levels of aggression appeared to be lower for girls. In addition, trajectory memberships were not as consistently associated with later anti-social outcomes for girls as they were for boys. Without specific empirical tests of these apparent gender differences, these findings are inconclusive. In the present study, we expected that, although the hypothesized trajectories for girls would be analogous to those found for boys, the absolute level of aggression-disruption over time within these trajectories would be lower than those found for boys (based on the results of Broidy *et al.*, 2003). Also consistent with the existing research, we expected that, although girls with chronic high or moderate aggression-disruption would be more at risk for antisocial outcomes than would more aggressive-disruptive girls, their level of risk would be lower then that of boys with analogous early-starter patterns.

Studies thus reveal that gender of the child is an important factor in the development of disruptive behaviour.

Increases in the number of children suffering from emotional and behavioural problems have implications for the Child and Adolescent Mental Health Services (CAMHS) which are currently being restructured to conform to a '4-tier model'.

- Tier 1 consist of 'direct contact' services provided by non-specialists such as GPs, health visitors, school nurses, social services, teachers, etc., who can identify problems at an early stage, offer general advice and treatment, and take on preventative work.
- The first specialized layer is Tier 2, which consist of a network of a individual specialists, (e.g. psychologists, psychiatrists, pediatricians, psychiatric nurses) offering a range of services including assessment, treatment, training, consultation and outreach work.
- More severe, complex or persistent disorders require Tier 3 services, which involve multi-disciplinary terms made up of Tier 2 specialists augmented with other experts such as psychotherapists, occupational therapists, etc.
- Finally come the highly specialized Tier 4 services, (e.g. out-patient, day or in-patient) units of the severely mentally ill or those at risk from suicide.

The complexity of this structure means that there are many challenges in ensuring that the system works as intended, that so many professionals (with many different perspectives) work together (rather than in competition), and that produces do not become so unwieldy and bureaucratic as to be both expensive and ineffective.

References

Adams, E.K., Gunnar, M.R., and Tanaka, A. (2004). Adult attachment, parent emotion, and observed parenting behaviour: Mediator and moderator models. *Child Development*, 75, 110-122.

Amato, P.R. (2000). The consequences of divorce for adult and children. *J Marriage Fam*, 62: 1269-1287.

Belsky, J. (1984). The determinants of parenting: A process model. *Child Development*, 55, 83-96.

Broidy, L.M., Nagin, D.S., Tremblay, R.E. Bates, J.E., Brame, B., Dodge, K.A., *et al.* (2003). Developmental trajectories of childhood disruptive behaviours and adolescent delinquency: A six-site, cross nation study. *Developmental Psychology*, 39, 222-245.

Conger, R.D., Conger, K.J., Elder, G.H., Jr., Lorenz, F., Simons, R., and Whitbeck, L. (1992). A family process model of economic hardship and adjustment of early adolescent boys. *Child Development*, 63, 526-541.

Conger, R.D. and. Elder, G.H., Jr (1994). *Families in troubled times*: Adapting to change in rural America. New York: De Gruyter.

Cowan, P.A., Cohn, D.A., Cowan, C.P., and Pearson, J.L. (1996). Parents' attachment histories and children's externalizing and internalizing behaviours: Exploring family systems models of linkage. *Journal of Consulting and Clinical Psychology*, 64, 53-63.

Crowell, J.A., Trebaux, D., Gao, Y., Fyffe, C., Pan, H., and Waters, E. (2002). Assessing secure base behaviour in adulthood: Development of measure, links to adult attachment representations, and relations to couples' communication and reports of relationships. *Developmental Psychology*, 38, 679-693.

Cummings, E.M., and Cicchetti, D. (1990). Toward a transactional model of relations between attachment and depression. In M.T. Greenberg and D. Cicchetti (Eds.), *Attachment in the Preschool Years: Theory, Research and Intervention* (pp. 339-372). Chiago: University of Chicago Press.

Cummings, E.M., and Davies, P.T. (1994). Maternal repression and child development. *Journal of Child Psychology and Psychiatry*, 35, 73-112.

Cummings, E.M., Keller, P.S., and Davies, P.T. (2005). Towards a family process model of maternal and parental depressive symptoms: Exploring multiple relations with child and family functioning. *Journal of Child Psychology and Psychiatry*, 46, 479-489.

Davies, P.T., Dumenci, L., and Windle, M. (1999). The interplay between maternal depressive symptoms and marital distress in the prediction of adolescent adjustment. *Journal of Marriage and the Family*, 61, 238-254.

Downey, G, and Coyne, J.C. (1990). Children of depressed parents: An integrative review. *Psychological Bulletin*, 108, 50-76.

Du Rocher Schudlich, T.D., and Cummings, E.M. (2003). Parental dysphoria and children's internalizing symptoms: Marital conflict styles as mediators of risk. *Child Development*, 74, 1163-1681.

Fauber, R., Forehand, R., Thomas, A., and Wireson, M. (1990). A mediational model of the impact of marital conflict on adolescent adjustment in intact and divorced families: The role of disrupted parenting. *Child Development*, 61, 1112-1123.

Forehand, R., Thomas, A.M., Wierson, M., Brody, G., and Fauber, R. (1990). Role of maternal functioning and parenting skills in adolescent functioning following parental divirce. *Journal of Abnormal Psychology*, 99: 278-283.

Hammen, C. (1997). *Depression*. London: Psychology Press.

Harold, G.T., Shelton, K.H., Goeke-Morey, M.C., and Cummings, E.M. (2002). Relations between interparental conflict, child emotional security, and adjustment in the context of cognitive appraisals. In P. Davies, G. Harold, M. Goeke-Morey, and E.M. Cummings (Eds.) *Child Emotional Security and Interparental Conflict. Monographs of the Society for Research in Child Development*, 67, (3, Serial 270).

Harold, G.T., Shelton, K.H., Goeke-Morey, M.C., and Cummings, E.M. (2002). Marital conflict, child emotional security about family relationships and child adjustment. *Social Development*, 13, 350-376.

Hart, S., Aaron-Jones, N., and Field, T. (2003). A typical expressions of jealousy in infants of intrusive and withdrawn depressed mothers. *Child Psychiatry Human Development*, 33: 193-207.

Hetherington, E.M. (1987). Family relations six year after divorce. In: *Remarriage and Stepparenting Today: Current Research and Theory*, ed. Palsey K, Inhinger-Tollman. New York: Guilford, 185-205.

Hetherington, E.M., Chingempeel, W.G. (1992). Coping with marital transitions: A family systems perspective. *Monogr Soc. Res. Child Dev.*, 57: 35-73.

Kane, P., and Garber, J. (2004). The relations among depression in fathers, children's psychopathology, and father-child conflict: A meta analysis. *Clinical Psychology Review*, 24, 339-360.

Larson, R.W., Gillman, S. (1999). Transmission of emotions in the daily interactions of single mother families. *J Marriage Fam*, 61: 21-37.

Leinonen, J.A., Solantaus, T.S., and Punamaki, R.L. (2003) Parental mental health and children's adjustment: The quality of marital interaction and parenting as mediating factors. *Journal of Child Psychology and Psychiatry*, 44, 227-241.

Low, S.M., and Stocker, C. (2005). Family functioning and children's adjustment: Associations among parents' depressed mood, marital hostility, and children's adjustment, *Journal of Family Psychology*, 19, 394-403.

Miller, N.B., Cowan, P.A., Cowan, C.P., Hetherington, E.M., and Clingempeel, W.G. (1993). Externalizing in preschoolers and early adolescents: A cross-site replication of a family model. *Developmental Psychology*, 29, 3-18.

Misra, G., Srivastava, A., Gupta, S. (1999). The cultural constructions of childhood in India, some observation *Indian Psychological Abstracts and Reviews*, 62, 191-218: New Delhi, Sage.

Neki, J.S. (1976). An examination of the culture relation of dependence of social and therapeutic relationships. Social development. *British Journal of Medical Psychology*.

Oyserman, D., Bybee, D., and Mowbray, C. (2002). Influences of maternal mental illness on psychological outcomes for adolescent children. *Journal of Adolescence*, 25, 387-602.

Roberts, J.E., Gotlib, I.H., and Kassel, J.D. (1996). Adult attachment insecurity and symptoms of depression: The mediating roles of dysfunctional attitudes and low self-esteem. *Journal of Personality and Social Psychology*, 70, 310-320.

Simons, R.L., and Jhonson, C. (1996). Mother's parenting. In: *Understanding Differences between Divorced and Single Intact Families: Stress, Interaction, and Child Outcome*, (eds.) Simons, R.L. & Associates. Thousand Oaks, CA: Sage, pp. 81-93.

Srivastava, A.K., Banerjee, J. and Tripathi, A.N. (1995). *Role of acculturation in development of values among children: Maternal views*, New Delhi NCERT.

Whiteside, M.F., and Becker, B.J. (2000). Parental factors and the young child's post-divorce adjustment: A meta-analysis with implications for parenting arrangements. *Journal of Family Psychology* 14: 5-26.

Woodward, L., Fergusson, D.M., and Belsky, J. (2000). Timing of parental separation and attachment to parents in adolescence: Results of a prospective study from birth to age 16. *Journal of Marriage and Family*, 62: 162-174.

7

Childhood Technoholism

A Matter of Grave Concern

Shivali Sharma and *Supriya Chaturvedi*

The term "Technoholism" was conceived by the First author to describe the excessive dependence upon/addiction to the technological gadgets of various types. It is a matter of grave concern for Psychologists, Mental health workers and all responsible adults as the situation is turning grim and totally out of control. The present generation is turning a blind eye towards the repercussions of this uncontrolled use of technology. In today's world machines and gadgets have definitely received a much greater edge over human beings. This addiction now has its beginning in early childhood. The parents are using their television sets as baby sitters unaware of the consequences. The addiction for cartoon and media games gets transformed into addiction for mobiles and Internet during adolescence. This compulsive urge for technological gadgets continues throughout the life span. Though, the children and youth around the world including our nation are becoming more techno savvy than their previous generations but their excessive dependence upon technological gadgets is slowly and steadily turning into an addiction. This addiction is becoming as severe as drug dependence or alcoholism. In this chapter the authors had tried to discuss the forms and consequences of this new age addictive disorder.

Childhood Technoholism: T.V. and Media Game Addiction

Television during the recent years has become the most popular form of mass media as a result of cable connection and availability of programmes round the clock. The channels like cartoon network, Nick *et al.*, are especially designed to lure the young minds. The nuclear family set up has made it difficult for mothers to look after their small children all the time. The grandparents are unavailable and the benefits of extended family are absent. Though, the American Association of Pediatrics bans the T.V completely below the age of two, regular T.V. viewing typically begins between two to three years. The mother's start using it as a baby sitter to keep the baby distracted for some time. This apparently harmless act becomes a bigger headache when their children remain glued to the T.V. set, neglecting important tasks.

Television introduced in the United States of America in late 1940s was rapidly adopted especially by families with children. Now-a-days T.V. viewing and media games is becoming an epidemic not only in developed countries but in developing countries as well. Available studies (Singer and Singer, 2001, Strasburger and Wilson, 2002) and statistics (Livingstone, Bovill and Gaskell, 1999; Nielson Media Research, 2000) have shown that with the onset and advancement of electronic media like satellite/cable T.V. and the Internet, there has been an upsurge in the media consumption of children and adolescents (Comstock and Scharrer, 2001; Groebel, 2001; Von Feilitzen, 1999). Time spent watching T.V. is remarkably similar across developed nations and young people in developing nations are not far behind (Comstock and Scharrer, 2001; Scharrer and Comstock, 2003). For far too many children the time spent on T.V. watching is out of all proportions to the amount of time devoted on other forms of play (Hurlock, 1997). For several years, researchers have been concerned about the possibility that the large amount of time spent in viewing T.V. has displaced the time that would ordinarily be spent in other activities (Comstock and Scharrer, 2001). This idea is generally known as the Displacement Hypothesis. The Displacement Hypothesis suggests that if T.V. viewing increases, the amount of time spent in other activities correspondingly decreases (Sparks, 2002). The average North American 2-6 years old watches from one and a half hours to two hours a day. In the middle childhood, viewing increases to an average of three and a half hours a day for U.S. children and two and a half hours a day for Canadian children.

In a study in Pakistan, Ahmed (1980) found that children who viewed T.V. devoted less time to academic homework than non-viewing children. According to the statistics by indiantelevision.com 2004, the majority of households spent between 3-6 hours a day watching T.V. A market research agency which conducted a survey in India found that 7- 14 years old rated cartoons, music videos, serials and sports as their favourite programme. Studies have shown that late night T.V. viewing is becoming a common phenomenon even in families with small children.

Media game addiction is also becoming rampant in this population. The children are becoming addicted to mobile, video and computer games. This addiction is becoming a very serious behavioural disorder. Douglas Gentile, an Iowa state Associate Professor of Psychology and International Research Team (2011) conducted a study on video game addiction. The researchers report that the percentage of pathological youth gamers in Singapore is similar to other recent video game addiction studies in other countries, including the United States (8.5%), China (10.3%), Australia (8.0%), Germany (11.9%) and Taiwan (7.5%).

Children in the present times are more vulnerable as the outdoor activities are being restricted by the parents to ensure safety of their wards. More the time spent indoors, greater the chances of it being spent on video games and T.V. Most computer games emphasize speed and action in violent plots. The children greatly enjoy simulation games that involve entering virtual realities and role playing characters. Prof. Gentile reached his conclusions about the prevalence of video game addiction after analyzing data that had been collected during a 2007 survey of 1,178 American young people (boys and girls between the ages of 8 and 18). Prof. Gentile's research had yielded the following statistics:

- Just under 90 per cent of survey respondents reported playing video games.
- The average boy in the survey spent 16.4 hours a week playing games, while the average for girls was just over nine hours every week.
- The average "addicted" gamer played 24 hours a week — twice as much as casual gamers.
- 8.5 per cent of the young gamers exhibited "pathological patterns of play," which was described as the presence of at least six of the 11 clinical symptoms (as defined by the American Psychiatric Association).
- One-fourth of the surveyed gamers reported turning to video games in an attempt to escape problems, and nearly as many said they played instead of doing homework.
- Twenty per cent of the young video game enthusiasts said that their schoolwork had suffered because of the time they spent playing the games.

Consequences of Childhood Technoholism

There is a widespread concern among parents, teachers, psychologists and academicians regarding the impact of this excessive consumption of T.V. and media games on children. In an unusual investigation residents of a small Canadian town were studied just before T.V. reception became available in their community and two years later school age children showed a decline in their reading abilities and creative thinking, a rise in gender stereotypes, beliefs and an increase in physical and verbal aggression (William, 1986). The theory of Differential investment of mental effort (Salomon, 1983-84) posits that T.V. is an easy medium and T.V. viewing is an activity requiring little mental effort when compared to other forms of media, such as radio or print. The more preschool and school age children watch prime time shows and cartoons, the less time they spend reading and interacting with others and the poorer their performance on academic tests (Huston *et al.*, 1999; Wright *et al.*, 2001). Studies have shown that late night T.V. viewing and the consequent poor sleep patterns were reasons of academic underachievement of students (Sleepless, 2004, March 15). Another study observed that children who viewed T.V. for more than two hours a day began to behave like small screen characters (Dastur, 2004, November 25).

Rao (1984) studied 122 families in Hyderabad and noted that majority of parents (74%) were greatly concerned about the undesirable influence of T.V. on their children's study habits. A number of studies have been done on the negative impact of T.V. on the school going children and adolescents (Joy and Shejwal, 2005). Children devote more time to watching T.V. than to any other activity including playing, meeting friends, engaging in physical activities, reading or doing homework. Dieticians point out that children who sit in front of the T.V. have their metabolic systems almost switched off. T.V. also increases the consumption of junk food and mindless eating. This has contributed to an increase in childhood obesity and related diseases.

Most media games emphasize speed and action in violent plots. The children greatly enjoy simulation games that involve entering virtual settings and role playing characters. An increasing number of studies show that playing violent games like watching violent T.V. increases hostility and aggression (Anderson *et al.*, 2003). Furthermore, Video games are full of ethnic and gender stereotypes (Dietz, 1988). Compared with infrequent users "passionate" game players tend to be withdrawn young people who use games to escape from unpleasant family and school experiences. It has been found that those who spend several hours a day playing these games become addicted and constantly think about playing when they are not, believe that they play too much but cannot stop or cut back. Excessive playing of simulation games risks blurring of the distinction between virtual and real life (Turkle, 1995).

When such games are violent, they may contribute along with disengaged parents, anti-social peers and alienation from school to commission of heinous acts by young addicts. Columbine High school, teenage murderers Eric Harris and Dylan Klebold were obsessed with a game called 'Doom' in which players rack up most kills (Subrahmanyam, *et al.*, 2001).

The two-year longitudinal study of 3,034 third through eighth grade students in Singapore found approximately nine per cent of gamers to be pathological players according to standards similar to those established by the American Psychiatric Association for diagnosing gambling addiction. Some serious problems—including depression, anxiety, social phobias and lower school performance—seemed to be outcomes of their pathological play. Among this sample, pathological gamers started with an average of 31 hours of play per week. Using the American Psychiatric Association's "Diagnostic and Statistical Manual of Mental Disorders" as a guide to define the addictive condition, the researchers found between 7.6 and 9.9 per cent of the student sample could be defined as pathological gamers over the two-year period. Eighty-four per cent of those subjects who were first classified as pathological gamers were found to still be classified that way two years later. Yet in that same two-year window, only one per cent of the sample became new pathological gamers. (Douglas Gentile, 2009). This study also reported that when children stopped being addicted, depression, anxiety and social phobias decreased as well.

At an addiction treatment centre in Amsterdam, in the Netherlands, teenagers and young adults begin detox by admitting they are powerless over their addiction. But these addicts aren't hooked on *drugs* or alcohol. They are desperate to break their dependence on video games. Detox for video game addiction may sound like an exaggeration, but addiction experts believe that the concept makes sense. It's a clinical impulse control disorder, an addiction in the same sense as compulsive gambling (Kimberley Young). Young says compulsive gaming meets these criteria, and she has seen severe withdrawal symptoms in game addicts. "They become angry, violent, or depressed. If parents take away the computer, their child sits in the corner and cries, refuses to eat, *sleep*, or do anything."

The lure of a fantasy world is especially pertinent to online role-playing games. These are games in which a player assumes the role of a fictional character and interacts with other players in a virtual world. As Young puts it, an intelligent child who is unpopular at school can "become dominant in the game." The virtual life becomes more appealing than real life.

Children who play four to five hours per day have no time for socializing, doing homework, or playing sports, that takes away from normal social development. You can get a 21-year-old with the emotional intelligence of a 12-year-old (Keith Bakker).

According to the Centre for On-Line Addiction, warning signs for video game addiction include:

- Playing for increasing amounts of time.
- Thinking about gaming during other activities.
- Gaming to escape from real-life problems, anxiety, or depression.
- Lying to friends and family to conceal gaming.
- Feeling irritable when trying to cut down on gaming.

In addition, video game addicts tend to become isolated, dropping out of their social networks and giving up other hobbies. There definitely seems to be a correlation between violent video game use and aggressive behaviour in kids (Kimberley Young). Modern day video games may be even more addictive, he added, because they are open-ended and allow players to save their place and pick back up again, unlike the older generation games. Experts believe that violent video games can be as addicting as drugs. "It affects the same pleasure centers in the brain that make people want to come back," said Dr. Michael Fraser.

The consequences of this addiction are many and varied. This "technoholism" is plaguing the minds of our younger generation. The children are becoming highly materialistic and violent. They believe in instant gratification of needs. T.V., Internet and Media games are preferred over friends and neighbours. Obesity, Diabetes and many other life style related problems are on a steep rise. Suicidal tendencies and depression is becoming rampant in the society. As Educationists and concerned adults we need to catch hold of the situation before it ravages the life of the younger generation.

References

Ahmed, A. (1980). Effect of television on study hours of Pakistani children. *Psychological Abstracts*, 66(3), 1414.

Anderson, D.M. (2001). Early childhood television viewing and adolescent behaviour. *Monographs of the Society for Research in Child Development*, 66 (1, Serial No. 264).

Comstock, G., and Scharrer, E. (2001). The use of television and other film directed media. In D.G. Singer and J.L. Singer (Eds.), *Handbook of Children and the Media* (pp. 47-72). Thousand Oaks, CA: Sage Publications.

Dietz, T.L. (1998). An examination of violence and gender role portrayals in video games. Implications for gender socialization and aggressive behaviour. *Sex Roles*, 38, 425-442.

Groebel, J. (2001). Media violence in cross cultural perspective: A global study on children's media behaviour and some emotional implications. In D.G. Singer and J.L. Singer (Eds), *Handbook of Children and the Media*, pp. 255-268, Thousand Oaks, CA: Sage Publications.

Hurlock, E.B. (1997). Play Development. In *Child Development* (pp. 310-311), 6th eds. Tata McGraw Hill, New Delhi.

Huston *et al.* (1999). How Young Children Spend Their Time: Television and other activities. *Developmental Psychology*, 35, 912-925.

Joy, P., and Shejwal, B.R. (2005). Impact of T.V. viewing on adolescent lives: Cognitive processes and adjustment. *Psychological Studies* 50, 90-97.

Livingstone, S., Bovill, M., and Gaskell, G. (1999). European kids in a transformed media world: Findings of the U.K. study. In P. Lohr and M. Meyer (eds), *Children, television and the new media. A reader of research and documentation in Germany* (pp. 8-24). Luton, U.K.: University of Luton Press.

Lowa State University (2011). ISU'S Gentile contributes to study identifying risks, consequences of video game addiction, *http://www.highbeam.com/doc/1G1-246721940.html*.

Mental Health Centre (2006) Video Game Addiction No Fun: Compulsive video gaming is a modern-day psychological disorder that experts tell WebMD is becoming more and more popular, *http://www.webmd.com/mental-health/features/video-game-addiction-no-fun*.

Neilsen Media Research (2000). *2000 Report on television*. New York.

Salomon, G. (1983). The differential investment of mental effort in learning from different sources. *Educational Psychologist*, 18(1), 42-50.

Salomon, G. (1984). Television is "easy" and print is "tough": The differential investment of effort in learning as a function of perceptions and attributions. *Journal of Educational Psychology,* 76, 647-658.

Scharrer, E., and Comstock, G. (2003). Entertainment televisual media: Content patterns and themes. In E.L. Palmer and B.M. Young (eds.), *The Faces of Televisual Media: Teaching Violence Selling to Children* (pp. 161-193) Mahwah, NJ.

Singer, D.G. and J.L. Singer (Eds), (1984). *Handbook of Children and the Media* (pp. 47-72) Thousand Oaks, CA: Sage Publications.

Sparks, G.G. (2002.) *Media Effects Research: A Basic Overview*. Belmont, CA: Wadsworth.

Strasburger, V.C. and Wilson, B.J. (2002). *Children, Adolescents and Media.* Thousand Oaks, CA: Sage Publications.

Subrahmanyam, K., Greenfield, P., Kraut, R., and Gross, E. (2001). The impact of computer use on children's and adolescents development. *Applied Developmental Psychology,* 22, 7-30.

Turkle, S. (1995). *Life on the Screen: Identity in the Age of Internet*. New York: Simon & Schuster.

von Feilitzen, C. (1999). Children's amount of TV viewing: Statistics from 10 countries. In C. von Feilitzen and U. Carlsson (Eds), *Children and Media: Image, Education, Participation* (pp. 61-67). Goteborg, Sweden: Goteborg University, UNESCO International Clearinghouse.

Wright, J.C., Huston, A.C., Piemyat, S. (1994). Young Children's perception of television reality: Determinants and Developmental differences. *Developmental Psychology,* 30, 229-239.

8

Child Abuse, Neglect, School Refusal and Suicide Ideation in Children and Adolescents

Neelam Verma

Child abuse, a condition characterized by persistent exposure to rejection, lack of attention, loneliness or unavailability of loved ones in times of need, lack of emotional support, feeling of unloved and feeling of helplessness in conditions of being tormented by caregivers. Usually adults who have faced some form of emotional abuse or maltreatment during childhood may be seen mentioning about the emotional hurt when facing physical pain. The messages of not being loved or unaccepted are usually conveyed by gestures, tone of voice, lack of approval, their intensity and frequency. Usually, the unavailability of care giver in times of need, lack of support either physical or psychological/emotional, rejection, lack or absence of approval when deserved and expected by the child and highly critical attitudes have been found to be a part of emotional abuse and neglect towards the child.

Abuse may take a form of physical abuse, sexual abuse or neglect.

Physical Abuse: Physical Abuse has been defined as any act which results in a non-accidental physical injury. Mostly it results unreasonably and an unjustifiable punishment in form of deliberate assault to an individual. Majorly the affected areas include damage to skin, damage to skeleton or head and damage to other internal organs.

Sexual Abuse: The condition of sexual abuse involves child molestation or sexual act that can be reasonably being expected to trouble or offend a child. Such acts usually involve incest, sodomy, lewd and lascivious acts with the child, oral copulation and penetration of genital or anal opening by foreign objects leading to rapes whether alone or in group. Sexual exploitation is also a related condition and involves activities related to pornography depicting minors, promoting prostitution of minors and coercion of minors to participate in the obscene acts.

***Neglect*:** Neglect is a condition of harming children by being ignorant for their physical emotional and educational needs. Physical neglect is related to ignoring health care issues of the child. Emotional neglect involves harsh and punitive behaviours with the child stemming from inadequate nurturance and affection. The educational neglect is a form of neglect that holds not providing educational facilities to children and also permitting truancy behaviours from school. Overall the educational matters are neglected and not paid attention.

As mentioned in the common phrases, physical pain is easy to bear but the psychological one is difficult to deal. Owing to the same notion, other types of abuse may become faded with time; however, neglect is a condition which is far more difficult to manage both for the sufferer and for the treatment professional. Review of articles has shown presentations of this condition that are common among most of the sufferers:

- There is persistent unhappiness;
- Lack of emotional and social support;
- Loneliness and isolation;
- Disturbances of behaviours reflected by distress and turmoil;
- Insecure attachment style with regard to primary caregivers;
- Harsh and punitive behaviour or caregivers along with tendency for rejection, criticism, neglect and hostility;
- Feelings of worthlessness and helplessness resulting in low self-esteem;
- Prolonged anxiety, stress and uncertainty;
- Lack of assertiveness in required situations like peer group and social gatherings; and
- Submissive tendency interrupting overall psychological, academic and social growth.

Essential feature of emotional abuse and neglect is associated with quality of relationship between the abused and caregiver. Generally, it has been linked with disturbed attachment patterns with the parent/ caregiver. In many circumstances a parent may become aggressive, hostile and indifferent toward the child; however, only the frequency and intensity of such behaviours lead to the conclusion of condition of abuse. If the relationship exhibits unfriendly behaviours, lack warmth, increased hostility, critical and indifferent behaviour for prolonged period it usually results in emotional deprivation and neglect and subsequently the state of abuse. If the behaviours performed by caregiver are occasional and result in the condition where such behaviours are required or situation specific, then the relationship should not be termed as abusive.

According to the "Guidelines for the Psychosocial Evaluation of Suspected Psychological Maltreatment In Children and Adolescents" of the American Professional Society on Abuse of Children (APSAC, 1995): "Psychological maltreatment means a repeated pattern of care-giver behaviour or extreme incidents that convey to children that they are worthless, flawed, unloved, unwanted, endangered, or only of value in meeting another's needs". It includes:

- ***Spurning***: May involve verbal and non-verbal behaviours, such as belittling children, shaming or ridiculing them and general degrading or rejecting or abandoning them.
- ***Terrorizing***: Refers to acts of placing children in danger, threatening them, someone or something they care for, or generally creating a climate of fear.
- ***Isolating***: Imposing severe restrictions on the child, preventing developmentally appropriate social interactions and separating a child from the rest of family.
- ***Exploiting/Corrupting***: Encouraging children to develop inappropriate and/or antisocial behaviours or values such as stealing, abusing others verbally, breaking into houses, and hurting older people or younger children.
- ***Denying Emotional Responsiveness***: Being emotionally unavailable, ignoring the child, failing to express affection, becoming distant physically and emotionally and being dismissive or children's needs of warmth and affection.
- ***Mental Health, Medical and Educational Neglect***: Failing to provide and attend to the psychological, medical and cognitive and developmental needs of the child.

In cases of emotional abuse and neglect, the specified behaviours performed by caregivers may not be necessarily intentional. In many cases, the parent may be completely unaware of the neglect behaviours. They may not realize that behaviours performed by them may be harmful for the child. Parents or caregivers who consistently rebuke or threaten the child, humiliate and put down in the social situations, induce anxiety and fear in the child and never satisfied with their performances are said to be emotionally abuse and negligent. The condition usually results in poor relations with caregiver and interpersonal difficulties outside home also. Such individuals have been found to be engaged in drug taking behaviours and engaged in other disruptive behaviours.

Risk Factors for Child Abuse and Neglect

Researches have identified a number of risk factors related to child abuse and neglect; however, no single cause of abuse could be identified that explains the etiology of these conditions. The condition persists across cultures and may occur in any religion or ethnic group. The factors which have been identified as associated with child abuse and neglect are not definite causes or predict the condition to occur necessarily in those conditions; rather they have been found present in most of the studies cases of child abuse and neglect. It has been noted that child abuse does not result from a single factor; it rather is a resultant condition of multiple interactive factors. Different factors may contribute to different types of child abuse whether it is in the form of physical abuse, sexual abuse or neglect.

Factors Related to Caregivers

It has been found that caregivers of abused children may have been going through emotional and behavioural disturbances with extreme external locus of control where the adversities are perceived to be caused by external factors. The frustration caused by the same may take form of hostility, anxiety, poor impulse control, depressive mood and cruel forms of behaviour. Substance abuse has been found to be an added condition which is frequently seen among those being abused by their caregivers. Researchers also found that the maltreatment of the child may be governed by parent's own maltreatment by their caregivers or life partner. Frequent findings have supported the fact that such parents had been a victim or sufferer of the same condition at some point or the other.

Familial Factors

Usually the victims of child abuse or neglect have been found to be raised in dysfunctional families with number of problems existing between the parents or the family members in form of marital conflict, poor communication, domestic violence, unemployment, divorce and faulty parenting styles. Sometimes inadequate information about child's developmental process may lead to misunderstanding of child's behaviours and it may result in harsh and punitive behaviour. The cause of the same may be high expectation from the children beyond their age and development. Single parenting also is an important issue that increases the likelihood of child maltreatment and neglect. Reason for the same may be burden of the child and lack of support from partner. Absence of father figure is highly related to this condition and it increases the rate of physical abuse, sexual abuse and neglect of the children. It has been found that children with neglect issues usually have increased number of siblings; however, not all researches have supported the findings. It is also noted that usually the condition of abuse occurs during stressful life events where the impulses of parents become irresistible and child suffers from abuse. Attachment patterns and communication between child and caregivers is also an important part of these factors and studies have advocated that those who suffer from neglect or abuse do not have adequate communication with caregivers and lack attachment and intimacy. Such parents usually adopt harsh strategies of discipline rather than setting a healthy communication pattern.

Child Related Factors

It has been noted that there are factors related to child's condition and developmental status at the time of abuse. Researchers and survey have demonstrated that child's developmental condition may contribute to the type of abuse. Usually younger children suffer more from physical abuse or neglect but those who have entered in puberty and adolescence are at higher risk of sexual abuse. Some of the studies have indicated that children with any kind of disability are at risk of abuse as they are not able to defend themselves during that time. Many children with intellectual disability suffer from the condition multiple times. Also, children who have physical disabilities and dependent on others to perform routine activities suffer from the abuse frequently. Any psychological/psychiatric condition with child may work as an indirect factor contributing to abuse and neglect as it may decrease caregiver's tolerance to those conditions. Due to this reason a parent may lack warmth towards the child resulting in anger outburst and may not be able to understand child's condition.

Socio-Cultural Factors

Poverty and unemployment of caregiver has been frequently related to child neglect. The condition occurs due to unavailability of resources and frustration induced by the same. Surveys have indicated that parents whose children suffer from neglect usually report lack of social support, isolation and loneliness in community. Few factors related to violent community are also important for these conditions. A hostile and violent neighbourhood increases the risk of child to be abused. In current era media is playing an important in displaying violent acts. Excessive watching of such acts on television has been found to be associated with abusers performing such acts.

School Refusal

The condition of school refusal is characterized by severe emotional stress about attending school and the distress is usually shown or exhibited in form of anxiety, temper tantrums, depression and somatic symptoms. The condition may appear similar to truancy as the school avoidance behaviour is common in both the conditions, yet it differs from truancy as the children with truancy frequently display behavioural problems and lack of associated anxiety caused by absenteeism. They also lack willingness to meet academic expectation at home. Contradictorily, children with school refusal show willingness to complete home assignments of school and also the behavioural problems are absent. The condition is not characterized by presence of physical illnesses, absence motivated by parents, chronic runaways or homelessness. Generally, children with school refusal avoid school as they seek security at home and want to be closer to the parental figures and complain of multiple somatic symptoms when discussed about attending school. Somewhere separation anxiety leads to the condition of school refusal as it includes distress when the child assumes separation from the parental figures. There can be different groups of children displaying refusal symptoms in different ways:

- Some would never attend school or completely absent from there.
- Some would attend the school initially but may leave or come back home during the school hours.
- Some would go to school but only after a psychological reaction of anxiety displayed by vomiting or pain symptoms.
- Some would show consistent unusual distress during school hours and seek support for non-attendance.

Refusal behaviour may vary in severity and its persistency for a certain amount of time. Three major levels of severity of school refusal have been explained by Kearney and Silverman (1996):

1. ***Self Corrective School Refusal:*** Children who belong to this level reach remission within a week.
2. ***Acute School Refusal***: At this level refusal/absenteeism persists for about a period of two weeks.
3. ***Chronic School Refusal***: Children who belong to this level refuse going to school and are absent for the whole year and overlapping is found between the two academic sessions.

Individuals with school refusal frequently display physical symptoms like dizziness, headache, stomachache, nausea, vomiting, palpitations, joint pain, etc. in absence of organic basis. Behavioural symptoms may include physical protest before going to school so that the parents or caregivers allow them to stay at home or there may be oversleeping and missing the school vehicle due to being late in order to avoid school.

Symptoms of school refusal are generally displayed in two ways:

1. *Internalizing Symptoms*: These symptoms mainly include anxiety, low mood, negative affectivity, and somatic complaints.
2. *Externalizing Symptoms*: These symptoms are usually displayed as palpitations, clinging, threats of self harm etc.

There can be following reasons due to which an individual persists with school refusal behaviour:

- Refusal may be performed in order to avoid anxiety provoking objects related to school,
- The behaviour may also be continued to escape the conditions of academic tests, oral presentations and peer interactions, and
- Refusal may be a part of attention seeking behaviour or pursuing tangible rewards outside school.

School refusal leads to significant impairments in individual's academic growth resulting in poor grades and awkward condition among peers. The conditions results in anxiety and low self-esteem. In severe cases, there may be possibility of developing maladaptive coping mechanisms like substance abuse.

Etiology of School Refusal

Familial Factors

Usually, the children being brought in the dysfunctional families are more likely to refuse school. Stressful events at home may compel the child to stay at home. Young children usually refuse to attend school as they perceive that something catastrophic will occur at home in their absence. Older children may have fear of happening something wrong to a parent who is ill or is a drug abuser. Researches have also indicated that children of anxious parents are more likely to display such behaviours as school refusal have been found to be highly correlated with separation anxiety which has a cause lying behind the anxious parenting style. Many times first allowance by the parent to let the child stay at home makes the response conditioned and the child frequently asks to stay at home. Since the physical symptoms of nausea and body aches are related to the condition children may continue the refusal to gain attention by the parents that they usually provide when the child complains of the multiple pain symptoms. The association of attention seeking behaviour has also been found to be important in the condition as it has been found to increase when children gain extra attention of parents in the given condition.

Genetic Factors

The genetic factors usually represent the genetic susceptibility for a given condition. In cases of school refusal anxiety and emotional disturbances have been found to play a key role and many times school refusal occurs as a response to anxiety provoking situation. Temperamental characteristics such as emotional reactivity, adaptability to mood etc. are again related to the vulnerability factors. Separation anxiety is the major part of this disorder and it increases the likelihood that if somebody in the family has a history of anxiety disorder, child may develop separation anxiety which might result in school refusal.

School Related Factors

Many times the refusal may result from the tendency to avoid duties or the anxiety provoked by tests, examinations and presentations at school. Children who attend school initially but refuse later usually start behaving in such manner due to the mentioned reasons most of the time. There is consistent worry about the performance at school and worry of being judged. Sometimes, a child who has ever faced bullying by the classmates due to any reason such as poor test result, inability to speak properly infront of the class or late home assignment may also reject to attend school after some time. Few surveys have also found an association between inadequate teaching methods and harsh classroom discipline and school refusal.

Learning Factors

There is an obvious content of fear related to school refusing behaviour that can be learned either through modelling by observation or can be transmitted by others in form of wrong messages. Many times when younger children observe their older siblings crying during the pre-school hours or watch them discussing the punishment procedures at school. It may create an anxiety and fear causing negative attitude towards school related stimuli resulting in school refusal.

Suicide among Children and Adolescents

Suicide has been found to be one of the leading causes of death among adolescents. As explained by Rosenberg in his work that suicide is a condition characterized by the act or behaviour with the intention to kill oneself. Suicide, to be explained as suicide should be a personal intention to kill oneself and must not be executed by the other person. Also, the intention should be implemented in order to achieve death rather than harming oneself. Every person with the intention to commit suicide may not achieve complete suicide. In cases of incomplete suicide, intentionality and lethality of the suicidal attempt come under the questionable area. Usually those with actual intention to perform this behaviour would plan the act adequately so that it gives intended results. Suicide generally has a thought behind the act which may be cause by depressive life events such as academic failure, lack of career opportunities, familial problems, and issues with parents or closed ones and most importantly lack of Will-power to overcome life hazards. Those who had history of depression, substance use and had attempted suicide in past also, may have actual intention to die and also at high risk.

In cases of suicide the intention to kill oneself is very certain; however, on the other hand others may not attempt the act with the same intention, rather there is some other purpose of doing such behaviours, for example, seeking attention or help of others. This is known as "non-fatal suicide behaviours". If there is some or minimal intention to die is found (based on injuries resulted from the act) the condition is regarded as "instrumental suicide related behaviours". On the other hand if the suicidal attempt is found to be fully fledged non-fatal suicide behaviour the condition is termed as "parasuicide". Here, the intention of performing such act is totally achieving the other goal rather than death. Among adolescents, self-destructive behaviours are very common like cutting or carving the wrist, burning a part of body etc. on a superficial level. Usually the report is given by them as feeling of satisfaction and stress relief. The condition differs from suicide and parasuicide and termed as "self mutilation".

It has been found difficult to differentiate suicide from other related aspects; however, careful history review and interview can resolve the problem. Two major components of suicide behaviour have been identified as key factors:

1. *Intentiality*: is related to the severity of acts like the deepness of cut, amount of pills taken etc.
2. *Lethality*: is related to the planning of performing such act like ensuring the privacy while planning the act, taking complete care that nobody can make out that what is being planned.

Presence of high/low intentiality and lethality determine the severity of suicide. If the intent to die is high and the attempt is lethal enough, it is likely to be said as suicidal attempt; on the contrary, if the intentiality and lethality are low then the attempt may be categorized under other aspects of suicide.

The instrumental suicide related behaviours have been classified in the following subcategories by Silverman, Berman, Sanddal, O'Corroll and Joiner (2007a, 2007b):

1. When the act is performed in the absence of suicidal intent it is termed as *Self harm*.
2. If somehow the intent and lethality of the act are difficult to establish or determine it is labeled as *undetermined suicide related behaviour.*
3. If the intent to commit suicide was present indeed it would be termed as *suicide attempt*.

The authors further classify each of the categories with regard to the presence or absence of medical injuries. Thus the category expands in

Type I and Type II. Those who face no injuries are kept under Type I and those with injuries are categorized under Type II. The complexity of lethality is yet to be explored and decided on the basis of research evidences.

Many times the person who attempts suicide suffers through periods of recurrent thoughts of being dead or thinking that death may end all the worries of life. The thought related to death or wish to die is termed as "*suicidal ideation*" and is common among those who have suffered with major depressive symptoms. As discussed earlier, all who attempt suicide may not intent to commit that and also in some cases the purpose of doing such acts may be achieving or serving a different cause. In such cases it can be communicated to the family members or loved ones through verbal or non-verbal gestures that the suicidal act is likely to be performed in near future. These behaviours can be explained as suicidal threats with intention to seek attention or to make demands fulfilled.

In cases of history with depression or adverse life events it may not be difficult to identify the intent and lethality of the attempt; however, those suffering from impulse control disorder, borderline personally disorder and dissociative disorder are difficult to judge as all the other mentioned conditions may have depressive co-morbidity. Adolescence is the age of crises and rapid changes in physiological, emotional and psychological states of the individual. During this period the mind flows with lot of curiosities and myths and adolescents do not leave any single chance to explore them. Those who get adequate resources, appropriate family and social support get through the conditions easily and adapt in the environment. On the other hand those who lack the support of family and friends face more hazards in difficult situations and subsequently slip in to the clinical conditions like depression and substance abuse and in extreme cases suicide. It is found that usually people with complete suicide suffer from phases of maladjustment due to poor coping ability and lack of resources. Stress can also be contributing factors in this situation.

Etiology

Biological/Genetic Factors

Researchers have proved the importance of genetic factors in suicide. It has been found that monozygotic twins are at higher risk of attempting or complete suicide as compared to dizygotic twins. The risk has also been found to be high among first degree relatives. Altered serotonin functions mostly in favour of decreased serotonin levels have been found to be associated with increased risk of suicide. Researchers have also advocated that those who have a family history of suicide or major depressive disorder are likely to attempt suicide in future.

Psychodynamic Factors

The psychodynamic factors explain suicidal behaviour as redirecting of aggressive impulse towards oneself which was initially directed towards a significant other. Meninger (1938) postulated three motives behind it: (1) a wish to kill, (2) particularly to kill those who are loved ones, and (3) a wish to be killed. The third motivation is usually governed by the former two that is wish to be killed is generally induced by the guilt due to wish of killing the loved ones. It has also been described by Wade (1987), as an inability to love and a wish to transcend separateness feeling by returning to the position of infant and being merged with the caregiver.

Cognitive Factors

Beck has major contribution in exploring these factors. The cognitive factors play an important role in this condition and importance of schemas and belief system has been found to be an important aspect of these factors. Self-schemas containing negative beliefs, dysfunctional assumptions and cognitive distortions have been identified as diathesis for depressive and suicidal symptoms. The cognitions characterized by helplessness, hopelessness and worthlessness have been found to play a key role in cases of suicide. Hopelessness has been identified as a risk factor in cases of complete suicide. The term "suicidal mode" has been found to be a triggering factor for activation of affective, behavioural and motivational sources of suicide. A variety of dysphoric emotions influence the conditions of suicide. Marsha Linehan (1993) presented two major characteristics of those who attempt suicide and advocated that people with suicidal tendency lack skills in two areas which lead to suicidal attempts. First the ability to accept experiences completely, and second they lack use of means to regulate impulsive and self-destructive emotions for example difficulty in tolerating emotional distress and excessively passive attitude.

Social Factors

These factors explain the suicidal behaviours to be learned by modelling either through direct or indirect means. These factors stem from the concept of "Cluster" given by *O'Carroll, Mercy, and Steward (1988)*. The *Centres for Disease Control and Prevention* explains the concept as a group of suicides or suicide attempts that occur closer together in time and space that would normally be expected. Clusters are primarily a phenomenon among those running in the adolescence and early adulthood. Usually, the clustering is identified if the suicidal attempts share common features. Other types of clustering involve suicide following a suicide which is not necessarily located geographically but well publicized in media. The novel written by Goethe's (1774) "*The Sorrows of Young Werther*" comprised such imitated behaviours and it was thought to be precipitating an increased rate of suicides in Europe at that time. Many times fictional characters doing such acts, dramatization in stories and other TV shows containing similar behaviours have been found to result in increased suicidal behaviours among adolescents.

Psychological and Interpersonal Factors

These factors explain suicidal behaviours based on internal psychological processes and interpersonal dynamics. These factors are related to two basic orientations of human beings. People with intra-psychic orientation are mainly focused on their personal/psychological distress, least likely to seek support and may be at higher risk of complete suicides than attempted suicide. On the contrary, those with the inter-psychic orientation are more oriented towards the relational aspects of their problems and obstructions, more likely to seek support and at higher risk for attempted suicide than complete suicide. It is said that males tend to have the intra-psychic orientation and females tend to have inter-psychic orientation. Some of the researches have shown that those who have been exposed to extreme violence and threats at home feel less pain and face the suicidal situation without any fear. Some have the temperament to react and behave aggressively and engage in the risk taking behaviours repeatedly. Not all cases support that all who attempt suicide are fearless because many of the attempts are made under the influence of drug where the pain would be less but the injuries would be obvious.

Psycho-Social Factors

Edwin Shneidman (1996) coined a concept of "Suicidal Cubelet" and explained that suicide occurs only when there is a synergistic interaction among three major components, i.e. pain, press and perturbation. Pain is explained by intense emotional distress resulting in pain, press has been defined as either positive or negative environmental influence/pressure and finally perturbation which refers to one's level of emotional agitation cognitive constriction or narrowing of thoughts contributing to impulsive and potentially lethal attempt of suicide.

Biopsychosocial Factors

Biopsychosocial factors of suicide include interaction of biological, psychological and social factors. These factors explain the suicidal behaviours as an interaction of temperamental characteristics or personality traits (such as low frustration tolerance, sensitivity to criticism, poor coping mechanisms, impulsivity etc.), psycho-social and environmental factors (such as recent major stresses or stressful life events, exposure to suicide or any medical condition), genetic predisposition towards suicide and other biological causes (such as decreased level of serotonin) and psychiatric illnesses (like affective disorder, mood disorder or alcohol abuse).

Developmental Factors

The developmental factors are explained under three major contexts. The social context of this condition explains the development at different places including home, family, peers, schools etc. and its association with cognitive processing. For example, an adolescent who has been seeing the depressed attitude of parents may develop depressive attitude and act accordingly on the other hand s/he may behave differently among the peer group. Studies have indicated that healthy interactions with peers enhance quality of mental health. *Multifinality* and *Equifinality* context advocate the idea that risk conditions of childhood may influence the later conditions of life such as "poor attachment pattern with parents in childhood may negatively influence adolescence with depression, suicidal behaviour, anxiety and aggression. This is basically the multifinality". On the contrary, "equifinality explains the suicidal symptoms may be a common end product of different problems that varies with individual differences and life experiences of youngsters". For some there may be loss of hope for family acceptance, for some there may be dissociative walling off of the situation to avoid emotional pain and also a function of difficult temperament such as lack of impulse control and self-destruction. Another context of the etiology is termed as developmental transitions and trajectories that explain the suicidal behaviours on the basis of rapid reorganizations of biological, emotional and cognitive states during adolescence. Early puberty among girls and excessive delays in achieving physical growth among boys is often marked by embarrassment, rejection in the peer group, lack of popularity and low self-esteem. It may lead to feelings of depression, subsequently suicidal thoughts resulting in suicidal behaviours.

Any kind of abuse and emotional negligence during childhood have been found to be a strong predictor of defiant behaviours during adolescence such as cruel behaviour towards family members, antisocial acts in society, bullying behaviour among peers and many times school refusal. Also, the condition has been found to be associated with suicidal attempts in adulthood. Explanation of the same may be given as, abuse by close relatives leads to traumatic experiences especially when the abuse is repeated for a long time. Traumatic experiences faced by the individual negatively influence the emotional state and weaken the coping mechanisms increasing the risk of intra-psychic conflicts; a state where an individual is unable to take adequate decisions and take a step towards ending the life for ever.

A study published on line in a journal *"Suicide and life threatening behaviour: copyright 2014, American Association of Suicidology"* indicated that children who suffered from childhood abuse were at higher risk of suicidal behaviours as compared to those who had no history of such abuse. In a systematic review study a strong link was found between suicidal and self-harming thoughts/behaviours during adolescence and a history of physical and sexual abuse during childhood (Evans and Colleagues; 2005). A similar review of literature advocated that all types of maltreatment are associated with adolescent suicide behaviours; however, sexual and emotional abuse might be more correlated with such condition than physical abuse and neglect (Miller & Colleagues, 2013). Another study in the same field advocated sexual abuse to be the strongest factor behind suicidal ideations and attempted suicides as it was found to be closely associated with feelings of shame and internal attributions of blame (Brodsky and Stanley, 2008).

There is a group of research conducted to identify the protective factors in such conditions where role of parenting and quality of parent-child relationship has been found to be one of the major protective factors.

Rather than the child resorting to harmful behaviours and suicidal gestures after abuse, parents can model the child to overcome the situation and find more adequate coping mechanisms.

Like childhood abuse, school refusal is a major public health issue and a challenging situation for mental health professional and educationists. It has been found to be associated with violent behaviours, self-harming acts, threats to harm self and accidental suicides during impulsive emotional states. Literature indicates that such children have an automatic pressure from family and society to attend school; however, they have different psycho-social reasons to avoid schooling. So far, there are hardly researches in the literature that directly correlate school refusal and suicidal behaviours; however, there is a link between both the phenomena that might relate them indirectly. As mentioned above, there are different variants of school absenteeism such as adverse family atmosphere, faulty parenting, peer bullying, involvement in anti-social acts and substance abuse, depression, oppositional tendencies, etc. All the conditions somewhere correlate with the negative emotional state of the individual and at some point of time in life may lead to impulsive attempts of self-harm and sometimes ending up of life.

There is a scope for further researches to establish more sound correlational studies along with a comprehensive preventive and rehabilitative programme. Future researchers may give a direction to budding professionals in order to work on such critical and major issues of society and prevent the problems of youth that have a path down the lane in their childhood experiences.

References

Brodsky, B., and Stanley, B. (2008). Adverse childhood experiences and suicidal behaviour. *Psychiatric Clinics of North America*, 31, 223-235.

Evans, E., Hawton, K., and Rodham, K. (2005). Suicidal phenomena and abuse in adolescents: A review of epidemiological studies. *Child Abuse and Neglect*, 29(1), 45-58.

Miller, A.B., Esposito-Smythers, C., Weismoore, J.T., and Renshaw, K.D. (2013). The relation between child maltreatment and adolescent suicidal behaviour: A systematic review and critical examination of the literature. *Clinical Child and Family Psychology Review*, April 2013.

Thompson, R., Litrownik, A.J., Isbell, P., Everson, M.D., English, D.J., Dubowitz, H., and Flaherty, E.G. (2012). Adverse experiences and suicidal ideation in adolescence: Exploring the link using the LONGSCAN samples. *Psychology of Violence*, 2(2), 211-225.

9
Management of Dyslexia

A Case Study

Anubhuti Dubey and *Shalini Gupta*

Learning disorders refer to a child's or adolescent's deficits in acquiring expected skills in reading, writing speaking, use of listing, reasoning, or mathematics, compared with the children of the same age and intellectual capacity. In simple words, children and adults with learning disabilities see, hear, and understand things differently. This can lead to trouble with learning new information and skills, and putting them to use. The most common types of learning disabilities include problems with reading, writing, maths, reasoning, listening, and speaking. Learning Disabilities (LD) vary from person to person. One person may have trouble with reading and writing. Another person with learning disabilities may have problems with understanding math. Still another person may have trouble in each of these areas, as well as, with understanding what people are saying. Researchers think that learning disabilities are caused by differences in how a person's brain works and how it processes information. Children with learning disabilities are not "dumb" or "lazy". In fact, they usually have average or above average intelligence. Their brains just process information differently. Of all students with specific learning disabilities, 70 per cent to 80 per cent have deficits in reading.

Dyslexia

The term "Developmental Dyslexia" is often used as a synonym for reading disability; however, many researchers assert that there are different types of reading disabilities, of which dyslexia is one. Dyslexia can be defined as a neuro-developmental disorder with a biological origin and behavioural signs which extend far beyond problems with written language. At the cognitive level, putative causes of the behavioural signs and symptoms of the condition can be specified (Firth, 1999; Ramus, Pidgeon and Frith, 2003). Like many other scientific words the term dyslexia is originated from Greek. The prefix 'dys' means 'difficulty' or 'malfunction' and root word 'lexis' suggest the problems with reading, spelling, writing and other aspects of language.

The Hindi movie '*Tare Jameen Par*' directed and produced by actor Amir Khan illustrated the problems of dyslexic child and his parents had brought the issues of such learning disorders into focus of educationists, psychologists, health professionals and parents as well.

Signs and Symptoms of Dyslexia

There is no one sign that demonstrates that a person has any learning disability. Dyslexics' have difficulties in reading and spelling. The condition is wide-ranging, genetically based, neuro-developmental syndrome (Stein and Telcott, 1999; Stein, Talcott and Witton, 2001). Experts look for a noticeable difference between how well a child does in school and how well he or she can do, given his or her intelligence or ability. There are also certain clues that may mean a child has a learning disability. Most of the clues relate to elementary school tasks, because learning disabilities tend to be identified at elementary school level. A child probably won't show all of these signs, or even most of them. However, if a child shows a number of these problems, then parents and the teachers should consider the possibility that the child has a learning disability. After a child begins school, the signs of dyslexia include:

- Problems reading single words, such as a word on a flash card.
- Problems linking letters with sounds.
- Confusing small words, such as "at" and "to".
- Reversing the shapes of written letters such as "d" for "b". For example, the child may write "dat" instead of "bat".
- Writing words backward, such as "tip" for "pit".

If a child has one of these signs, it does not mean that he or she has dyslexia. Many children reverse letters before age 7. But if the child has several signs and reading problems, or if one have a family history of dyslexia, such child should be checked and assessed.

Phonological Deficit

Phonological awareness deficits in dyslexia have been documented by many researchers in many languages (e.g. Snowling, 1980; Bruck and

Treiman, 1990; Olson *et al.*, 1990; De Gelder and Vroomen, 1991; Bowey, Cain and Ryan, 1992; Wimmer, 1993; Elbro, 1996; Elbro, Borstrom, and Petersen, 1998); Lundberg, 1994; Goswami, 2000; Silani, Frith, Demonet, Fazio, Perani, Price and Paulesu, 2005). There is also a small amount of evidence that is consistent with the idea that lexical restructuring is delayed in dyslexia. Dyslexics' have difficulty working with the sounds in words e.g., identifying beginning and end sounds in aword, producing a word that rhymes and problems learning phonic (letter/sound association) skills.

Poor auditory short-term memory leads to difficulty with blending sounds together, taking in verbal information, remembering instructions, and learning lists of facts (Oyler, 2009; Jenkins and O'Connor, 2002). The findings with reading disability adolescents indicated that such adolescents learned significantly fewer list items and did so at a slower rate than the control group. Although they were equally able to retain information once learned, they did demonstrate inefficient elaborative rehearsal strategies. They also recalled fewer words in both the semantic and phonetic cued-recall conditions, but the effect size was significantly greater in the latter. These students have less efficient rehearsal and encoding mechanisms but typical retention. Retrieval also appears typical except under conditions that require information to be recalled based on phonetic codes (Oyler, Obrzut, and Asbjornsen, 2012).

Slower naming speed leads to difficulty recalling names and words, less fluent oral reading, and trouble with basic sight words (Bowers and Wolf, 1993;Wolf and Katzir-Cohen, 2001). Katzir *et al.* (2006) reported that children's performance in spelling recognition was significantly associated with their skills in word reading and reading comprehension regardless of their reading disability status. Furthermore, spelling recognition contributed significant variance to reading comprehension for both dyslexic and non-dyslexic children after the effects of phonological awareness, rapid naming, and word reading proficiency had been accounted for.

Orthographic processing difficulties lead to reading and spelling problems (Attaining automaticity in underlying and component skills needed for reading and written language. They may be able to perform the required skills but the process is slow, effortful and mechanic and can only do one thing at a time (e.g., can't focus on spelling and ideas when writing, can't decode words and take in the meaning of the text), reading/ comprehension difficulty, written language difficulty, listening/note-taking difficulty (Manis, Custodio, and Szeszulski, 1993; Valdois, Bosse and Tainturier, 2004).

Difficulty in multi-tasking as they have problems in organization and time management (Moody, 2010). In a study in U.K. by Morris, and Turnbull (2007) found that dyslexia provided a challenge to the everyday work of registered nurses, which was often met successfully using a range of individualized strategies. Career progression was achievable but compared with peers, was perceived to take longer. People with the learning disability developmental dyslexia characteristically have difficulties in processing written language. There is some evidence that they may also have talents in other areas such as visuospatial processing. This pattern of strengths and weaknesses may predispose people who have dyslexia towards adopting certain occupations and away from others. Adults with symptoms of dyslexia were much less likely than adults not reporting such symptoms to be involved in professions such as science/ computing, management and finance. They were more likely to be involved in people-oriented professions such as nursing or sales (Taylor and Walter, 2003).

Challenges for Parents

For many parents it is quite difficult to accept that their offspring may have any learning disability or disorder. Denial, blaming each spouse, emotional turmoil is the common reactions of parents. If the parents accept, then the question arises before them 'Now What'? If a parent suspect that his/her child has some learning difficulties which may require special assistance, then the question is how, where and when in finding support. The sooner the parent moves forward, the better chances for the child in attaining his or her full potential. An important part of treatment is educating the parents about the condition of their children. It is important to know dyslexia is a lifelong condition. Even though early treatment during childhood can help, so it is important to consult the pediatrician if the parents are concerned about child's development. Additionally, meeting with the teachers of the child is an important step towards.

Learning disabilities look very different from one child to another. One child may struggle with reading and spelling, while another loves books but can't understand math. Still another child may have difficulty understanding what others are saying or communicating out loud. The problems are very different, but they are all learning disorders. It's not always easy to identify learning disabilities. Because of the wide variations, there is no single symptom or profile that you can look to as proof of a problem. However, some warning signs are more common than others at different ages. Children who do not grasp basic reading and writing skills in their first year of school are at risk of ongoing learning difficulties. At the end of reception, most children can give the sound and write each of the letters of the alphabet when presented in jumbled order.

Management of Dyslexia

Management uses a number of teaching methods to help your child read better. These methods include:

- Teaching how letters are linked to sounds to make words.
- Having the child read aloud with a teacher's help.
- Teaching the child to listen to and repeat instructions.

There is no cure for dyslexia, but dyslexic individuals can learn to read and write with educational support. There are techniques and technical aids that can manage or even conceal symptoms of the disorder. Removing stress and anxiety alone can improve written comprehension. For *dyslexia intervention* with alphabet writing systems the fundamental aim is to increase a child's awareness of correspondences between *graphemes* and *phonemes*, and to relate these to reading and spelling. It has been found that training focused towards visual language and *orthographic* issues yields longer-lasting gains than mere oral phonological training. There is some evidence that the use of specially tailored fonts may provide some measure of assistance for those suffering from dyslexia. Intervention early on while language areas in the brain are still developing is most successful in reducing long-term impacts of dyslexia.

A Case of Dyslexia

Master A.T. aged 13, Hindu male child studying in class 7th from High Socio-economic status referred by his doctor for psychological intervention having no significant prenatal and postnatal history and normal developmental milestones. The chief complaints were—Delayed Speech, Poor Reading and Writing (writing Deficits) and Impaired in abstraction.

Assessment of Adaptive Behaviour

Independent toilet skills; partially dependent dressing, washing, bathing and brushing; dependent eating.

Basic Concepts

3 R's

Reading: read only alphabets and identify normal pictures.
Writing: scribble, draw Strokes, Can write alphabets.
Arithmetic: knows only simple arithmetic.
Socialization: Oriented towards parents and siblings and partially oriented to peers.

Behavioural Observation and Mental Status Examination

Physical Presentation	:	Neat
Manners	:	Absent
Dressing	:	Neat
Psychomotor Activity	:	Hyper
Eye Contact	:	Fleeting
Orientation	:	Less
Attention	:	Less
Vocabulary	:	50-300 Words
Memory	:	Poor
Abstraction	:	Absent
Thinking	:	Yet to be developed

Psychological Tests used for Master A.T.

- Seguin Form Board: First trail takes 30 sec., second trail takes 28 sec., and third trail take. 24 sec., Impression: Average IQ 72.
- Bender Visual Motor Gestalt Test: Impression: Average IQ 72.
- Vineland social maturity scale: Impression: Average SQ SA–6.4 year.

***Provisional Diagnosis*:** Diagnosed as child with specific learning disorder (Dyslexia).

***Diagnostic Formulation*:** He was observed and assessed by Clinical

Psychologist, Special educator, Doctor and Occupational Therapist. He is diagnosed as child with Specific Learning Disorder (Dyslexia). After the assessment part he joined the regular therapy session of occupational therapy and special education part.

According to special educator his problems were: Poor oral expression, poor listening comprehension, poor written expression, poor basic reading skill, poor reading fluency skills, poor reading comprehension, and poor mathematical calculations.

Activities Planned for Master A.T.

Physical Activities: Exercise with physio-boll, Taking 4-5 rounds of balancing, Bicycling, Martial arts, Weight lifting, Camping, Swimming etc.

Education: Special education with the help of his school collaboration.

Management: Management of the case can be discussed in two sub-topics; they are short-term goal and long-term goal.

> *Short-term goals*: Master A.T. has improved a lot and we can recognize the changes in him. But still he requires an intense regular therapy. Short-term goal planned for him and started working on it; it includes physical activity, socialization skills and basic concepts. And also removing stress and anxiety for improve written comprehension.
>
> *Long-term goals*: As we know dyslexia can't fully manage with short-term goals it requires long-term intervention is inclusive education like copy writing, self-initiated writing and reading skills. When the child became adult at that time he should be independent for that he needs vocational training, it is must for the child so that he can start some business which can help him out in future.

Conclusion

Dyslexia is characterized by difficulty in learning to read fluently and with accurate comprehension despite normal intelligence. This includes difficulty with phonological awareness, phonological decoding, processing speed, orthographic coding, auditory short-term memory, language skills/verbal comprehension, and/or rapid naming. Master A.T.

is suffering from Special Learning Disorder (Dyslexia). Certain exercise intervention to counselling, copy writing, dictation, writing and self initiated writing were done with him for the intermittent year and he has shown remarkable improvement in writing skills. Similarly, remedial work was done on his reading skills and these skills too are satisfactory. He has been recommended for long-term rehabilitation programme and Disability certification.

How to Help Children with Dyslexia

There is no cure for dyslexia. But early intervention can give children with dyslexia the encouragement and tools they need to manage in school and compensate for their disability. If a parent or teacher suspects that a child has dyslexia or another learning disability, talk with his/her pediatrician as soon as possible. The doctor can rule out any physical issues — such as vision problems in the child. They may then refer him/ her to a learning specialist, educational psychologist, or speech therapist. The first step will be to have the child evaluated only then appropriate steps can be taken at school and at home. An assessment by educational/ developmental psychologist will provide information about child's learning abilities and his/her particular strengths and weaknesses as well as current literacy/numeric levels, and identify whether or not the child might have a specific learning difficulty such as dyslexia. If there are also speech and/or language concerns a speech and language assessment by a speech pathologist, for a hearing assessment by an audiologist can also be organized. Further concerns, e.g. sleep problems or behavioural issues may benefit from an appointment with a pediatrician. Occupational therapy assessment and intervention can assist children who have coordination difficulties, attention difficulties and sensory issues.

References

Bowey, J.A., Cain, M.T. and Ryan, S.M. (1992). A reading-level design study of phonological skills underlying fourth grade children's word reading difficulties. *Child Development*, 63, 999-1011.

Bruck, M. and Treiman, R. (1990). Phonological awareness and spelling in normal children and dyslexics: the case of initial consonant clusters. *Journal of Experimental Child Psychology*, 50, 156-178.

De Gelder, B. and Vroomen, J. (1991). Phonological deficits: beneath the surface of reading acquisition. *Psychological Research,* 53, 88-97.

Elbro, C. (1996). Early linguistic abilities and reading development: A review and a hypothesis. *Reading and Writing*, 8, 453-485.

Elbro, C., Borstrom, I. and Petersen, D.K. (1998) Predicting dyslexia from kindergarten: The importance of distinctness of phonological representations of lexical items. *Reading Research Quarterly,* 33, 36-60.

Frith, U. (1999). Paradoxes in the Definition of Dyslexia1. *Dyslexia*, 5, 192-214.

Goswami, U. (2000). Phonological representations, reading development and dyslexia: Towards a cross-linguistic theoretical framework. *Dyslexia*, 6(2), 133-151.

Jenkins, J.R., and O'Connor, R.E. (2002). Early identification and intervention for young children with reading/learning disabilities. *Identification of Learning Disabilities: Research to Practice*, 99-149.

Katzir, T., Kim, Y., Wolf, M., O'Brien, B., Kennedy, B., Lovett, M., and Morris, R. (2006). Reading fluency: The whole is more than the parts. *Annals of Dyslexia*, 56(1), 51-82.

Lundberg, I. (1994) Reading difficulties can be predicted and prevented. In C. Hulme and M. Snowling (Eds), *Reading Development and Dyslexia*, (pp. 180-199). London: Whurr Publishers.

Manis, F.R., Custodio, R., and Szeszulski, P.A. (1993). Development of phonological and orthographic skill: A 2-year longitudinal study of dyslexic children. *Journal of Experimental Child Psychology,* 56, 64-86.

Morris, D.K., and Turnbull, P.A. (2007). The disclosure of dyslexia in clinical practice: Experiences of student nurses in the United Kingdom. *Nurse Education Today*, 27(1), 35-42.

Olson, R., Wise, B., Connors, F. and Rack, J. (1990) Organisation, heritability and remediation of component word recognition and language skills in disabled readers. In T. Carr and B.A. Levy (Eds), *Reading and its Development: Component Skills Approaches,* (pp. 261-322). San Diego, CA: Academic Press.

Oyler, J.D. (2009). *Verbal Learning and Memory Functions in Students with Reading Disabilities*. ProQuest.

Oyler, J.D., Obrzut, J.E., and Asbjornsen, A.E. (2012). Verbal learning and memory functions in adolescents with reading disabilities. *Learning Disability Quarterly*, 35(3), 184-195.

Ramus, F., Pidgeon, E., and Frith, U. (2003). The relationship between motor control and phonology in dyslexic children. *Journal of Child Psychology and Psychiatry*, 44(5), 712-722.

Silani, G., Frith, U., Demonet, J.F., Fazio, F., Perani, D., Price, C., and Paulesu, E. (2005). Brain abnormalities underlying altered activation in dyslexia: a voxel based morphometry study. *Brain*, 128(10), 2453-2461.

Snowling, M.J. (1980). The development of grapheme–phoneme correspondence in normal and dyslexic readers. *Journal of Experimental Child Psychology*, 29, 294-305.

Stein, J., and Talcott, J. (1999). Impaired neuronal timing in developmental dyslexia}themagnocellular hypothesis. Dyslexia. *An International Journal of Research and Practice*, 5, 59-77.

Stein, J., Talcott, J., and Witton, C. (2001). The sensorimotor basis of developmental dyslexia. In A.J. Fawcett (Ed.), *Dyslexia. Theory and Good Practice*. London: Whurr Publishers.

Taylor, K.E. and Walter, J. (2003). Occupation choices of adults with and without symptoms of dyslexia. *Dyslexia*, 9: 177-185. doi: 10.1002/dys.239.

Valdois, S., Bosse, M.L., and Tainturier, M.J. (2004). The cognitive deficits responsible for developmental dyslexia: Review of evidence for a selective visual attention disorder. *Dyslexia,* 10, 1-25.

Wolf, M., and Katzir-Cohen, T. (2001). Reading fluency and its intervention. *Scientific Studies of Reading*, 5(3), 211-239.

10
Emotional Disturbance and Parenting

Sarita Joshi and *Aradhana Shukla*

The family has been an essential institution throughout the centuries, evolving from humans' co-dependent tendencies and need for nurturing relationships. It's importance to humanity is unquestionable. It lays the foundation for an individual's future, having the power to influence either positively or negatively. There is much debate as to what equals a complete family. Ideally family "consists of a father, mother and their children living in a state of greater geographical, economic and social independence from other relatives and kin". Under this definition, a single-parent home would not be categorized as a true family. While analyzing parenting, Children unbeatably need both of the parent or complete family to develop into mature and productive adults. Parenting can be viewed as transaction a task involving two parties the parents and the child. As an old Jewish proverb says "more than the calf wishes to suck, the cow wishes to give suckle." This proves the fact that the parent-child relationship involves reciprocity, the parent provides love and material support while the child responds with affection and obedience. Parenting constitutes key process in any, civilization. It is an intentional or deliberate process ensuring familial and societal continuity. In general, parents wish to ensure the well-being of societal offsprings. They want their children to be successful in the different walks of life, to take pride in their heritage, to be respectful towards elders and to live happy and healthy lives both physically and mentally. However, when children are reared in the single parent family or in an abusive or neglectful household, the negative effect on the individual's self-esteem and method of relating to others, obviously manifests itself. Thus, the family is a strong determining factor in the outcome of an individual's success and happiness in life. Over the past two decades or so, a significant literature has developed on the impact of parenting and family structure on child well-being. This literature documents an accumulating body of evidence that children raised in different family contexts display differential patterns of outcomes across a wide range of developmental domains. Single parenting has been found to be associated with an array of adverse outcomes for child. Parental separation has been reported in the literature as being associated with a wide range of adverse effects on children's well-being, as a short-term consequence of the transition and in the form of more enduring effects. Effects reported include adverse impacts on cognitive capacity (Fergusson, Lynskey and Horwood, 1994), schooling (Evans *et al.,* 2001), physical health (Dawson, 1991), mental and emotional health (Chase-Lansdale, *et al.,* 1995), social conduct and behaviour (Morrison and Coiro, 1999), peer relations (Demo and Acock, 1988), criminal offending (Hanson, 1999), cigarette smoking (Ermisch and Francesconi, 2001).

There is a considerable range of functioning within both groups of children from divorced and intact families. Among children whose parents have divorced are many who are functioning quite well, while among children from intact families are many with major adjustment problems. In short, there is no one-to-one relationship between divorce and psychological adjustment problems in children. Children also benefit where a parental separation provides release from an aversive family situation; for example, where the parental relationship is highly conflicted and the children are drawn into the conflict (Booth and Amato, 2001). Further where children may benefit from a parental separation is where a parent exhibits antisocial behaviour, despite all these it remains true that children who are reared by single parent do less well, on average, across a range of measures of well-being. In present study the attempt is made to find out the emotional disturbance as effected by parenting type, sex of the parent and sex of the child. The objectives and hypothesis were as follows:

- To find the impact of parenting type on emotional disturbance of the child. It was hypothesized that variation in parenting type would cause variation in emotional disturbance.
- The second objective of this study was to ascertain the impact of parents' sex on emotional disturbance of the child. It was proposed that the sex of the parent would lay difference in emotional disturbance.
- The third objective of this study was to find out the impact of sex of the child on emotional disturbance of the child. It was hypothesized that the magnitude of emotional disturbance would vary in boys and girls.

Method

Sample

Three hundred-twenty children were taken in consideration and they were arranged according to the requirement of 4×2×2 of factorial design with four type of parenting (Double parenting, single due to divorce and familial clash, single due to job of partner or spouse, single due to death of spouse), sex of the parent (male/female) and sex of child (boy/girl), i.e. 20 participants per cell, i.e. 20 participants per cell. The schematic presentation of experimental design is presented in Table 10.1

Table 10.1: Schematic presentation of experimental design

		A1		A2		A3		A4	
		B		B		B		B	
		B1	B2	B1	B2	B1	B2	B1	B2
	C1	20	20	20	20	20	20	20	20
C									
	C2	20	20	20	20	20	20	20	20

Legends:

A = Types of parenting
Al = Two parent
A2 = One parent due to divorce or familial clash
A3 = One parent due to the job of parent/spouse.
A4 = One parent due to the death of the spouse.

B = Sex of parent   C = Sex of the child
Bl = Male   Cl = Boy
B2 = Female   C2 = Girl

Tools: Emotional Disturbance Scale (EDS), modified version of Dhaundhiyals (1993) and constructed by Shukla and Dhami (2002). It deals with many areas where emotional disturbance can be seen or at least felt. It was, 90 five point items and it used for children as well as for adults. It covers 10 areas of life, where emotional disturbance is seen or felt, They are: Withdrawal from the society, Isolation, Rejection, Day dreaming, Guilt Feeling, Inferiority complex, Conflict, Low confidence, Nervousness, Anxiety.

Procedure: Data collection was made individual and in group and best attempts was made to avoid external distractions.

Results

Obtained data were analyzed by three-way analysis of variance and the findings are presented below in Table 10.2.

Table 10.2: Summary table of analysis of variance showing the impact of types of parenting, sex of the parent and sex of the child on emotional disturbance

Sources of variations	*SS*	*df*	*MS*	*F*
A	5.25	3	1.75	3.36
B	5.58	1	5.58	10.74
AB	17.01	3	5.67	10.91
AC	18.18	3	6.06	11.66
C	1.76	1	1.76	3.38
BC	4.31	1	4.31	8.29
ABC	18.69	3	6.23	11.99
Error Within	158.08	304	.52	

A close perusal of the table indicates that the main effect of type of parenting was significant (F, 3,304 = 3.36 $p < .01$). It was found that the magnitude of emotional disturbance in their children varied with their types of parenting. Mean values pooled across sex of the parents and sex of the child were 169.29, 173.95, 184.21 and 184.70 respectively for double parents, single divorce parents, distant parent and widow or widower. It was noticed that children of widows/widower were highest regarding emotional disturbance as compared to children of single parents and double parents. The main effect of sex of parent was significant (F, 1,304 = 10.74 $p < .01$) and it was seen that children reared by father were less emotionally disturbed (X = 142.11) than the children reared by mother (X = 212.97). The third main effect of the sex of the child was also significant (F, 1,304 = 3.38 $p < .01$). It was resulted that boys were less emotionally disturbed (X = 171.31) than girls (X = 183.76).

The main effect of type of parenting X sex of the parents was significant (F, 3,304 = 10.91 $p < .01$) and it is appeared in Fig. 10.1.

Figure 10.1 reveals that differences in the level of emotional disturbance were highly prominent in distant parents and widower rather

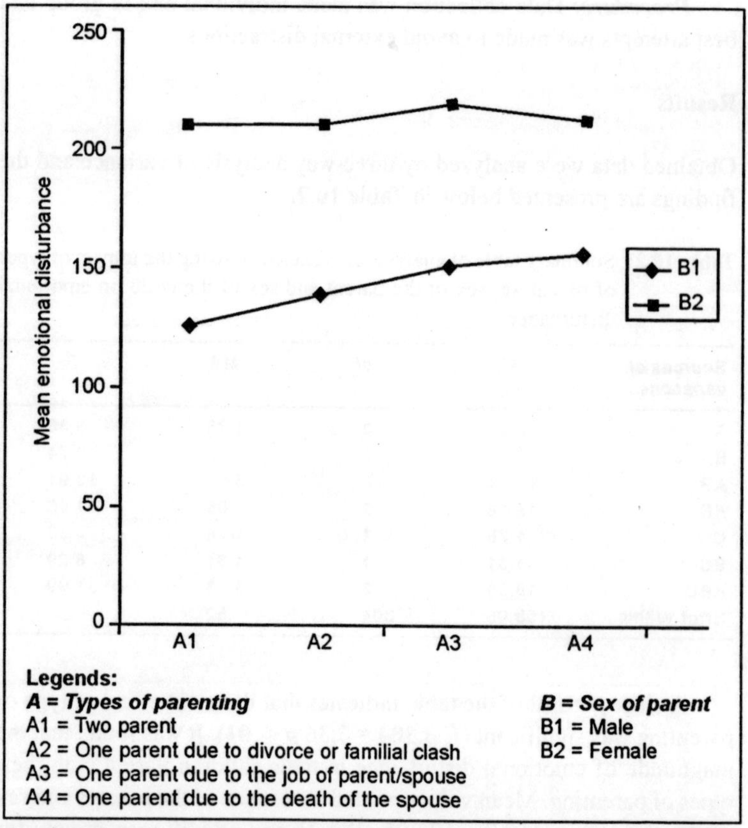

Fig. 10.1: Impact of types of parenting and sex of parents emotional disturbance

than double parents and divorces. The type of parenting X sex of child interaction was also significant (F, 3,304 = 11.66 $P < .01$) and it is appeared in Fig. 10.2.

The sex of the parents X sex of the child interaction was significant (F, 1,304 = 8.29 $p < .01$) and it is appeared in Fig. 10.3.

The three way interaction of type of parenting X sex of the parents X sex of the child was significant (F, 3,304 = 11.99 $p < .01$) and it is appeared in Fig 10.4 and it was found that all variables laid their impact on the dependent variable.

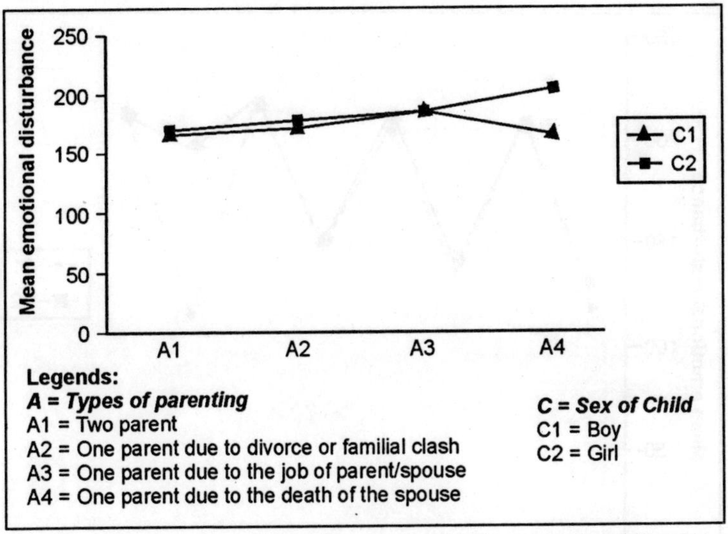

Fig. 10.2: Impact of types of parenting and sex of child on emotional disturbance

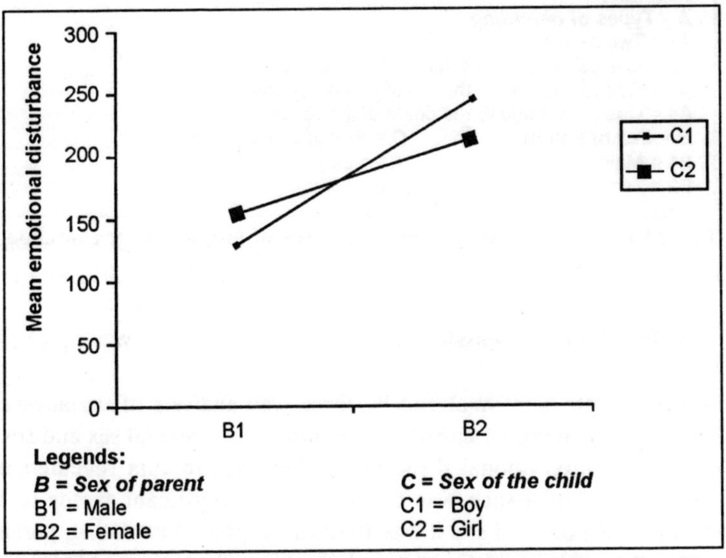

Fig. 10.3: Impact of sex of parents and sex of the child on emotional disturbance

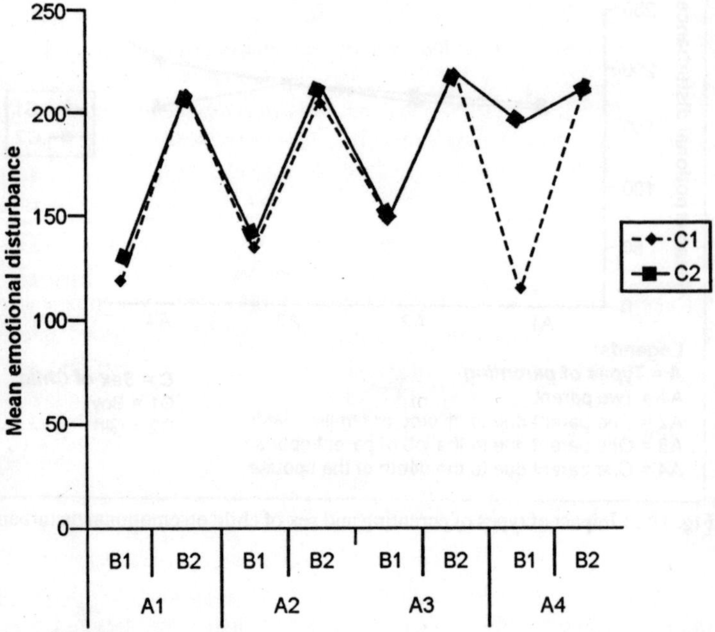

Legends:
A = Types of parenting
A1 = Two parent
A2 = One parent due to divorce or familial clash
A3 = One parent due to the job of parent/spouse.
A4 = One parent due to the death of the spouse.

B = Sex of parent	***C = Sex of Child***
B1 = Male	C1 = Boy
B2 = Female	C2 = Girl

Fig. 10.4: Impact of types of parenting, sex of parents and sex of child on emotional disturbance

Conclusion and Discussion

Obtained data were analysed by three way analysis of variance and interpreted in terms of impact of parenting type, parental sex and sex of the child on emotional disturbance. Findings in sum revealed that emotional disturbance was found to be a significant factor to the development of child and it was affected by types of parenting, parental sex and sex of the child. Emotion is derived from the Latin world "*Emover*" which means the spirit that moves us. That energy is the transmitter and recorder of all feelings, thoughts and action. In other words, emotions are the currents of energy that are within us. It activates our lives, shapes our perceptions and behaviour, which then emanate outward and influence others. The Oxford English Dictionary defines motion as "*any agitation or disturbance of mind, feeling, passion, and any vehement or excited mental state.*" Emotions are primarily motivating forces; they are processes which, arouse, sustain and direct activity. Emotions are reported to influence learning, in addition to influence a range of behaviours such as helping, negotiating, altruism, risk-taking, and compliance (Isen, 1983).

Every emotion has a cognitive component and every thought is influenced by emotional factors. Both emotion and thought are basic attributes, which in the human being are intimately mashed, in a dialectical unity. Differentiated psychological traits of older children and adults clearly state the interaction processes that involve emotion and thought. Feelings reinforce ideas and ideas in true reinforce feelings. When we remember incidents that made us feel angry and sad when we thought about these incidents, our moods are also changed and recalling memories of these events influence the way we felt and our thoughts seems to exert strong effects on our emotions. This relationship works in the other directions as well. Being in a happy mood often causes us to think happy thoughts, while feelings sad tends to bring negative memories and images to mind. In short, these appear to be important links between emotion and cognition—between the way we feel and the way we think. Most researchers on the relationship between emotion and cognition indicate that: Our moods, or emotional states, strongly influence our perception of ambiguous stimuli. In general, we perceive and evaluate these stimuli more favourably when we arc in good mood then when we are in a negative one. Positive and negative moods exert a strong influence on memory. In general, information consistent with our current mood is easier to remember. Our current moods often influence the process of decision-making. Would any one be more willing to adopt relatively risky course of action when in a good mood or when in a bad mood? Informal observation suggests; when in a good mood. The emotions or feelings we experience are strongly determined by the interpretation or cognitive labels we select. According to Dunn (1964) "a child is emotionally disturbed when his relations to life-situations are so personally unrewarding and so inappropriate as to be unacceptable to his peers and adults". Emotionally disturbed children have also been characterized as having unusual difficulty in maintaining satisfactory inter-personal relationship (Magary and Eichorn, 1964). Telford and Sawrey (1967) have mentioned that emotionally disturbed children are children with emotional problems severe enough to prevent them from making necessary adjustments for effective functioning in the culture.

Telford and Sawrey (1967) mentioned that when socially or personally unsatisfactory modes of behaviour are acquired in the course of living and the manner of acquisition is relatively easy to discern, we generally refer to this as '*social maladjustment*'. While, when the reinforcements are subtle and the behaviour not obviously adaptive, the individual is said to be emotionally disturbed. Thus, emotional disturbance is a psycho-emotional state of withdrawal, isolation, fear, anxiety and pessimism. In this way we can say that emotional disturbance is the key of behavioural disturbance and it can be seen in many sorts of behaviour like withdrawal, guilt, fear, and pessimism, etc. Parenting is the way that the parents employ in upbringing their children. In case of single parenting either due to divorce or death of spouse, the income declines, place mother headed family at risk of material and economic deprivation this in turn leads to compromised parenting effecting emotional well-being of the child. Present study is consistent with other studies. Amato (1993) outlined a range of ways in which the economic position of a single parent family might exert-effects on child well-being. Financial hardship may negatively affect children's nutrition and health; it reduces parental investment in books, educational toys, computers, private lessons; it constrains choice of residential location, which means that the family may have to live in a neighbourhoods where school programmes are poorly financed, services are inadequate and crime rates are high; children are more likely in such neighbourhoods to associate with delinquent peers. As Amato (1993) notes, the absence of one parent means a deficit in terms of parental time available to do the work of parenting and all the other work in the household, which further restricts the available time for parenting and create stress. Increased parenting risk has been repeated identified as a risk factor for higher level of child disruptive behaviour problems (Barry, Dunlop, Cottoen, Lackman and Wells, 2005; Podolski and Nigg, 2001); as well as maladaptive parenting practices The stress associated with economic hardship can have negative impacts on parental mental health, which can in turn impair the quality of parenting. Hetherington *et al.* (1978) showed not only that separation effect mental health of custodial mothers, in the form of higher rates of anxiety, depression, anger and self-doubt, but also that this in turn impacted on their parenting, exemplified by less affectionate, less communicative, more punitive and more inconsistent disciplinary interactions with their children. Such suboptimal parenting behaviours, in turn, have adverse consequences for children's well-being through which single parenting exerts effects on children's well-being. The separation can take a toll quality of parenting. Block *et al.* (1986) noted that divorced mothers describe themselves in terms indicating low self-esteem and that a failed or failing marriage affects mothers more strongly than father. So Parent should balance their family life or modify their parenting behaviour to increase positive outcomes with their children.

References

Amato, Paul, R. (1993) "Children's adjustment to divorce: Theories, hypotheses, and empirical support", *Journal of Marriage and the Family*, 55:23-38.

Block, J.H., Block, J.Q., Gjerda, P.F. (1986). The personality of children prior to divorce. A prospective study. *Child Development,* 57, 827-840.

Booth, Alan and Paul R. Amato (2001) "Parental predivorce relations and offspring postdivorce well-being". *Journal of Marriage and Family,* 63:197-212. (1): 109-126. *Journal of Marriage and Family*, 63: 197-212.es, 76(3): 905-936.

Barry, T.D., Dunlap, S.T., Cotten, S.J., Lochman, J.E., and Wells, K.C. (2005). The influence of maternal stress and distress on disruptive behaviour problems in boys. *Journal of the American Academy of Child and Adolescent Psychiatry*, 44, 265-273.

Chase-Lansdale, P. Lindsay, Andrew J. Cherlin and Kathleen E. Kiernan (1995). "The long-term effects of parental divorce on the mental health of young adults: A developmental perspective". *Child Development*, 66: 1614-1634.

Demo, David, H. and Alan, C. Acock (1988). "The impact of divorce on children" *Journal of Marriage and the Family,* 50(3):619-648.

Dawson, Deborah A. (1991) "Family structure and children's health and well-being: Data from the 1988 National Health Interview Survey on Child Health". *Journal of Marriage and the Family,* 53:573-584.

Dunn, L.M. (1964), *Exceptional Children in the School.* Holt, Reinehart and Winston, New York, p. 242.

Evans, M.D.R., Kelley, J. and Wanner, R.A. (2001). Educational attainment of the children of divorce: Australia, 1940-90. *Journal of Sociology*, 37(3): 275-297.

Ermisch, John F. and Marco Francesconi (2001) "Family structure and children's achievements", *Journal of Population Economics*, 14: 249-270.

Fergusson, David M., Michael T. Lynskey and L. John Horwood (1994), "The effects of parental separation, the timing of separation and gender on children's performance on cognitive tests", *Journal of Child Psychology and Psychiatry*, 35(6): 1077-1092.

Hanson, Thomas L. (1999). 'Does parental conflict explain why divorce is negatively associated with child welfare?" *Social Forces*, 77(4):1283-1315.

Hetherington, E.M., Cox, M., and Cox, R. (1978). The aftermath of divorce. In J.J. H. Stevens and M. Matthews (Eds.), *Mother-child, father-child relations*. Washington, DC: National Association for the Education of Young Children.

Isen, A.M. (1987). Positive affect, cognitive processes and social behaviour, Advances in *Experimental Social Psychology.* 20, 203-253. DC: National Association for the Education of Young Children.

Magary, J.F. and J.R. Elichoon (1964). *The Exceptional Child: A Book of Reading*, Holt, Rinechart & Winston, New York.

Morrison, Donna Ruane and Mary J. Coiro (1999). "Parental conflict and marital disruption: Do children benefit when high-conflict marriages are dissolved?" *Journa/of Marriage and the Family*, 61:626-637.

Podolski, C., and Nigg, J.T. (2001). Parent stress and coping in relation to child ADHD severity and associated child disruptive behaviour problems. *Journal of Clinical Child Psychology*, 30, 503-513.

Telford, C.W. and J.M. Sawney (1967). *The Exceptional Individual: Psychological and Educational Aspects.* Prentice-Hall, Englewood Cliffs, New Jersey.

11
Parenting, Ecological Conditions and Psychological Complications in Runaway Children and Adolescents

Pragya Tripathi and *Anubhuti Dubey*

Researches on the street children pointed that the influence of family factors such as abuse, parent-child conflict, and child stress on an adolescent's decision to leave home. This paper offers evidence for the ecological conditions, role of parenting and psychological complications of runaway children. Using the survey method of 200 participants aged between 6-19 years living on streets, different area of railway stations, near temples and *durgahs*, in markets, under bridges, near bus deports and stops of Gorakhpur district, a main business city of eastern Uttar Pradesh as a data collection. Content analysis used for the analysis of data. Findings of the studies revealed that teenage participants, males who belong to the uneducated and rural area were easily affected by the external environment (Curiosity, fun and friendship) and leave their home in compared to the urban and educated children and females. In the other side specific reasons were also emerges like as substance abuse, sexual abuse, lacking control on anger, lacking control on coping skills, curiosity, parental negligence, parental beating, drinking of guardian, broken homes, loss of parents, poverty and domestic violence are the major reasons for run away from home. The factors emerging can be useful for identifying high-risk families with children in pre-adolescent age and hence for prevention and rehabilitation.

The poverty rate in India is very high. India is thought to be a poor developing country although its economy is growing very rapidly. However, the number of running away children living in both rural and urban areas is also rising alarmingly. Earlier running away children were thought to the problem associated with physical or sexual abuse, family problems, substance abuse, effect of parenting, separation or divorce, problem with friends or at school. But now researchers are gradually becoming aware of the gravity of the risk that this problem may have long-term repercussions that running away children may indulge in anti-social activities and suffer with a number of psychosocial problems and psychopathology, like abusive behaviour, addiction, maladjustment, etc. Nevertheless, it is also very difficult to count the number of street children living in India because of their floating (moving often) nature, but it is estimated that more than 400,000 street children in India exist.

The most common reasons for running away found so far are beating by parents/relatives, followed by a desire for economic independence. Other reasons were maltreatment by step parent/s, being both parents died, arguments with parents etc. The factors emerging can be useful for identifying high-risk families with children in pre-adolescent age and hence for prevention and rehabilitation. Mathur (2009) conducted a study on 200 street children of Jaipur city and had made the profiles of their background, incidence of migration, familial contacts, clothing and food, work experiences, play and entertainment, personal habits, peer interaction, attitudes towards self, family and society; and aspirations and expectations. She found that majority of street children were boys (71%) and in 8–12 years age group. Incidence of migration was observed and 70.5 per cent of these children lived with their families. Gambling, watching films and television; smoking and drinking, and taking drugs were common modes of entertainment and relaxation for these children. Aptekar (1994) reviewed the literature on street children and pointed out the reasons why there are street children in certain cultures and not in others and reported that the reasons for their existence are related to poverty, abuse, and modernizing factors.

Street children are defined and distinguished from working and refugee children. Kombarakaran (2004) conducted a research on street children of Bombay and found that children face several challenges in their search for food, safety, employment, shelter and medical care. They commonly depend on their peers, non-governmental agencies, and their own resourcefulness to survive on the streets. While the majorities use positive mechanisms to cope with their daily stresses, some children also employ maladaptive strategies such as using alcohol, drugs, and visiting prostitutes. Agencies that work with street children may need to recognize these challenges and strengths to provide needed services to improve their condition.

Mainly because of family conflict, they come to live on the streets and take on the full responsibilities of caring for themselves, including working to provide for and protecting themselves. Tiwart, Gulati, Sethi, and Mehra (2002) reported that majority of children (55%) had left home between 10-12 year of age. They were more from "Joint" families. A higher percentage had literate fathers. A higher percentage had no parent earning and a higher proportion of "Not Runaways" had only the mother earning. Presence of a step parent, guardian other than the parents and intra-familial physical abuse were found associated with "Runaway".

Ecological conditions and family factors are important issues related to street children (Plan and Hotaling, 1995). "Research into the etiology of running away has long provided evidence for the influence of family factors such as abuse, parent-child conflict, and child stress on an adolescent's decision to leave home. Possibility that running away may be deeply entrenched in patterns of family interaction those extend across generations." Melissa, Meade and Slesnick (2002), argued that in many circumstances, requiring parental consent may not be in the youth's best interest and may preclude his or her participation in treatment and research programmes. Safyer *et al*. (2004) had compared between adolescents' and parents' reports of family functioning demonstrated significant discrepancies and found that few parents assumed any responsibility for the runaway behaviour or change efforts. More adolescents blamed themselves or cited difficulties in parent-child relationships and offered ideas that entailed altering their attitudes and behaviours or family relationships.

Running away home of children's is a growing global problem and to kept in mind that the first legislation on juvenile justice in India come in 1850 with the Apprentice Act which required that children between the ages of 8-10 convicted in courts to be provided vocational training as part of their rehabilitation problems. Section 29 of the Act provides constituting five member district level quasi-Judicial bodies "Child Welfare Committee". The committee shall have the final authority to dispose of cases for the care protection, treatment, development and rehabilitation of the children.

The reasons why street children live on the street vary. However, there is one explanation that holds true for both developed and developing countries is poverty. Most street children go onto the streets to look for a better way of life. A study was conducted on the Iranian children byVameghi, Sajjadi, Rafiey, and Rashidian (2010) found the relationship between poverty and becoming street child. The high prevalence of economic factors are one of the pertinent reasons for becoming street child.

The following are some of the reasons, both social and psychological, which are found responsible for running away of children from their homes—

Poverty and Illiteracy: They lack basic resources to sustain a healthy living. They usually have no financial means to buy decent clothing (which may be necessary in cold places), and no money to buy food, which is crucial for their development. Because of the costs of services most street children cannot afford to go to school. Even where schools are free, many children cannot afford to buy uniforms, shoes and books. Street children live in places where they are not adequately protected from the environment. They rarely have access to facilities that they need for hygiene and sanitation, such as toilets and clean and safe water supply. They are, therefore, more vulnerable to health problems resulting from poor sanitation.

To Earn Money and Support Families: Street children work on the streets to earn money for themselves. Some children need to work to support their families. Some children may have been denied a chance to go to school or have dropped out of school and have nothing to do. They can earn money by begging, carrying or bearing, car washing, drug trafficking, juggling, performing music, running errands, scavenging, sex work, shoe shining or vending.

To find Shelter: In overcrowded households, children may decide to leave home to make room for younger siblings and elderly family members. Others are on the streets because they do not have an alternative. They may have become separated from their families during civil unrest or their Parents/caretakers may have died from illnesses such as AIDS or killed during armed conflict. Other children may have nowhere else to go when they are released from institutions such as a jail or a detention centre.

To Escape from Family Problems including Rejection: Many children feel that living on the streets is better than coping with problems in their homes. These problems can include conflicts with parents, physical or sexual abuse or neglect (e.g. an abandoned disabled child). Some children are forced to leave home by their families because the family does not approve of a child's behaviour or its consequences, e.g. pregnancy, homosexuality or substance use.

To Escape from Work Demands in the Home: In many cultures, children are expected to participate in routine family tasks. At times the demands on children may be more than they can take. This leads to the child feeling that he or she is a slave or a servant. Such children leave home in search of freedom from adult demands.

To Escape from a Children's Institution: Street children may feel that children's homes are 'like prisons'. They cannot adjust to rules after experiencing the freedom of the streets. At times the personnel in these institutions may abuse children.

Psychological and Behavioural Problems

Previous research has indicated that homeless children exhibit high rates of behavioural and emotional problems and come from families characterized by conflict and rejection. Further, some evidence exists to show that family variables may relate to adolescent distress differently for homeless males and females. The study of homeless children by Dadds, Baraddock, Cures, Elliot, and Kelly (1993) reported that the highest incidence of all behavioural and emotional problems, parental marital discord, overprotection, and the lowest levels of parental care and acceptance. Sex effects were not evident in reported levels of personal or family problems. However, substantially more variance in the adolescent's level of behavioural and emotional disturbance was predictable from family measures for females than males.

Khurana, Sharma, Jena, Saha, and Ingle (2004) reported that 20.7 per cent of children were found to have high hopelessness and 8 per cent of children had depression. Two per cent of children revealed that they had attempted suicide at any point of time in life. Among children with high hopelessness, 3.2 per cent had ever attempted suicide. 8.3 per cent of the depressed children gave history of suicidal attempts. 38 per cent of children gave history of physical abuse, 14.6 per cent of sexual abuse and a large number reported substance abuse. 69.33 per cent were found to have behavioural problems (i.e. scored above the recommended cut off score of 9). 81 per cent of children had antisocial behaviour, 7.8 per cent were neurotic and 10.5 per cent remained undifferentiated and concluded that runaway adolescents suffer from a wide array of mental health problems and there is a need for a broad based psychosocial intervention programme.

Most of the time street children encounter the psychological problems in their daily life such as—

A Stressful Past: Many situations and events that pushed these children onto the street in the first place (like natural disasters, man-made disasters, exploitation and conflicts) may have a lasting impact on their well-being. For example, the family conflict that pushed the child onto the streets continues to deprive the child of emotional and material support for years afterwards. When the child has his or her own baby, neither the new parent nor the baby will have the benefit of the previous generation's support.

A Transitory Lifestyle: Street children in some large cities move frequently from district to district or between cities. Sometimes they do this by choice, but at other times they are forced to move to hide from the police, welfare authorities, gangs, and drug syndicates. This type of lifestyle leads to problems of social isolation and loneliness and difficulties in developing emotional attachments to special individuals.

Mental Health: The stresses that street children experience make them vulnerable to emotional problems, psychiatric disorders and learning difficulties. They do not receive adequate care for these conditions.

Substance Use: Many street children are involved in harmful use of psychoactive substances. This can lead to overdose, increase the chance of accidents, violence, unwanted pregnancy and unprotected sex. Over time, the continued use of substances can lead to complications such as brain and liver damage.

Discrimination and Lack of Accessible Resources: When the community makes plans, it does not take into consideration the plight of street children. Street children tend to be excluded from participating in most of the activities and facilities of other children. This is one reason why street children often do not have access to medical, educational, recreational and vocational resources. They face problems such as lack of vaccinations, poor health, illiteracy and they cannot acquire skills needed for finding jobs.

Violent Environment: The street is an unprotected environment and street children are exploited frequently. In some places, street children may even face the possibility of physical injuries or death from violence. Common sources of violence are: the police, gangs, and drug syndicates, those who operate commercial sex businesses, death squads, other street children, families and sexual partners.

Stigmatization: Society usually perceives street children as difficult children who are out there to cause trouble. In general, the public thinks that street children are uncontrollable and violent, have substance use problems, have no morals, have lost all the ability to feel emotions such as love and that they turn into terrorists and revolutionaries. They tend to be unsympathetic to the street children's plight. This negative attitude may be a result of the society's inability to care for its people.

Lack of Adequate Nutrition: Even though some street children can usually get enough to eat, they do not have nutritious diets. This leads to malnutrition, anaemia and vitamin deficiencies.

Injuries: Injuries may be caused intentionally (including injuring self while intoxicated or when depressed) and unintentionally, e.g. due to use of tools which have been designed for adults. The rate of injuries is usually higher for male than for female street children.

Sexual and Reproductive Health Problems: Sexual and reproductive health problems affect both girls and boys. However, street girls are more vulnerable to physical and sexual abuse and exploitation. Common sexual and reproductive health problems include sexually transmitted diseases, HIV/AIDS, unwanted pregnancies and unsafe abortions. Pregnant street girls do not receive adequate antenatal care.

Common Diseases: Street children experience many common diseases such as tuberculosis, skin diseases, dental problems and parasitic diseases which can be prevented easily if these children have enough resources and their basic needs are met.

The studies ıeviewed are mainly focused on epidemiologic properties, etiological factors and outcomes of problems of street children.

Some Survey Reports on Street Children

For child protection and rights in India child line was founded by Ms. Jeroo Billirnornia, who was then a professor of the Tata institute of Social Sciences (TISS), member initiated in June 1996 as an experimental project of the Department of Family and Child Welfare of TISS, child line come long way today to becoming a nationwide emergency helpline for children in distress.

The survey of child line (2002-2003) indicated that child line counselled (20%) contacted in children about physical or sexual abuse sometimes both. Over 22,000 of children counselled (20%) contacted us about physical or sexual abuse and sometimes both. Nearly, 21,000 of children counselled (18%) contacted about bullying more than 16,000 children counselled (13%) contacted is about family problems. Children also contacted us about substance abuse, running away, bereavement the effect of parents, separation or divorce, pregnancy worries about sex or suicide and problems with friends or at school.

UNICEF (2003) estimated that there were at least 100 million street children in the world, but though this figure is commonly found it is not seen to be based on any actual studies or surveys. UNICEF (1994) estimated that there were 11 million street children in India. This number is said to be a drastic under-estimation. The Indian embassy estimated 314,700 street children in cities like Bombay, Calcutta, Madras and

Kanpur, Bangalore and Hyderabad and around 100,000 street children in Delhi.

The MWCD (2007) report on child abuse, found 65.9 per cent of the street children lived with their families. Out of these children, 51.84 per cent slept on the side-walks, 17.48 per cent slept in shelters and 30.67 per cent slept in other locations such as under flyovers and bridges, railway platforms, bus stops, parks, market places, etc. 66.8 per cent of children reported being physically abused by family members and others. To download the full report please visits the Abuse and Violence section.

Objective of Present Study

The present study is planned to track the psychological, social and environmental factors associated with the running away from home by Children of eastern part of Utter Pradesh. Present study is the further step in this area (child protection and rights) because this includes the concept of parenting negligence, socio-economic status, fun and friendship, illiteracy, substance abuse, family environment, social and psychological factors associated to it. The main focus of the study will be to create a psychosocial profile of runaway and street children.

Sample: Sample consisted of 200 participants (male and female) aged between 6 to 19 years living on streets, different area of railway stations, near temples and *durgahs*, in markets, under bridges, near bus deports and stops of Gorakhpur district, a main business city of eastern Uttar Pradesh. All the participants were at the age of 6 to 18 years.

Materials: For assessing the reasons of runaway from home we have conducted an open-ended interview and survey method as a tool of research.

Procedure: The data collected from the participants with the help of survey method and open-ended interview of street children. The children living on streets, different area of railway station, near temples and durgahs, in markets, under bridges, near bus deports and stops of Gorakhpur district. Rapport was established to the children and some incentives were also given to the children after data collection.

Results and Discussion

Some of the earlier studies indicated that most of the street children in India are over 6 years, and majority are over 8 years of age. But our research revealed that there is a high incidence of running away occurs in between 13 to 18 years. This is the stage of teenage in which the children feel high level of emotionality and lack of coping strategies. The present study illustrated that the majority of street children are boys with little or no education. Lesser number of girls is on streets as they are much less likely to break family ties and live alone; even though facing all types of abuse including physical and sexual abuse. Another possible explanation is that boys may leave home more because of the conflict-filled dynamics that sometimes exist between a stepfather and male step children that do not exist with female step children.

Table 11.1: Demographic Details of Runaway Children

Demographic Details		*Frequency*	%
Age	9 to 11 years	36	18
	11 to 13 years	62	31
	13 to 18 years	102	51
Gender	Male	180	90
	Female	20	10
Occupation of children	Student	52	26
	Labourer	148	74
Religion	Hindu	143	71.5
	Muslim	57	28.5
Education of parents	Educated	28	14
	Uneducated	132	66
Ecological settings	Rural	130	65
	Urban	70	35

A study of street children in Bombay (1989) found that 54.5 per cent had never been enrolled in school and 66 per cent of the children were illiterate. Another study of street children in Bombay (2004) revealed that circumstances were largely the same: 60 per cent of the children had never attended school and approximately two-thirds were illiterate. There is also a large number of participants were labourer not students and most of the parents were also uneducated. Being a poor and uneducated parents, parents never motivates their children for studies even they provokes their children for work. Despite the fact that some children's accepts that they were not interested in studies and when their parents pressurize they left home. Ecological settings indicating that there were large number of street children comes from rural area because of that the children's of rural area are more curious about the cities and urban sectors.

This study illustrated the trend found by most researchers that most children leave their families to live on the street because of the family problems. Family problems include such things as death of a parent, alcoholism of father, strained relationships with step parents, parent separation, abuse, and family violence. Most children who leave home to

Table 11.2: Reasons for runaway from home

Major Themes	*Sub-themes*	*Frequency*	*Exemplars*
Child related Variables	Substances abuse	10	I like to drink alcohol and tobacco.
	Sexual abuse	11	My uncle or my relative sexually assaults me.
	Lacking control on impulses	16	I cannot control my impulses.
	Lacking control on anger	18	I cannot control my aggression.
	Lack in coping skills	12	I am not satisfied with my family and life.
	Curiosity	7	I like to live in big city.
Parental factors	Parental negligence	37	My parents never care of me.
	Parental beating	18	My father always beats me without any mistake of me.
	Drinking of father and guardian	32	My father always beats and abuses me after taking alcohol.
	broken homes	15	My step mother is not good.
	Loss of parents	14	I leave home after death of my mother because my father is not good.
	Domestic violence	13	My father abuses me and beats me.
Contextual factors		6	
Pressure of early marriage on girls		8	My parents want to marry me in early age of 9 years.
extreme poverty		28	
Pressure of social gangs		5	I like the company of my friends more than my family.

live on the streets come from slums or low cost housing, both which is areas of high illiteracy, drug use, and unemployment. Children usually transfer their lives to the streets through a gradual process; they may at first only stay on the street a night or two. Gradually they will spend more time away from home until they do not return. Once on the streets, children sometimes find that their living conditions and physical and mental health is better than at home; however, this fact speaks to the poor conditions of their homes rather than good conditions in the street. Street conditions are far from child-friendly. Once they leave home, many street children move around often because of the fear that their relatives will find them and force them to return home.

The reason why children leaving their home? There are lots of child related factors associated with like as many children said that "I like to drink alcohol and chewing tobacco". Our findings of research is also indicating that some children's involved in substance abuse (Alcohol, marijuana, plus, drugs and other substances) while some children's complaining of sexual abuse by their relatives and family members while there are high rate of female participants in the case of sexual abuse. Early identification of and intervention for runaway youth can decrease the risk of harm that may result from sexual assault while the teen is away from home (Saewyc and Edinburgh, 2010). Many girls participant admits that "My uncle or my relatives sexually assaults me". So she run away from home because of that they sexually abused, touched or sexually assaulted by their family members and relatives and sometimes due to pressure of early or mismatches marriage. Even some children's said that " I cannot control my anger and impulses", as we have already discussed that this is the age when children feels high level of emotionality, so many times they fails to coping and anger management that is why they use to run away from home.

Some factors are associated with their Receiving health care after a sexual assault is important to help prevent or reduce the negative consequences of such trauma (Edinburgh, Saewyc, and Levitt, 2008; Adams *et al.*, 2007). In most instances, the teen's parents and family, Parental negligence and parental beating is one of them like the statement (given by street children), "*My parents never cares of me*", is showing the parental negligence of the parents. Parental negligence also may be four type medical neglect, supervisory neglect, emotional neglect and complete abandonment, many children's comes from poor and labourer family where medical neglect and supervisory neglect is a very common issue.

Table 11.2 indicated that approximately 64.5 per cent children's runaway due to their parental factors and its play an important role in runaway the case of runaway children. Children in single-parent families may be at higher risk of physical abuse and neglect, although the effects of poverty, stress, social isolation, and lack of support are all contributing factors. Risk is reduced for the children of single mothers when the children have a relationship with their fathers. In two-parent families, the risk of maltreatment is greater if marital conflict or domestic violence is also present. Domestic violence is also a causal factor of runaway children's like many children's complaint that "My father beats me always without my mistake". Studies suggested that children who have been neglected are prone to internalizing problems such as low self-esteem, depression, social withdrawal, apathy, passivity and helplessness. They are often delayed in their cognitive and language development and have poor communication skills. They have difficulty with interpersonal relationships.

Poverty is also a prime cause of the street children. Children from well-off families do not need to work, or beg. They live in houses, eat well, go to school, and are likely to be healthy and emotionally secure. Families living in areas challenged by poverty and unemployment, particularly when coupled with the individual and family factors described above, are at higher risk of child abuse and neglect. The degree of social support available to parents, along with community attitudes about raising children and using punishment, can also contribute to the risk of child maltreatment. Many children lost their home or misguide during in search of work. Our Findings of Research are also showing that poverty is also a prime cause of street children. Beyond this there are other reasons of leaving home like pressure of marriage and peer pressure.

Conclusion

The findings of the present study revealed that teenage males who belong to the uneducated and rural area were easily affected by the external environment (Curiosity, fun and friendship) and leave their home in compared to the urban and educated children and females. In the other side specific reasons were also emerged like as substance abuse, sexual abuse, lacking control on anger, lacking control on coping skills, curiosity, parental negligence, parental beating, drinking of guardian, broken homes, loss of parents, poverty and domestic violence are the major reasons for run away from home.

References

Adams, J.A., Kaplan, R.A., Starling, S.P., Mehta, N.H., Finkel, M.A., Botash, A.S., Kellogg, N.D., and Shapiro, R.A. (2007). Guidelines for medical care of children who may have been sexually abused. *Journal of Pediatric and Adolescent Gynecology,* 20, 163-172.

Aptekar, L. (1994). Street Children in the Developing World: A Review of Their Condition. *Cross-Cultural Research,* Vol. 28(3), 195-224.

Catherine Panter-Brick. (2002). Street Children, Human Rights, and Public Health: A Critique and Future Directions. *Annual Review of Anthropology*, Vol. 31, 147-171.

Edinburgh, L., Saewyc, E.M., Levitt, C. (2008). Caring for young sexual abuse victims in a hospital-based children's advocacy center. *Child Abuse and Neglect: The International Journal,* Vol. 32, 1119-1126.

Francis, A. Kombarakaran (2004). Street children of Bombay: their stresses and strategies of coping. *Children and Youth Services Review,* Pages 853-871.

Khurana, S., Sharma, N., Shivanandan, J., Saha, R, Ingle, G.K. (2004); Mental health status of runaway adolescents. *The Indian Journal of Pediatrics,* Volume 71(5), pp. 405-409.

Mathur, M. and Monika, M. (2009). Incidence, type and intensity of abuse in street children in India. *Child Abuse and Neglect*: 33907-913.doi:10.1016/ i.chiabu.2009.01.003.

Mark R. Dadds., David Baraddock., Simone Cures., Amanda., Amanda Elliot., Adrain Kelly *M. Clin. Psych. Community Mental Health Journal.* Volume 29(5), pp. 413-422.

Melissa A. Meade and Natasha Slesnick, (2002), Ethical Considerations for Research and Treatment with Runaway and Homeless Adolescents. *The Journal of Psychology: Interdisciplinary and Applied*, DOI:10.1080/ 00223980209604171, 449-463.

Mathur, M. (2009). A Socio-economic Profile. *Psychology Developing Societies*, (21), 299-325.

Patel, Sheela (October 1990). "Street children, hotel boys and children of payment dwellers and construction workers in Bombay—how they meet their daily needs."*Environment and Urbanization*: 9-26.doi.10.1177/ 095624789000200203.

Peggy S. Plass, Gerald T. Hotaling. (1995), The intergenerational transmission of running away: Childhood experiences of the parents of runaways. *Journal of Youth and Adolescence*. Volume 24(3), 335-348.

Singh, A. and Puroht, B. (2011). Street Children as a Public Health Fiasco. *Peace Review* (23) 102-109.doi:1080/10402659.2011.548270.

Swart J Malunde. (1990). The Street Children of Hillbrow. Johannesburg, *Witwatersrand University Press* (ISBN 1-86814-1225).

Tiwart, P.A., Gulati, N., Sethi, G.R. and Mehra, M. (2002). Why do some boys run away from home? *The Indian Journal of Pediatrics*, Volume 69(5), 397-399.

Vameghi, M., Sajjadi, H., Rafiey, H., Rashidian, A. (2010). Systematic Review of Studies on Street children in Iran in recent Decade: Poverty, a Risk Factor for Becoming A Street Child. *Social Welfare. 9* (35): 337-378.

12

Emotional Disturbance as Affected by Residential Locale, Gender and Family Type

A Developmental Analysis

Pooja M. Galiakoti and *Aradhana Shukla*

Children with Emotional Disturbance (ED) are one of the most under identified and untreated child clinical subpopulations (Wagner, 1995; Forness and Kavale, 2001; President's New Freedom Commission, 2003). As indicated in the Surgeon General's report on mental health (U.S. Department of Health and Human Services, 2000), one in five children display a diagnosable mental disorder each year and approximately 5 per cent have an ED that significantly impacts their daily functioning at home and school. Similarly, children with ED represent about 5 per cent of youth diagnosed with mental disorders and about 1 per cent of those children diagnosed with ED are treated (Oswald and Coutinho, 1995; Walwarth, Nickerson, Crowel, and Leaf, 1998). Research has found that the number of students classified as ED varies by state and school district. For example, in a study representing over 14,000 school districts, Coutinho and Oswald (2005) found that state and local variations in ED classification are due, in part, to the child's gender with males overrepresented as ED (e.g., male : female odds ratios ranged from approximately 2 to 6 for ED in comparison to 1.7 to 2.7 for LD students). It is unknown whether gender differences are due to a higher prevalence rate of ED among males and/or under diagnosis of ED among females. The identification of children with ED is hindered by vague diagnostic/eligibility criteria which impacts access, to effective school based interventions (Forness and Kavale, 2001; Reddy, 2001). Scholars have attributed the identification problem, in part, to the Individual Disability

Education Act definition (IDEA, 1997, 2005). According to IDEA, ED is one of 12 disability categories that is defined as "a condition exhibiting one or more of the following characteristics over a long period of time and to a marked degree which adversely affects school performance: (a) an inability to learn which cannot be explained by intellectual, sensory, or health factors, (b) an inability to build or maintain satisfactory interpersonal relationships with peers and teachers, (c) inappropriate types of behaviour or feelings under normal circumstances, (d) a general pervasive mood of unhappiness or depression, (e) a tendency to develop physical symptoms or fears associated with personal or school problems", (IDEA, 1997, 2005). The five ED criteria in IDEA are not supported by research on the subtypes of children with emotional and behavioural disorders (Schroeder and Gordon, 2002). In addition, there is a clause requiring "adverse educational performance" (e.g., poor grades) which may be interpreted by some professionals to exclude children who have "marginal grades" (e.g., D's), but who exhibit social and behavioural difficulties at school. Also, IDEA includes an exclusionary criterion of "social maladjustment" which is not fully defined and thus may misled some professionals to exclude children diagnosed with conduct disorder. Research has found that conduct disorders often co-occur 'with attention deficit hyperactivity disorder' (ADHD), reading disabilities, depressive disorders, and anxiety disorders (Hinshaw, Lahey, and Hart, 1993; Reddy and DeThomas, in press). Nelson (1992) asserted that the field does not have evidence to differentiate between conduct disorders and other emotional and behavioural disorders. In fact, students with ED who exhibit disruptive behaviour or symptoms of conduct disorder constitute the largest subgroup of youth placed in ED classrooms (Greenbaum *et al.*, 1996; U.S. Department of Health and Human Services, 2000; Wagner, 1995). Historically, there has been a reliance on restrictive educational and out-of-home placements (e.g., residential care) for children with ED. However, with the advent of managed care, the use of restrictive placements has decreased, and as a result, schools and community agencies have increasingly become the "system of care" for children with ED (Reddy and Savin, 2000). Treatment outcomes (e.g., reduced aggressive and disruptive. behaviours) acquired in restrictive placements are often temporary and limited in scope (e.g., behavioural control and containment).

Many restrictive placements also do not successfully transition children back into their homes, schools, and neighbourhoods (Epstein, Kutash, and Duchnowski, 1998; Hansen, Litzelman, March, and

Miispaw, 2004). Despite national initiatives (e.g., President's New Freedom *Commission,* 2003), parents and schools struggle to educate and treat children with ED (U.S. OSEP, 2001). Described by some as "mad, bad, sad, and can't add" (Friedman and Kutash, 1986), these children are prone to academic failure, family/peer rejection, restricted educational placements, and in some cases out-of-home placements and hospitalizations. As Osher, Osher, and Smith (1994) stated, educating children with ED "is one of the most stressful, complex, and difficult challenges facing public education today, and perhaps one of our greatest failures" (p. 7). Research has shown that children with ED have lower grades than other disability groups, significant academic and language deficits, and high grade retention and absenteeism rates (Armstrong, Derick, and Greenbaum, 2003). Research has also shown that children with ED are more likely to drop out of school, receive school suspensions and expulsions, fail one or more courses, not graduate, and have difficulties socially integrating at school than other disability groups (Duchnowski, 1994; U.S. OSEP, 2001; Wagner, 1995). Numerous personal, diagnostic, and organizational barriers interfere with treatment success for children with ED in school and home (Reddy, 2001). For example, youngsters with ED represent a complex mix of emotional, behaviour, educational, and medical/neurological difficulties that make the diagnostic, teaching, and learning process difficult. School and family treatments are further complicated by high rates of family psychopathology, inadequate parenting skills, and limited support systems and resources. In addition, lack of knowledge of services and programmes offered by other agencies (e.g., schools, social service, and juvenile justice), differential use of terminology between agencies, and ineffective interagency collaboration often interfere with treatments. Limited or poor school preserves and in-service training on internalizing and externalizing symptoms in the classroom and behavioural techniques (e.g. use of aversive techniques, physical restraints, positive behavioural techniques) are also found. Other barriers may include, limited placement options (e.g. access to intermediate levels of care) and support services (e.g. respite for parents and teachers) (Ready, 2001). Despite these barriers, innovations in school-based programming continue. In the past decade, new school prevention and intervention programmes have emerged from school, agency, and/or university partnerships and offer promising new approaches for educating and treating children with ED.

Objectives and Hypotheses

In this study an attempt was made to trace the pattern of emotional disturbance in children and adolescents as affected by their locale, grade, gender and family type. The objectives and hypotheses were as follows:

- The first objective of this study was to ascertain the impact of locale on emotional disturbance. It was contended that variation in locale would cause variation in emotional disturbance.
- The second objective of the study was to explore the impact of grade on emotional disturbance. It was contended that variation in grade would cause variation in emotional disturbance.
- The third objective of this study was to study the impact of gender on emotional disturbance. It was contended that variation in gender would cause variation in emotional disturbance.
- The last but not the least, fourth objective of this study was to ascertain the impact of family type emotional disturbance. It was contended that variation in family type would cause variation in emotional disturbance.

Keeping these views in consideration study is planned in factorial perspective.

Method

Sample: Two hundred and forty participants ranging between 10-12 grade will serve as participants and they were be arranged according to the requirements of 4-way factorial design with three locale (City, Town and Village), two grades (X and XII), two genders (Boy and Girl) and two types of family (Joint and Nuclear), i.e., 10 participants per cell. A schematic presentation of experimental design is as follows:

Measure of Emotional Disturbance: This scale is developed by Shukla and Dhami (2000). It consists of 90 five-point items which represent the area of life when a person can feel are 10 domains of emotional disturbance in this scales, namely:

- ***Withdrawal from the Society:*** It is defined is a defence mechanism with which we protect ourselves and escape from the society.
- ***Isolation:*** Separation from others of the same species, used for

Table 12.1: Schematic presentation of experimental design

	A											
	A1				A2				A3			
	B				B				B			
	B1		B2		B1		B2		B1		B2	
	C		C		C		C		C		C	
	C1	C2	C1	C2	C1	C2	C1	C2	C1	C2	C1	C2
D1	10	10	10	10	10	10	10	10	10	10	10	10
D2	10	10	10	10	10	10	10	10	10	10	10	10

Legends:

A = Locale
A1 = City
A2 = Town
A3 = Village

B = Grade
B1 = 10th
B2 = 12th

C = Gender
C1 = Boys
C2 = Girls

D = Family Type
D1 = Joint
D2 = Nuclear

groups or organism existing separate from other groups of the same species either geographically, or with respect to reproductive maturity, in either case with the effect of preventing interbreeding.

- *Rejection:* A type of avoiding behaviour on the part of an organism, throwing out something that has already been taken into the body; mentally negative attitude a judgment, of belief.
- *Day dreaming:* Type of phantom, in which the individual allows his mind to wonder aimlessly among pleasant imagery, wishes which are ungratified in real life.
- *Guilt feeling:* Sense of wrong-doing, as an emotional attitude, generally involving emotional conflict, arising out of real or imagined contravention of moral or social standards, in act of thought.
- *Inferiority Complex:* A hypothetical complex arising from conflict between the impulse to seek recognition (positive self impulse), and fear of the hurt arising from frustration frequently experienced in similar situation in the past, resulting in defensive, compensatory, or often aggressive behaviour, unconsciously determined.
- *Conflict:* Opposition between contradictory impulses or wishes, a rule producing emotional tension, often disagreeable. According to psychoanalytic theories, to repress of one of the impulse.

- ***Low Confidence:*** Less determination of a person over himself/herself for any activity termed as low confidence. It is deferent with inferiority complex.
- ***Nervousness:*** Nervousness is a state of perplex ion and sorer which blackness the behaviour of a person, as a result, he either hesitates to express himself or wrong response are produced by him.
- ***Anxiety:*** A chronic complex emotional state with apprehension or dread as its most prominent component, characteristic of various nervous and mental disorders.

Scores range between 90-450. Low score indicates low emotional disturbance and high score *vice versa.*

Procedure: Data collection was done with individually and best attempts were made to avoid external distractions.

Results

Obtained data were analyzed by 4-way analysis of variance and they are appeared in Table 12.2.

Table 12.2: Summary table of ANOVA showing the impact of locale, grade, gender and Family type on emotional disturbance

Sources of variation	*Ss*	*df*	*MS*	*F*
A	14.48	2	7.24	4.78
B	5.09	1	5.09	3.36
C	15.90	1	15.90	10.50
D	1.09	1	1.09	0.72
AB	29.09	2	14.54	9.60
AC	30.18	2	15.09	9.96
AD	30.36	2	15.18	10.02
BC	13.15	1	13.15	8.68
BD	13.81	1	13.81	9.12
CD	13.03	1	13.03	8.60
ABC	26.06	2	13.03	8.60
ABC	27.16	2	13.58	8.96
ACD	29.15	2	14.57	9.62
BCD	11.56	1	11.56	7.60
ABCD	35.21	2	17.60	11.62
Error within	327.28	216	0.66	
		239		

A close perusal of the table indicates that the main effect of locale was significant (F, 2,216 = 4.78 $p < .05$). Mean values pooled across grade, gender and family type were 307.87, 306.82, 318.48, respectively for city town and village. I was found that well-being was higher in the residents of city as compared to the participants of town and village. The next main effect was grade significant (F, 2,216= 3.36 $p < .05$). It was found that the well-being of XII grade (M = 314.29)/washigher than X grade (M = 307.87). The third main effect of gender was significant (F, 1,216 = 10.50 $p < .01$). It was found that boys (M = 332.65) and girls (M = 289.48) were almost equal in relation to their scores on emotional disturbance. The last main effect of family type was insignificant (F, 1,216 =.72 $p > .05$) *r*evealing the fact that participants living in joint family (M = 312.89) were almost equal with the participants who live in nuclear family (M = 309.27).

The two way interaction of locale and grade was significant (F, 2,216 = 9.60 $p < .01$). It was found that the trend of emotional disturbance was entirely different in X and XII grades. The second interaction of

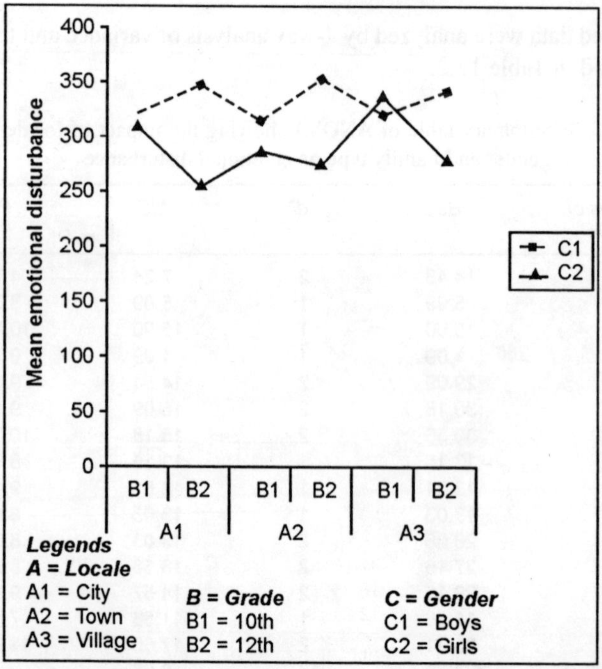

Fig. 12.1: Mean values showing the impact of locale, grade and gender on Emotional Disturbance

locale and gender was also significant (F, 2,216 = 9.96 $p < .01$) and it was found that the pattern of well-being was entirely different in boys and girls. The locale x family type interaction was also significant (F, 2,216 = 10.02 $p < .01$) and it showed same pattern as it was evident in locale and gender interaction.

The grade x gender interaction was also significant (F, 2,216 = 8.68 $p < .01$) showing the reverse trend in emotional disturbance. The grade x family type interaction was also significant (F, 2, 216 = 9.12 $p < .01$) and it was found that different pattern of well-being was show by the participants both type of family. The gender x family type interaction was also significant (F, 2,216 = 8.60 $p < .01$) and it shared prior trend.

The three way interaction of locale x grade x gender was significant (F, 2, 216 = 8.60 $p < .01$) and it is appeared in Fig. 12.1.

The locale x grade x family type interaction was also significant (F, 2,216 =8.96 $p < .01$) and it is appeared in Fig. 12.2.

Similarly the locale x gender x family type interaction was also significant (F, 2,216= 9.62 $p < .01$) and it is appeared in Fig. 12.3.

The grade x gender x family type interaction was also significant (F, 1,216= 7.60 $P < .01$) and it is appeared in Fig. 12.4.

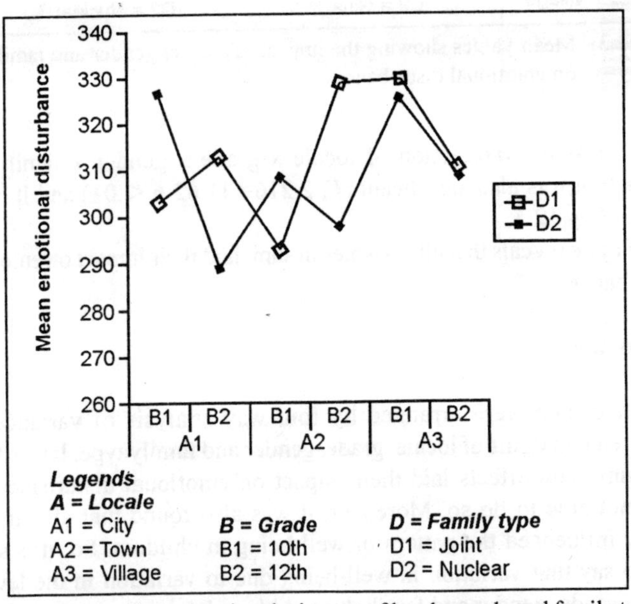

Fig. 12.2: Mean values showing the impact of locale, grade and family type on emotional disturbance

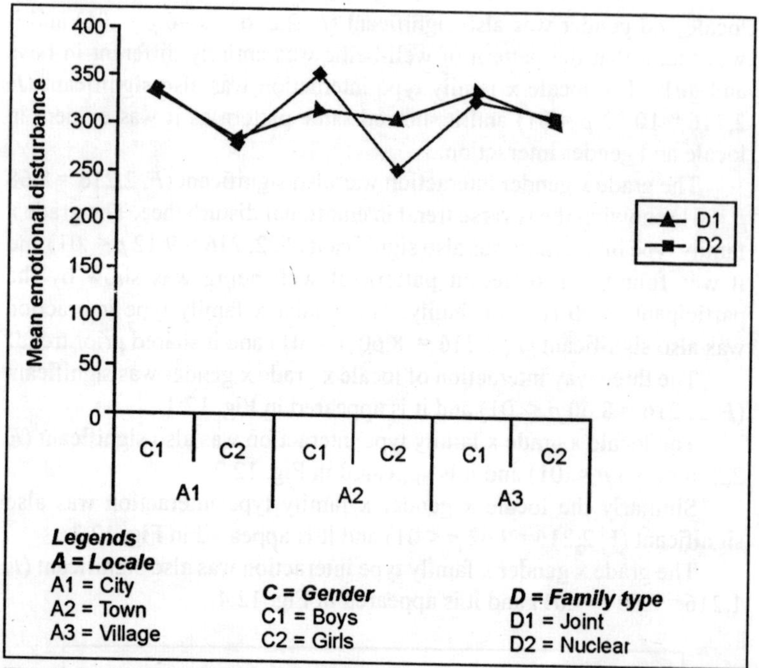

Fig. 12.3: Mean values showing the impact of locale, gender and family type on emotional disturbance

The 4-way interaction of locale x grade x gender x family type interaction was also significant (F, 2,216= 11.62 $p < .01$) and it can be seen in Fig. 12.5.

Figure reveals that all variables in sum, laid their impact on emotional disturbance.

Discussion

Obtained data were arranged by four-way analysis of variance and interpreted in terms of locale, grade, gender and family type. It was found that sum main effects laid their impact on emotional disturbance sum were not able to do so. Moreover, it was also found that all variables jointly influenced the pattern of well-being in children. So, it is surely fear to say that variation in well-being due to variation in the level of locale, grade, gender and family type. Although it was not equal at every place. At the turn of the 20th century, emotional disturbance was a

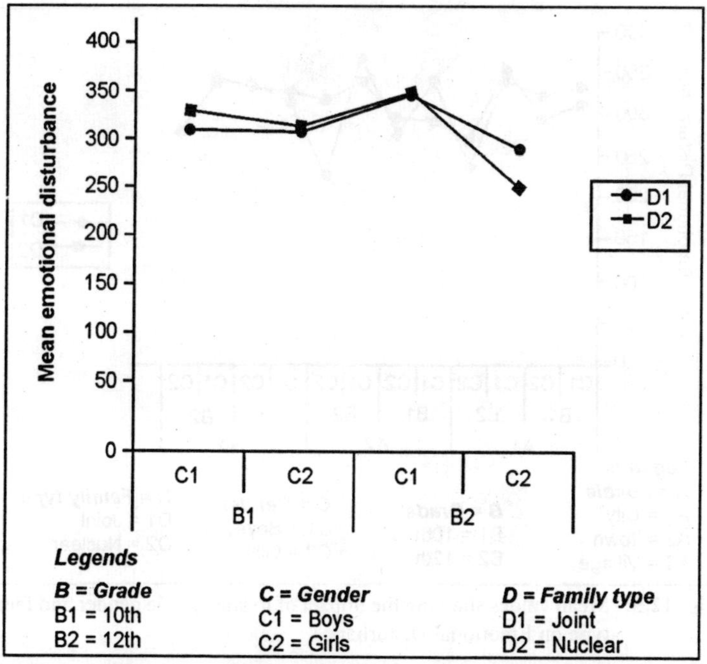

Fig. 12.4: Mean values showing the impact of grade, gender and family type on emotional disturbance

tentative, barely recognizable idea. It was not yet legitimate enough to have its own journal, place inlegislation, or diagnostic criteria. Emotional disturbance was instead a loose and vague idea appearing randomly and infrequently in writings. It was conceptually indistinguishable from the concepts backward, merely backward, deviant, maladjusted, delinquent, incorrigible, disruptive, and bizarre, and the only clear concept holding all of these various ideas together was that troubled and troubling children were *atypical*. How has emotional disturbance moved from a tentative idea to one of legitimacy in special education? Through what mechanisms has "legitimate" meaning been assembled for this idea? Emotional disturbance has come to be "real" through its asserted resemblance to the *natural* world. For example, emotional disturbance has been understood as a weather system; daily "emotional thunderstorms" in which families argue, wrangle, and finally break apart has been proposed as a cause or instigator for the child's emotional and behavioural responses. A child has been seen to be like a plant that needs sunshine, warmth, and gentle rain to grow and flourish. A dearth of these essential elements (such as a

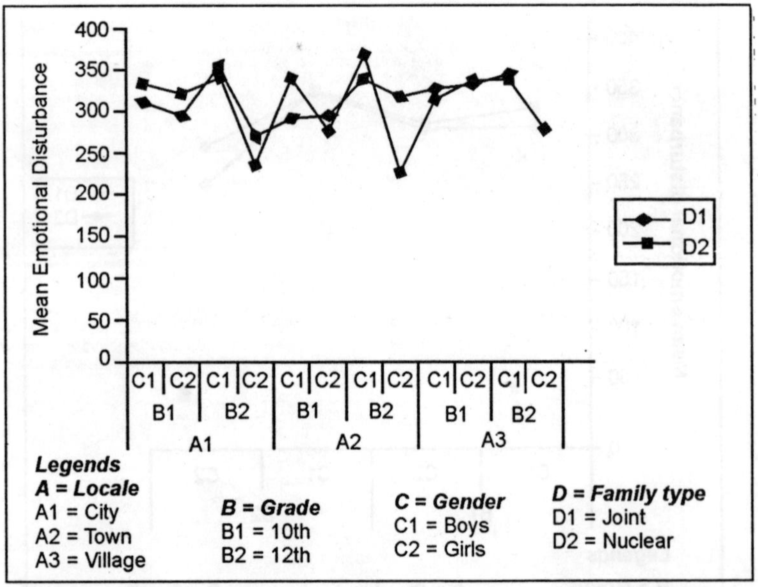

Fig. 12.5: Mean values showing the impact of locale, grade gender and family type on Emotional Disturbance.

lack of love, attention, and gentle conflict) or the excess of these elements (such asover whelming attention, overprotection, or harsh conflict) has been blamed for the presence of emotional disturbance. In addition to resemblance to the natural world, the child and his or her emotional development have been understood in relationship to the world of natural *living* beings. As part of an admonishment to treat the whole child rather than just a piece of the child's personality or behaviour, the child has been understood at a 80 "unified organism". Emotional developments have been likened to an amoeba that has no specialized organs. As with the amoeba, there has been no organ of emotion—rather, emotions have been seen to be pervasive and scattered throughout the body. Furthermore, emotional disturbance has been understood as directly analogous to the physical body of humans. Just as infants have ingested nutrition and air to develop, psychological selves "ingest, digest, and assimilate psychological foods which are the experienced feelings of other people towards us. If those are wholesome and in proper quantity we grow inio healthy psychological selves." The complex idea of emotional disturbance has been seen as similar to a cache tic body that wastes away due to a chronic disease. In an effort to distinguish between the concepts of socially maladjusted and emotionally disturbed, an analogy to a bellyache has been used. Just as a generalized bellyache has indicated only a manifestation of a problem rather than the true cause to the problem, the categories of socially maladjusted and delinquent have been critiqued for only indicating that there is a problem rather than explaining the nature of the whole student. Emotional disturbance, unlike a bellyache, has been understood as having the explanatory power that socially maladjusted and delinquent have not had. Students diagnosed with emotional disturbance are those students whose educational performance is adversely affected by one or more of the following characteristics:

(i) An inability to learn that cannot be explained by intellectual, sensory, or health factors.
(ii) An inability to build or maintain satisfactory interpersonal relationships with peers and teachers.
(iii) Inappropriate types of behaviour or feelings under normal circumstances.
(iv) A general pervasive mood of unhappiness or depression.
(v) A tendency to develop physical symptoms or fears associated with personal or school problems.

References

Armstrong, K.H., Dedrick, R., F., and Greenbaum, P.E. (2003). Factors associated with community adjustment of young adults with serious emotional disturbance: A longitudinal analysis. *Journal of Emotional and Behavioural Disorders,* 11(2), 66-76.

Barney Rabinow. "A proposal for a training programme for teachers of the emotionally disturbed and the socially maladjusted." *Exceptional Children* 26, no. 6 (1960): 287-293: 289.

Coutinho, M.J., and Oswald, D.P. (2005). State variation in gender disproportionality in special education: Findings and recommendations. *Remedial and Special Education,* 26(1), 7-15.

Duchnowski, A.J. (1994). Innovative service models: Education. *Journal of Clinical Child Psychology, 23,* 13-18.

Epstein, M.H., Kutash, K., and Duchnowski, A. (1998). *Outcomes for Children and Youth with Behavioural and Emotional Disorders.* Austin: Pro-Ed.

Fomess, S.R. and Kavale, K.A. (2001). Reflections on the future of prevention. *Preventing School Failure,* 45(2), 75-82.

Friedman, R.M., and Kutash, K. (1986). *Mad, bad, sad, can't add. Florida Adolescent and Child Treatment Study.* Tampa: Florida Mental Health Institute

Greenbaum, P.E., Dedrick, R.F., Friedman, R.M., Kautash, K., Brown, E.C., Lardieri, S.P., and Pugh, A.M. (1996). National adolescent and child treatment study (NACTS): Outcomes for children with serious emotional and behavioural disturbance. *Journal of Emotional and Behaviour Disorders,* 4, 130-146.

Hansen, M., Litzelman, A., Marsh, D.T., and Milspaw, A. (2004). Approaches to serious emotional disturbance: Involving multiple systems. *Professional Psychology: Research and Practice,* 35, 457-465.

Hinshaw, S.P., Lahey, B.B., and Hart, E.L. (1993). Issues of taxonomy and co-morbidity in the development of conduct disorder. *Development and Psychopathology,* 5, 31-49.

Individuals with Disabilities Education Act of 1997 20 U.S.C. 1400-1485 (1997).

Individuals with Disabilities Education Act of 2005 7. (118) U.S.C. 1221 (e-3).

Margaret, A. Winzer. (1993). *The History of Special Education: From Isolation to Integration.* Washington, D.C.: Gallaudet University Press.

Nelson, C.M. (1992). Searching for the meaning in the behaviour of antisocial pupils, public school educators, and lawmakers. *School Psychology Review,* 21

Osher, D., Osher, T., and 'Smith, C. (1994). Toward a national perspective in emotional and behavioural disorders. *Beyond Behaviour, 6,* 6-17.

Oswald, D.P., and Coutinho, M.J. (1995). Identification and placement' of students, with serious emotional disturbance. Part 1: Correlates of state child count data. *Journal of Emotional and Behavioural Disorders, 3,* 224-229.

Paul, W. Terry. (1939). "Contributions of psychology to special education." *Journal of Exceptional Children* 6 : 96-100.

President's 'New Freedom Commission on Mental Health'. (2003). *Achieving the promise: Transforming mental health care in America. Final Report* (DHHS Pub. No. SMA-03-3832). Rockville, MD: Author.

Reddy, L.A. (2001). Serious emotional disturbance in children and adolescents: Current status and future directions. *Behaviour Therapy,* 32, 667-691.

Reddy, L.A., and De Thomas, C. (in press). Assessment of co-morbid ADHD children and adolescents. In S.R. Smith & L. Handler (Eds). *The clinical 'assessment of children and adolescents: A practitioner's guide.* Mahwah, NJ: Lawrence Erlbaum Associates, Inc.

Reddy, L.A., and Savin, H. (2000). Designing and conducting outcome evaluations. In H. Savin and S. Kiesling (Eds). *Putting our Housein order: A- Provider's guide to Account Table: Sustains of Behavioural health care* (pp.' 132-158). San Francisco: Jossey-Bass.

Samuel, R. Laycock. (1940). "Mental health qualifications for special class teachers." *Journal of Exceptional Children* 7: 4-8, 23.

Schroeder, C.S., and Gordon, B.N. (2002). *Assessment and treatment of childhood problems: A clinician's guide* (2nd ed.) New York: Guilford Press.

U.S. Department of Health and Human Services. (2000). *Report of the surgeon general's conference on children's mental health: A national action agenda.* Washington, DC: Author.

U.S. Department of Education Office of Special Education Programmes (2001). *Twenty-third annual report to congress on the implementation of the Individuals with Disabilities Education Act: Results.* U.S. Department of Education, Office of Special Education Programmes (OSEP).

Wagner, M. (1995). Outcomes. for youth with serious emotional disturbance in secondary school and early adulthood. *The future of children: Critical issues for children, and youths,* 5, 90-112.

Walrath, C.M., Nickerson, K.J., Crowel, R.L., and Leaf, P. (1998). Serving children with serious emotional disturbance in a system of care: Do mental health and non-mental health agency referrals look the same? *Journal of Emotional and Behavioural Disorders, 6,* 205-213.

13

Suicide Risk and Mental Health Disorders

Muniram and *Arun Kumar*

Many people may be at risk of suicide at some time in their lives depending on circumstance, but the focus of this study was those with serious mental illness. Suicide refers to factors about a person's condition and/or in their environment that may provoke the action of suicide. Suicide can result from a range of factors, including, for example, psychiatric disorder, negative life events, psychological factors, alcohol and drug misuse, family history of suicide, physical illness, exposure to suicidal behaviour of others, and access to methods of self-harm. In any individual case multiple factors are usually involved. No one is immune to suicide. It should be noted that family history of suicide or self-harm is particularly important. There are also some factors which may offer some degree of protection against suicide. More than 90 per cent of all cases of suicide are associated with mental disorders such as depression, schizophrenia and alcoholism. Therefore, reducing the global suicide rate means effectively addressing the serious and growing burden of mental illness around the world. The majority of suicide victims suffered from mental disorders. This indicates that a strong relationship between suicide and the Mental Health Disorders.

There is considerable debate all over the world as to why people commit suicide, since self-destruction of human beings has always been a matter of curiosity. Since suicide is an act of killing oneself performed by the person with his/her full knowledge, and knowing fully well the results of the final outcome, it is always considered something very close to the person committing the act. The various causes for a suicide are by and large many and complex, ranging from social, economic, health, cultural, political, and religious and other areas of an individual's life. Recent research indicates that suicides are multidimensional in nature, cumulative due to number of causes which are progressive and operate over a period of time. A small percentage of impulsive suicides have been extremely difficult to understand. The field of suicide has attracted considerably attention in recent years. Several governments around the world have established suicide prevention programmes. The major reason for this has been the very large increase in suicide in young people especially males, seen in many countries. There is also increasing empirical interest in suicidal behaviour in the elderly. The increased attitude to suicide and attempted suicide has resulted in a massive expansion in research, which has occurred on all fronts, including, psychiatry, psychology, social sciences, biology and genetics.

Suicide: Nature and Incidence

There are differences in patterning and trends of suicide between Asian and Western countries. The sex ratio for suicide in Asia is smaller than that in the West, the occurrence of suicide in Asia tend to increase with age. There is new evidence suggesting that mental illness, especially depressive illness and alcoholism is a strange risk factor for suicide in both the East and West. More research in biological factors needed in Asia very low suicide rate is found in Islamic countries. The common methods of suicides seen in Asia indicate that these are society dependent. A number of culture specific types of suicide, such as burning or self-immolation. Many factors may contribute to suicidal ideation or suicidal behaviour, including stressors in the work situation, factors outside the work situation and personality dimensions, as well as the interaction between these variables (Schmidtke, Fricke and Lester, 1999). According to the holistic model of work wellness, suicide ideation can be regarded as an outcome of unwellness. Suicide (Latin Sui caedere, to kill oneself) is the act of intentionally terminating one's own life. Suicide occurs for a number of reasons such as depression, substance abuse shame, avoiding pain, financial difficulties or other undesirable situations (Meltzer and Howard, 2000). In recent years suicide has emerged as an important public health problem in many countries (Krug *et al.* 2000) internationally, approximately one million people die by suicide each year (WHO, 1999). The wish to die and thoughts of killing oneself, the wish to die and thoughts of killing oneself (suicide ideation) are a frequent phenomenon among the youth of today. Suicidal ideation is the fist link or lowest level of suicidal behaviour. Suicide is the third leading cause of death among adolescents in the United States (Anderson, 2002).

The rate of suicide rose in the 1970s–1990s in youth between age range of 15 to 19 years. This increase is attributable to rising rate depression, the increased availability of firearms and other means among adolescents (Commission on Adolescent Suicide Prevention, 2005). In India, more than one lakh persons lost their lives by committing suicides in year 2006 (National Crime Record Bureau, India). Similarly, in other Asian countries the certified suicide data confirm the general observation that suicide rated increase with age, but the recent increase in young suicides has not been paid much attention. However, in some of the Asians countries, adolescent suicide rate is relatively lower. In Taiwan, for instance, there has been a decline in adolescent suicide rates form 20 per 1,00,000 in 1964 to just under 5 per 1,00,000 in 1988. The corresponding rate was even lower in Hong Kong (1.8 per 1,00,000 in 1982-1986) and in Singapore (3.3 per 1,00,000 in 1986), this could reflect a general trend towards improvement in living conditions, or it could mean that adolescents in countries like Hong Kong and Singapore are less attracted to resorting to suicidal behaviour as a means of coping with stress (Cheng and Lee, 2000).

Although suicide was condemned in the Dharamashastras, yet there is also a chapter on allowed suicides. But the earlier scriptures, of Manu's and Kautilya's were against suicide, these sentiments were echoed for ages in India. Even though today, attempted suicide is also a crime in India under the Indian Penal Code system. The neighbouring country of Sri Lanka has removed attempted suicide as punishable offence in India, even the assisting and abetting suicide is also a punishable offence.

Suicide rates in India have shown a gradually increasing trend. The rate in 2005 was 10.3 per lakh. The striking aspect of Indian data is the large variation in different parts of India in relation to attempted/committed suicide. The states and cities with rapid social change are associated with higher suicide rates, such as the states of Kerela and Tripura, and cities like Pondicherry and Bangalore, the number of suicides in country during the decade (1995-2005) has recorded an increase of 27.7 per cent during the decade. The 35.3 per cent of suicide victims were the youth (15-29 years). There has been a slightly inverse of 0.1 per cent in suicide in the country in year 2004 as compared to 2003 (Accidental Deaths and Suicides 2005, NCRB).

In many studies it is reported that the exposure to model of suicidal behaviour can be a risk factor for suicide behaviour, suicide behaviour can be learn by imitation, especially among children, adolescents and adults (Schmidtke, 1998, 1998; Diestra, 1995). Suicide rates in India have shown a gradually increasing trend, the rate in 1999 was 11.2 per 1,00,000 (Accidental Deaths and Suicide in India 1999, published by

National Crime Record Bearue (NCRB, Ministry of Home Affairs, Government of India). States and cities with rapid social change are associated with higher suicide rates, such as the states of Kerala and Tripura, and cities like Pondicherry and Bangalore, the important association is alcohol dependence as a direct or indirect cause of suicide.

The Haryana state reported significant rise in suicide (43.1%) in 1999 over 1998. The average suicide rate of Haryana was 11.7 per lakh as compared to national suicide rate 11.2 per lakh (Accidental Deaths and Suicide in India, published by NCRB, Ministry of Home Affairs, and Government of India).

Suicidal behaviours often occur as response to a situation that the person views as overwhelming, such as social isolation, death of loved one, emotional trauma, serious physical illness, growing old, unemployment or financial problems, guilt feelings and alcohol or other drug dependence.

According to World Health Organization (WHO) estimates approximately on million people are likely to commit suicide in the year 2000. Suicide is among the top 10 causes of death in every country, and one of the three leading causes of death in the 15 to 35 years age-group.

The psychological and social impact of suicide on the family and society is immeasurable. On average, single suicide intimately affects at least six other people. If a suicide occurs in a school or workplace it has an impact on hundreds of people.

The number of suicides in India during the decade (2001-2011) has recorded an increase of 25.0 per cent (from 1,08,506 in 2001 to 2011, and 35,585 in 2010). The increase in incidence of suicides was reported each year during the decade. The population has increased by 17.8 per cent during the decade but the rate of suicides in 2011 was 11.2 which is marginally greater than 10.6 recorded in 2001. The rate of suicides has shown a declining trend since 2001 to 2003. An increasing trend is observed during 2007 to 2010. Young Indians are more likely to commit suicide than previously thought, especially those living in wealthier and more educated regions, according to a study on Friday that experts say suggests India's rapid development is driving many youth to despair. Opportunities that have come with two decades of economic boom and open markets have also brought more job anxiety, higher expectations and more pressure to achieve, mental health experts said. India has some of the world's highest suicide rates, with many believing the biggest risk group to be rural farmers facing debt after poor harvests. However, the study—published in the *Lancet Medical Journal* on Friday—says suicide rates are highest in the 15-29 age-groups, peaking in southern regions that are considered richer and more developed with better education, social welfare and health care. That puts the young at high risk, new phenomenon experts said, has happened recently as more middle-class youth strive to meet achievement expectations, and new technologies like cell phones and social networking sites help break down traditional family units once relied on for support.

The State/UT and City-wise information on the number of suicides reported its percentage share in total suicides and rate of suicides during the year. West Bengal has reported the highest number of suicides (16,492) accounting for 12.2 per cent of total suicides followed by Tamil Nadu (15,963), Maharashtra (15,947), Andhra Pradesh (15,077) and Karnataka (12,622) accounting for 11.8 per cent, 11.1 per cent and 9.3 per cent respectively of the total suicides in the country. These 5 States together accounted for 56.2 per cent of the total suicides reported in the country. The remaining 43.8 per cent suicides were reported in the rest of 23 States and 7 UTs. Uttar Pradesh, the most populous state (16.5% share of population) has reported comparatively lower percentage of suicidal deaths, accounting for only 3.6 per cent of the total suicides reported in the country. The States which have witnessed significantly higher cases of suicidal deaths during the year 2009 to 2011. These States have accounted for about 10 per cent or more of the total suicides reported in the country during 2009 to 2011. All the five States, viz. Tamil Nadu, West Bengal, Andhra Pradesh, Maharashtra and Karnataka have registered consistently higher number of suicidal deaths during the last few years. West Bengal reported the highest number of suicidal deaths in 2009, second highest in 2010 and again reported highest in 2011 accounting for 11.5 per cent, 11.9 and 12.2 per cent respectively of total such deaths in the country. Delhi has reported the highest number of suicides (1,716) among UTs, followed by Puducherry (557). Seven UTs together accounted for 1.9 per cent of total suicides in the country. 53 mega cities on the contrary, accounted for 13.5 per cent of the total suicides in the country. The States and UTs which have reported significant increase in Suicides in 2011 over 2010 were Nagaland (from 12 in 2010 to 33 in 2011, i.e. an increase of 175.0%) followed by Chandigarh (47.9%), Meghalaya (41.7%), Uttar Pradesh (33.5%), Odisha (23.2%), Uttarakhand (12.8%), Haryana (12.1%), Delhi (11.2%) and J&K (10.8) as compared to the National average of 0.7% while highest number of decrease was reported in Bihar (from 1,226 in 2010 to 795 in 2011).

The overall male:female ratio of suicide victims for the year 2011 was 64.8:35.2 represent a marginal decrease of male and marginal increase of female ratio as compared to year 2010. The proportion of Boys: Girls suicide victims (up to 14 years of age) were 52:48 in 2011, i.e. the same ratio as in the year 2010. The proportion of female victims was comparatively more under the heads 'Illegitimate Pregnancy' (100.0%), 'Dowry Dispute' (95.7%), 'Physical Abuse (Rape, Incest etc.)' (69.3%) and 'Barrenness/Impotency (Not having children)' (65.2%). It is observed that social and economic causes have led most of the males to commit suicide whereas emotional and personal causes have mainly driven females to end their lives. Youth (15-29 years) and lower middle-aged people (30-44 years) were the prime groups taking recourse to the path of suicides. Around 35.4 per cent suicide victims were youths in the age group of 15-29 years and 34.1 per cent were middle aged persons in the age group 30-44 years. Among the specified causes, 'Illness' (262), 'Family Problems' (344), 'Failure in Examination' (283) and 'Love affairs' (215) were the main cause of suicides among children (3,035). 'Family Problems' have driven 11,768 youth (15-29 years), 13,162 lower middle aged people (30-44 years) and 6,659 upper middle aged persons (45-59 years) to commit suicide. Nearly 37.8 per cent (4,073 out of 10,785) of suicides committed by senior citizens (60 years and above) were due to 'Illness'. Senior citizens have accounted for 8.0 per cent of the total victims.

In the U.S. suicide accounts for about 1 per cent of all deaths of each year. The highest rate is among the elderly, but there has been a steady increase in the rate among adolescent. Suicide is now the third leading cause of death for those 15-19 years old, after accidents and homicide. Suicide attempts that do not result in death for outnumber completed suicide. Many unsuccessful suicide attempts are carried out in manner that makes rescue possible. They often represent a desperate cry for help.

The method of suicide varies from relatively non-violent methods (such as poisoning or overdose) to violent methods (such as shooting one-self). Males are more likely to choose violent methods, which probably accounts for the fact that suicide attempts by males are more likely to be completed.

Suicide and Mental Health Disorders

In developed countries psychiatric illnesses are highly correlated with suicidal behaviour. In developing countries this relationship is less tenacious and more (or equal) emphasis has been placed on socio-cultural factors. But it has been argued that the low rate of diagnosis of mental illness in suicides in developing nations does not preclude the presence of psychiatric problems in the said population. It is believed that mental illness are under-diagnosed due to a variety of factors such as, mental activity of mental health professionals and resources, the tendency to view suicide as a consequence is some external factor such as domestic problems, a failure in academics or love affair etc., the perception that only psychotic disorders such as schizophrenia are mental illnesses. For example many people in developing countries often do not recognize symptoms of depression and rarely approach facilities for treatment, the stigma associated with mental illness also prevents many who need help form approaching appropriate centres, the relationship of mental illness with suicide is an area in which a growing body of research is now becoming available and many studies now conducted in developing countries especially in Asia show that a substantial number of people who commit suicide have had mental illness (60-80%). Suicide is now understood as multi-dimensional disorder, which results form a complex interaction of biology, genetic, psychological, sociological and environmental factors. Research has shown that between 40 per cent and 60 per cent of people who commit suicide had seen a physician in the month prior to suicide of these, many more had seen a general physician rather than psychiatrist, in countries where the mental health services are not well developed, the proportion of people in suicidal crisis consulting a general physician is likely to be higher.

Psychiatric disorders can lead to decrease in socio-economic status the breakup of a marriage or significant relationship, or the failure to form meaningful relationships, separating the effect of psychosocial adversity from that of psychiatric illness can be difficult (Mann, 2002). Psychiatric illness can lead to psychosocial adversity and both factors can combine to increase the person's level of stress and thereby potentially increase the risk for suicidal behaviours.

Most studies have found that suicide victims had a psychiatric disorder at the time of suicide, approximately half of all suicides occur in persons with a mood disorder, and the rest occur in persons with various other psychiatric condition, including schizophrenia and personality disorders, such as borderline or antisocial personality disorder, a combination of two psychiatric disorders. Especially alcoholism or drug addiction along with mood disorder, a personality disorder or schizophrenia, raises the risk for suicide. Although suicide in generally a complication of a psychiatric disorder usually depression, most persons with a psychiatric disorder never attempt suicide.

Nwosu *et al.* (2001) revealed that in Africa depressive disorders, (a major cause of suicides) is thought to be rare in Africa, is fairly common, it was generally present in a rather subtle form with features of somatization. A study by (Alem *et al.*, 1999) in Ethiopia reported that persons with mental illness attempted suicide more often than other. Similarly, a study in Cape Town, South Africa that compared patients with a history of previous parasuicide. Dirks, (1998) found that a six year study (1997-82) in a child psychiatric unit of Johannesburg hospital in South Africa that found psychiatric illness in the patient was a significant predisposing factor in adolescent suicidal behaviour. Cummins *et al.* (1984) seen that 10 per cent of all referrals to the psychiatry clinic had made suicidal attempts and threats. Okasha *et al.* (1979) revealed that depressive illnesses, hysterical reactions and situational disorders in that order of frequency were the main causes of suicide attempts identified by investigators in a study in Egypt.

Cheng *et al.* (2000) found that Major depressive episode, emotionally stable personality disorder and substance dependence were significantly correlated with suicidal behaviour in a study form Taiwan. Researchers in Taiwan (Liu *et al.,* 1996) investigated that 64 suicidal acts of 62 psychiatric inpatients over a ten year period. The findings indicated the frequency of suicidal behaviour of psychiatric inpatients was 0.91 per cent of total admissions; two-thirds of the patients who attempted suicide ware diagnosed with schizophrenia or depression. Patients suffering from depression, substance abuse, and personality disorders had a higher parasuicide rate, among whom. Those diagnosed bipolar disorder with depressive episode hade an extremely high rate.

Bhatia *et al.* (2000) found that In India tertiary care hospital on 373 subjects reported that in suicidal ideations, mixed anxiety and depressive disorder was the most common psychiatric diagnosis followed by the major depression and schizophrenia. Among suicide attempters, adjustment disorder with depression was the most common diagnosis, in another study (Latha, 1996) done in Manipal, India on 73 persons who attempted suicide a psychiatric diagnosis was possible in 93 per cent of the cases. The most common diagnosis was a mood disorder. Dysthymic disorders were associated with 42 per cent of the cases. Axis II diagnosis was possible in 12 per cent of the cases 21 per cent of the cases received more than one diagnoses.

A population based case control study (Vijaya Kumar and Raj Kumar, 1999) employing the psychological autopsy technique was conducted in

100 completed suicides in India, 88 per cent of the cases received a life time diagnosis for an Axis I disorder, 34 per cent of the cases were alcoholics, mood disorder was present in 25 per cent of the cases, personality disorders were present in 20 per cent of cases and co-morbidity was found in 30 per cent of cases (De Leo D., 2003). Other studies in India have shown that personality disorders such as schizoid, histrionic and antisocial type are high risk for suicide. Chang *et al.* 1990 found that 9 to 24 per cent of persons with schizophrenia will commit suicide even while under treatment. In India chronic mental illness contributes to 14 per cent to 30 per cent of total suicides.

A common finding in those who commit suicide is the presence of more than one disorder. The common disorders occurring together are alcoholism and mood disorder (i.e. depression), and personality disorder and other psychiatric disorders.

Psychiatric Illness and Suicide

Affective Illness

The overwhelming majority of suicide victims suffer a concomitment psychiatric illness at the time of this act with excellent diagnostically oriented, retrospective studies confirming figures as high as 93 per cent and 94 per cent (Barrachlough *et al.*, 1974). Affective illness, usually major depression, was identified in 4 per cent to 80 per cent of the victim in a consecutive series of suicides and alcoholism in 20 to 30 per cent. The increase correlation of suicide with schizophrenia, organic mental disorders, and other psychiatric diagnoses has been made as well.

Guze and Robins (1970) estimated the risk of suicide for patients with a primary affective disorder to be 25 times greater than the risk in the general population, and they estimate the lifetime risk of suicide at 15 per cent in the depression patients, suicide among depressed patients infrequently occurs in the early stages of affective complaints.

Weissman *et al.* (1973) separated a subset of depressed patients who had attempted suicide from those who had not. This separation was based on the patient's demonstration of greater open hostility during interviews with those patients who made suicide attempts. Several studies (Roy, 1983, 1984), which matched patients manic depressive illness who committed suicide with those who did not and so called neurotic depressive who committed suicide with those who did not, found additional risk factors beyond the illness *per se*. These studies revealed social and psychiatric risks including being depressed and suicidal on a previous hospital admission.

Substance Abuse

Substance Abuse, and more specifically alcoholism, is the second most frequently encountered psychiatric diagnosis found among patients who commit suicide (Evenson *et al.*, 1982). Major differences appear in the comparison of suicide, depression, and alcoholism when life circumstances and events are reviewed. Not surprisingly, the lives of alcoholism are marked by a considerable number of crises in the year preceding their death: Economics, financial, legal, occupational, and health problems are well represented in the list of disruptive events (Murphy *et al.* 1979). Although, the research focus relating substance abuse and suicide has been mainly on the alcoholic population, studies corroborate an assumption that non-alcohol drug abusers have similar suicide statistics (Viallent, 1966). One impressive similarity in the two populations does exist. In both categories suicide tends to results after many year of substance abuse.

Suicide in the schizophrenic patients is 15 per cent (Bleuler, 1978) similar to the risk for the patients with depression or alcoholism. As schizophrenia occurs at a rate of only one-tenth of that of affective illness, the overall number of suicide in any given period of time is small by comparison. Several studies by Roy (1982) tend to document that the highest suicide rate in this particular population is with young men who are in the earliest stages of their illness, principally the first four years (Waltzer, 1984). By statistical analysis alone it is the responsibility of the primary care physician to be mindful of the association among affective illness, alcoholism, and suicide, sleep, appetite, and concentration disturbances are nearly always present at some point in the history of the suicide victims, simply stated, a high index of suspicion to suicide is necessary at all times when dealing with the psychiatrically disturbed patients.

Genetics and Family Factors

The association between suicide and a family history of suicide has been recognized for some time (Rainer, 1984). Whether the act is produced from a genetic aberration passed from generation to generation or by the modelling of suicidal behaviour as a coping style by a family member is controversial. It is possible that suicide is not simply a symptoms of another disorder but may also be a genetic defect itself that found alone or to accompany certain of these clinical entities clearly not all who develop major psychiatric illness go on to complete suicide. Rainer (1984) stated succinctly "when it comes to determinants of overt behaviour, we tend to believe that genetic vulnerability interacts with other predisposing or precipitating factors such as stressful life events, developmental trauma, physiological, metabolic, neuralgic triggers, and sociological factors." Recent biological studies of psychiatric phenomena have focused on central nervous system metabolites particularly the catecholamine (nor epinephrine, dopamine and the serotonin transporter (5 – HTT) gene. Von Praag (1984) compared several different clinical groups featuring violent and suicidal behaviour and his results supported the hypothesis that low 5-hydroxy indoleacetic acid (5-HIAA) may be correlated with deregulation of aggression in suicidal behaviour. Stanley *et al.* (1982) earlier reported decreased triliated imipramine binding in the frontal cortex of patients who had completed suicide.

Suicide and Violence

Suicide and violence are not opposite and unrelated acts. They appear instead to be overlapping end point on a continuum of aggressive behaviour. This observation's evident from studies showing an increased risk of violence in suicidal psychiatric patients and an increased risk of suiçidal behaviour in those known to be violent. Murder suicide and suicide act events, in which both suicidal and violent behaviours are observed almost simultaneously, provide additional examples of the overlap between the two behaviours. The filled continues to await a testable, coherent explanation of why the link between violence and suicide exists. Both behaviours seem to stem from a predisposition to impulsive, aggressive behaviour which probably results from a combination of environment, psychiatric and neurological factors. The relative importance of factors governing the 'vector' of aggression (inward *vs.* outward) remains to be established. Some researchers for example Plutchik *et al.* (1989), developed models to address this issues the dated accumulating about the link between suicide and violence forces us to see suicide for what is really is, an act of aggression. Future research focusing on aggression, which we propose is the key element underlying both behaviours, will lead to better understanding, prediction and prevention of these destructive behaviours.

Mood Disorders

All types of mood disorders have been associated with suicide. These include bipolar affective disorder, depressive episode, recurrent depressive disorder and persistent mood disorders (e.g. cyclothymia and dysthymia), which form categories F31-F34 in ICD-10. Suicide is, therefore, a significant risk in unrecognized and untreated depression. Depression has a high prevalence in the general population and is not recognized by many as a disease. It is estimated that 30 per cent of patients seen by a physician are suffering from depression. Roughly 60 per cent of those who do seek treatment initially contact a general practitioner. It is a special challenge for the physician to work with both physical disease and psychological disorders simultaneously. In many instances, depression is masked and patients present only with somatic complaints.

Rutz *et al.* (1992) Depression is an important factor in suicide among both adolescents and the elderly but those with late onset of depression are at a higher risk. Recent advances in the treatment of depression are very relevant for suicide prevention in primary care. Education of the general practitioner in identifying and treating depression was found to reduce suicide in Sweden. Epidemiological data suggest that anti-depressants reduce suicide risk among the depressed. The full therapeutic dose of medication should be continued for several months. In the elderly it may be necessary to continue treatment for two years after recovery. Patients on regular lithium maintenance therapy have been found to have lower suicide risk (Schou, 1998).

Personality Disorders

Recent studies on young people who committed suicide have shown a high prevalence (20-50%) of personality disorder. The personality disorders that are more frequently associated with suicide are borderline personality and antisocial personality disorders (Işometsa, *et al.* 1996). Histrionic and narcissistic personality disorders and certain psychological traits such as impulsivity and aggression have also been associated with suicide.

Anxiety Disorders

Among anxiety disorders, panic disorder has been most frequently associated with suicide, followed by Obsessive-Compulsive Disorder

(OCD). Somatoform disorder and eating disorders (anorexia nervosa and bulimia) are also related to suicidal behaviour. The relationship between suicide attempts and other anxiety disorders has been less studied, again with conflicting results. Analysis of ECA data revealed elevated rates of suicide attempts in both comorbid and uncomplicated obsessive-compulsive disorders (Hollander *et al.*, 1996). Examination of social phobia using the same data set showed that the comorbid, but not the uncomplicated cases, had significantly elevated rates of suicide attempts (Schneier *et al.*, 1992). In the NCS, after controlling for comorbid disorders, post-traumatic stress disorder was the only anxiety disorder significantly associated with suicide attempts (Sareen *et al.*, 2005).

This paper primarily examines the association of mental health risk factors with suicide. Mental health disorders, which are among the most consistently reported risk factors for suicide. The increase in suicide rates may be viewed as the tip of the 'mental health iceberg'. While suicide remains a relatively rare event, its increase signals more prevalent underlying mental health problem. Mental disorders have a strong association with suicide. This meta-analysis, or statistical overview, of the literature gives an estimate of the suicide risk of the common mental disorders. All mental disorders have an increased risk of suicide excepting mental retardation and dementia. The suicide risk is highest for functional and lowest for organic disorders with substance misuse disorders lying between. Higher suicide rates among those with diagnosed mental health disorders suggest the importance of suicide prevention strategies, including identification, treatment and monitoring of major risk factors for suicide.

References

Alem, A.; Kebede, D.; Jacobsson, L.; Kullgren, G. (1999). Suicide attempts among adults in Butajira, Ethiopia. *Acta Psychiatrica Scandinavica*, 397, 70-76.

Allan, A.; Roberts, M.C.; Allan, M.M.; Pienaar, W.P.; Stein, D.J. (2001). Intoxication, criminal offences and suicide attempts in a group of South African problem drinkers. *South African Medical Journal.* 91(2), 145-150.

Anderson, R.N. (2002). Deaths: Leading causes for 2000. *National Vital Statistics Reports,* 50(16), Hyattsville, MD: National Centre for Health Statistics.

Angst, J., Angst, F., Stossen, H.M. (1999) Suicide risk in patients with major depressive disorders. *Journal of Clinical Psychiatry*, 60. 2: 57-62.

Barraclough, B.; Bunch, J.; Nelson, B. (1974). A hundred cases of suicide. *Clinical Aspects,* 125, 355-373.

Bhatia, M.S.; Aggarwal, N.K.; Aggarwal, B.B. (2000). Psychosocial profile of suicide ideators, attempters and completers in India. *International Journal of Social Psychiatry*, 46(3), 155-63.

Bleuler, M. (1978). *The Schizophrenic Disorders: Long-Term Patient and Family Studies.* Translated by S.H. Clemens.New Haven, CT: Yale University Press.

Chang, A.T.A. and Lee, C.S. (2000). Suicide in Asia and the far east. In Keith Hawton & Kees Van Heeringen (Ed). *The International Handbook of Suicide and Attempted Suicide* 29-48, New York: John Wiley and Sons Ltd.

Cheng, A.T.; Chen, T.H.; Chen, C.C.; Jenkins, R. (2000). Psychosocial and Psychiatric Risk Factors for Suicide. Case-control Psychological Autopsy Study. *British Journal of Psychiatry,* 177, 360-365.

Cheng, K.K.; Leung, C.M.; Lo, W.H. (1990). Risk factors for suicide among schizophrenics. *Acta Psychiatrica Scandinavica.* 81, 220-224.

Cheng, A. (1995). Mental illness and suicide. A case control study in Taiwan. *Archives of General Psychiatry.* 52, 594-603.

Cummins, R.R.; Allwood, C.W. (1984). Suicide attempts or threats by children and adolescents in Johannesburg. *South African Medical Journal*, 10, 66(19), 726-729.

De Leo, D. (2003). The interface of schizophrenia, culture and suicide. *Suicide Prevention Meeting the challenge together.* Ed Vijayakumar. L Orient Longman, 11-41.

Dirks, B.L. (1998). Repetition of parasuicide—ICD-10 personality disorders and adversity. *Acta Psychiatrica Scandinavica*, 98(3), 208-213.

Evenson, R.; Wood, J., and Nuttal, E. (1982). Suicide rates among public mental health patients. *Acta Psychiatrica Scandinavica,* 66, 244-254.

González Seijo, J.C. (1997). Poblaciones específicas de alto riesgo. (Population groups at high risk.) In: Bobes García J. *et al.*, eds. Prevención de las conductas suicidas y parasuicidas. (Prevention of suicidal and parasuicidal behaviours.) Masson, Barcelon, 69-77.

Gupta, S., (1998). Factors associated with suicide attempts among patients with schizophrenia. *Psychiatric Services*, 10: 1353-1355.

Guze, S.B. and Robins, E. (1970) Suicide and primary affective disorders. *Br J Psychiatry*; 117: 437-438.

Hollander, E.; Greenwald, S.; Neville, D.; Johnson, J.; Hornig, C.D., Weissman M.M. (1996-97). Uncomplicated and comorbid obsessive compulsive disorder in an epidemiologic sample. *Depress Anxiety*, 4:111-119.

Howard, M. (2000). *Non Fatal Suicidal Behaviour Among Adults Aged 16 to 74 in Great Britain.*

Isometsa, E.T. (1996). Suicide among subjects with personality disorders. *American Journal of Psychiatry*, 153: 667-673.

Krug, E.G.; Dahlberg, L.L.; Mercy, J.A. (2002). *World Reports on Violence and Health.* Geneva: World Health Organization.

Latha, K.S.; Bhat, S.M.; D.'Souza, P. (1996). Suicide attempters in a general hospital unit in India: their socio-demographic and clinical profile—emphasis on cross-cultural aspects. *Acta Psychiatrica Scandinavica*, 94(1), 26-30.

Liu, C.Y.; Bai, Y.M.; Yang, Y.Y.; Lin, C.C.; Sim, C.C.; Lee, C.H. (1996). Suicide and parasuicide in psychiatric inpatients – ten years experience at a general hospital in Taiwan. *Psychol Rep.* 79(2): 683-90.

Mann, J.J. (2002). A Current Perspective of Suicide and Attempted Suicide. *Annals of Internal Medicine*. 19 February, 136, 4, 302-311.

Meltzer, H.; Lader, D.; Corbin, T.; Singleton, N.; Jenkins, R. and Brugha, T. (2000). *Non-Fatal Suicidal Behaviour Among Adults Aged 16 to 74 in Great Britain.*

Murphy, G.E.; Armstrong, J.W.; Hermela, S.L.; Fihoscher, J.R. and Clendeniu, W.W. (1979). Suicide and alcoholism: International loss confirmed as a predictor. *Archieves of General Psychiatry*, 36, 65-69.

National Crime Record Bureau (2006). *Accidental Deaths and Suicides in India.* New Delhi: Ministry of Home affairs, Government of India.

Nwosu, S.O.; Odesanmi, W.O. (2001). Pattern of suicides in Ile-Ife, Nigeria. *West African Journal of Medicine*, 20(3), 259-62.

Okasha, A.; Lotaif, F. (1979). Attempted suicide. An Egyptian investigation. *Acta Psychiatrica Scandinavica.* 60(1), 69-75.

Plutchik, R.; Van Praag; H.M. and Conte, H.R. (1989). Correlates of suicide and violence risk: A two stage model of countervailing forces. *Psychiatry Research*, 28, 215-225.

Praag van, H.M.: (1983). Depression, Suicide and serotonin metabolism in the brain. In: *The Neurobiology of Manic Depressive Illness*. RM Post, JC Ballenger (eds). Williams and Wilkins, Baltimore.

Rainer, J.D. (1984). Genetic factors in depression and suicide. *American Journal of Psychiatry*, 38(3): 329-340.

Roy, A. (1984). Suicide in recurrent affective disorder patients. *Canadian Journal of Psychiatry*, 29, 319-322.

Roy, A. (1982). Suicide in chronic schizophrenia, *British Journal of Psychiatry*, 141, 171-177.

Roy, A. (1983). Suicide in depressives. *Comprehensive Psychiatry*, 24, 487-491.

Rutz, W.; von Knorring, L.; Walinder J. (1992). Long-term effects of an education programme for general practitioners given by the Swedish Committee for the Prevention and Treatment of Depression. *Acta Psychiatry Scand.*; 85(1): 83-8.

Sareen, J.; Houlahan, T.; Cox, B.J.; Asmundson, G.J.G. (2005). Anxiety disorders associated with suicidal ideation and suicide attempts in the National Comorbidity Survey. *J Nerv Ment Dis* 193:450-454.

Schneier, F.R.; Johnson, J.; Hornig, C.D.; Liebowitzm, M.R.; Weissman, M. (1992). Social phobia: Comorbidity and morbidity in an epidemiological sample. *Arch Gen Psychiatry*, 49: 282-288.

Schmidtke and Hafner (1998). The weather effect after television films. *Psychological Medicine*, 18: 665-676.

Schmidtke, A.; Fricke, S.; and Lester, D. (1999). Suicide among German Federal and state police officers. *Psychological Reports, 84*, 157-166.

Schou, M. (1998). The effect of prophylactic lithium treatment on mortality and suicidal behaviour. *Journal of Affective Disorders*, 50: 253-259.

Stanley, M. and Mann, J.J. (1982). Increased serotonin- 2 binding sites in frontal cortex of suicide victims. *lacent*, 1, 214-216.

Viallant, G. (1966). Twelve year follow-up of New York narcotic addicts. *American Journal of Psychiatry*, 122, 727-737.

Vijayakumar, L. (2003). Psychosocial risk factors for suicide in India. *Suicide Prevention – Meeting the Challenge Together*. Ed Vijayakumar. L Orient Longman. 149-162.

Vijayakumar, L.; Rajkumar, S. (1999). Are risk factors for suicide universal? A case control study in India. *Acta Psychiatrica Scondinavia.* 99, 407-411.

Weissman, M.; Fox, K.; and Keerman, G.L. (1973). Hostility and depression associated with suicide attempts. *American Journal of Psychiatry*, 130, 450-456.

WHO (World Health Organization). (1999). Figures and Facts Anput Suicide. Geneva: Department of Mental Health, World Health Organization. Simpson S.G., Jamison K.R. The risk of suicide in patients with bipolar disorder. *Journal of Clinical Psychiatry*, 1999, 60, Suppl. 2: 53-56.

WHO. (1992). International Statistical Classification of Diseases and Related Health Problems, Tenth Revision. (1) Geneva, World Health Organization.

14

Causes of Stress and Burnout in Doctors

Anubhuti Dubey and *Darshana Shahi*

Feelings of job dissatisfaction and job stress are problems shared by general practitioners in many countries (Bailie *et al.*, 1998; Burdi and Baker, 1998; Dowell, Hamilton and McLoad, 2000; Kirwan and Armstrong, 1995; Calnan *et al.*, 2001). General physicians' state lack of time and work overload as the most important causes for feelings of discontent and stress (Appleton, House and Dowell, 1998; Dowell, Coster and Maffey, 2002; Huby *et al.*, 2002; Sibbald, Bojke and Gravelle, 2003) and long-term negative feelings may lead to burnout (Van Dierendonck, Schaufeli and Sixma, 1994; Demerouti, Bakker, Nachselincr and Schaufeli, 2001). Unfortunately, many of the people who undergo from stress are the health-care providers themselves. Burnout may be the outcome of unrelenting stress, but it isn't the same as too much stress. Stress, by and large, involves '*too much*', *burnout,* on the other hand, is about '*not enough*' *and being* burned out means feeling empty, devoid of motivation, and beyond caring. While burnout is a defence characterized by disengagement, stress is characterized by over-engagement. In burnout emotions become blunt, whereas, the stress response is more likely to involve emotional over-reactivity. Burnout produces helplessness and hopelessness, stress produces urgency and hyperactivity. Both states can lead to depression; the depressions have distinct, etiologies. In burnout depression is secondary to the grief experienced over loss of one's ideals, however, in stress, depression is related to the physical needs to conserve energy and protect the body. And while stress can lead to panic, phobic and anxiety-type disorders, burnout is more linked to paranoia, detachment and depersonalization.

The contribution of Gil-Monte, Peiró and Valcárcel (1998) about the etiology, process and consequences of burnout syndrome, and an emphasis on reciprocity, or transaction is worth noting. The relationship between experiencing stress (because of mental overload, under-load, and conflict of role or role ambiguity) and its consequences (stress symptoms, health problems) may be mediated by the onset of burnout syndrome (stress response).

Stress

Work stress is more and more acknowledged as one of the gravest occupational health hazards reducing workers' satisfaction and productivity, and increasing absenteeism and turnover (Gianakos, 2001). Hospital staff in particular is subject to work related stress merely because they are harshly challenged by their rapidly changing environment (Al-Aameri, 2000). Earlier researches revealed that there were many causes correlated to work stress found within the workers' personality and within the work environment (Newman and Beehr, 1979). Studies reported that work overload and influenced home life; poor administration and resources; administrative responsibilities assumed; and dealing with patients' pain were perceived as sources of stress (Alphonsa, 2011; Xianyu and Lambert, 2006; Al-Omar, 2003), The strain of working day in and day out with too many patients, taking responsibility for critical decisions based on ambiguous information, facing the potentially serious consequences of these decisions, and the attendant pressure to avoid mistakes, are among the job conditions that render medicine inherently stressful career (Sanders, Suls, Maslach, and Jackson, 1982; McManus, Keeling, and Paice, 2004; Piko, 2006).

Burnout

Coined by Freudenberger (1974), the term burnout is most commonly used in the human service fields to "refer to a state of emotional exhaustion caused by excessive psychological and emotional demands made on people helping profession" (Jackson, Schwab, and Schuler, 1986). With growing assertion on professionalism increasing attention has been paid to the phenomena of burnout in human service professions. Burnout appears to be a response to interpersonal stressors on the job in which an overload of contact with people results in changes in attitudes and behaviours towards them. Paine (1982) has observed the Burnout Stress Syndrome (BOSS). It is the consequence of high levels of job stress, personal frustration, and inadequate coping skills which have major personal and social costs and these costs are probably increasing. BOSS is a debilitating psychological condition brought about by unrelieved work stress. Four types of consequences can arise from it— (a) depletion of energy reserves, (b) lowered resistance to illness, (c) increased dissatisfaction and pessimism, and (d) increased absenteeism and inefficiency at work.

Burnout is "an experience of physical, emotional, and mental exhaustion, caused by long-term involvement in situations that are emotionally demanding" (Mateen, and Dorji, 2009). Another valuable definition is "Burnout is the index of location between what people are and what they have to do. It represents erosion in values, dignity, spirit, and will and erosion of the human soul" (Cole and Carlin, 2009). It may manifest as depersonalization, low productivity, and feelings of low achievement.

Some occupations aim burnout to their holders, like consultancy. Allegra *et al.* (2003) found that the rate of burnout in the U.S. oncology community exceeded 60 per cent. The survey was administered to 1,740 oncologists, of which 22.6 per cent responded. The top three signs of burnout reported were frustration (78%), emotional exhaustion (69%) and lack of satisfaction with their work (50%). The most frequently cited causes for self-reported burnout included overwork, lack of time away from the office and reimbursement concerns. Brewer and Shapard (2004) stated that the environmental and organizational factors which have shown to effect burnout are work overload, role conflict, role ambiguity, the work environment, and support from the supervisors. Negative relationships exist between the burnout indicators—exhaustion, depersonalization, and diminished efficacy and various outcomes, such as job satisfaction (Mirvis, Graney and Kilpatrick, 1999), patient satisfaction (Leiter, Harvie and Frizzell, 1998) and self-assessed quality of care. Work overload contributes to predicting exhaustion and cynicism; professional values crises contribute to predicting exhaustion, cynicism, and low professional efficacy. The interaction of values and workload for women in particular has implications for the distinct work-life patterns of male and female physicians. Specifically, the congruence of individual values with values inherent in the health care system appeared to be of greater consequence for women than for men (Leiter, Frank and Matheson, 2009).

Goldberg *et al.* (1996) identified major correlates of burnout as negative perception of self, negative practice habits and attitudes, unhealthy life styles, lack of job involvement, dissatisfaction with career, high level of alcohol consumption, intent to leave practice within 10 years' and lower level of exercise. Symptoms of burnout can lead to physician error, and these errors can in turn contribute to burnout (Crane, 1998). Given the potential human costs of medical mistakes, the emotional impact of actual or perceived errors can be devastating for physicians. Some occupations aim burnout to their holders, like consultancy. Allegra *et al.* (2003) found that the rate of burnout in the U.S. oncology community exceeded 60 per cent. The survey was administered to 1,740 oncologists, of which 22.6 per cent responded. The top three signs of burnout reported were frustration (78%), emotional exhaustion (69%) and lack of satisfaction with their work (50%). The most frequently cited causes for self-reported burnout included overwork, lack of time away from the office and reimbursement concerns. High stress and low personal accomplishment were seen in Canadian gynaecologic oncologists (Elit *et al.*, 2004). Brewer and Shapard (2004) stated that the environmental and organizational factors which have shown to effect burnout are—work overload, role conflict, role ambiguity, the work environment, and support from the supervisors. Research shows consistently that mental challenge-assuming one is willing to respond to the challenge is a critical determinant of job satisfaction (Judge, 2000). Negative relationships exist between the burnout indicators—exhaustion, depersonalization, and diminished efficacy—and various outcomes, such as job satisfaction (Mirvis, Graney and Kilpatrick, 1999), patient satisfaction (Leiter, Harvie and Frizzell, 1998) and self-assessed quality of care. Identifying work engagementas a contrast to burnout Schaufeli and Bakker (2004) has broadened the question to encompass the vigour and dedication people bring to their work. Less than debilitating breakdowns can erode the quality of physicians' work (Gabbard, 1985). Burnout is common among American surgeons and is the single greatest predictor of surgeons' satisfaction with career and specialty choice (Shanafelt *et al.*, 2009).

Ozyurt, Hayran and Sur (2010) explored the predictors of burnout and job satisfaction among Turkish physicians and found that job satisfaction was inversely correlated with emotional exhaustion and depersonalization, and positively correlated with personal accomplishment. Under multilevel regression, the most significant and common predictors of all burnout dimensions and job satisfaction were the number of vacations at individual level, and public ownership of healthcare facilities at group level. Number of shifts per month was also a significant predictor of all burnout dimensions. Similarly, Jamal (2008) examined the relationship of job stress and burnout level and job satisfaction in two developing countries, namely Pakistan and Malaysia. After using regression analysis he found significant relationship between the job stress and job burnout with job satisfaction. Zhu *et al.* (2006) had investigated the status of job burnout in doctors of China and its relationship with occupational stress. Surgeon and doctors working in the internal medicine wards scored significantly higher in job burnout than their colleagues. The 30-40 years of age group scored highest in exhaustion. The score of professional efficacy decreased with age and increased with educational levels. Role overload, responsibility, physical environment, reaction and self-care were major predictors for exhaustion. Role insufficiency, role overload and responsibility were major predictors for cynicism. Role insufficiency, social support and rational/cognitive were major predictors for professional efficacy.

Bhugra, Bhui and Gupta (2008) had approached 100 members of Indian Medical Association and Dental College and found that on all three scales of Maslach burnout inventory the participants scored low. Key symptoms of depersonalization and emotional exhaustion each were present in less than half of the respondents. They concluded that being in private practice gives professional more control over their job style and may be responsible for low levels of burnout.

Consequences of burnout are visible in different areas of life, but first of all burnout disrupt family life, weaken the relationship with children and spouse, sometimes leading to its total severance. Health problems also appear and it may happen that a person with a syndrome of burnout simply runs away in a disease. Suicide attempts appear in extreme cases. The abuse of liquor, medicines, and drugs is not rare, all of which have consequences for work. Female physicians are more likely to experience work family conflict involving incompatible demands. The significant relationship between work-family conflict and emotional exhaustion indicate that physicians who experience greater conflict resulting from performing both work and family roles tend to experience greater emotional exhaustion (Ray and Miller, 1994; Bergman *et al.*, 2008; Fu and Shaffer, 2001). Similarly, many of the researchers found out, turnover intentions as the consequence of job burnout (Valentine *et al.*, 2006). Khudsen, Ducharme and Raman (2006) assessed the associations between job burnout turnover intention, and three aspects of organizational culture that are centralized decision-making, procedural justice, and distribution justice. Employee's turnover intentions were a concern for most types of organizations which have high turnover intentions of employees and may be more responsive in job burnout. Preventing burnout, a responsibility of all physicians and of the health care systems and organizations in which they work, entails the explicit promotion of physician well-being (Anderson, Gabbe and Christensen, 2002).

Objectives

Many recent studies have shown that increasing numbers of physicians and resident doctors are feeling stress and burnout and are feeling dissatisfaction with their professional life (Spickard, Gabbe, and Christensen, 2002; Linzer, Konrad and Douglas, 2002; Williams, Konrad and Scheckler, 2001). The first objective of the present study is to identify the sources of stress in health care professionals. The study will also emphasize to explore the factors other than workplace conditions and job pressure, which can further aggravate the intensity and frequency of their stress. The second objective of the present research work is that the prolonged stress renders these professionals susceptible to burnout. Several studies in western and oriental countries have been done which show a significant relationship between stress and burnout. But in Indian context this phenomenon has not been given ample attention in health care setup. Therefore, an attempt will be made to investigate the stress-burnout relationship specifically in Indian context in health care professionals.

Method

Sample: The sample consisted of 200 doctors (158 Male and 42 Female) aged between 30-60 years. They were from the districts of the urban area of Gorakhpur city and Kushinagar. The 100 participants have M.S./M.D. degree either in general surgery, E.N.T., gynaecology or in other emergency clinical branches of medicine. The other 100 participants were M.B.B.S. degree holder and are practicing as the general physicians. All the doctors were having degrees in Allopathic system of medicine. All of them were married and having children.

Materials: In the present investigation, six tools have been used. The detailed description of these tools have been given below –

Perceived Stress Scale (PSS): This questionnaire was developed by Cohen (1988). This is a widely used scale to assess perceived stress. It is a measure of the degree to which situations in one's life one appraises as stressful. The scale consists of 24 items. The responses were made on four point scale ranging from (1) does not apply to me to (4) does apply to me. PSS scores are obtained by reversing responses to the four positively stated items and then summing across all scale items. The validity and retest reliability was sought. The retest reliability after four weeks of interval was found 0.77.

Open Ended Interview Schedule for Sources of Stress: To find out the sources of stress amongst the doctors two open ended questions were framed—one is related to sources of stress at work place and other is sources of stress at home.

Burnout: Burnout was assessed by using Copenhagan Burnout Inventory (CBI). This scale was developed by Marianne Borritz (1999). The CBI is a 19-item self report inventory. The inventory is very easy and fast to respond. The responses were made on a five point scale ranged from (5) Always to (1) Never/almost never. The inventory measures three types of burnout, viz. personal burnout, work burnout and client burnout. The Cronbach's alpha for personal burnout was found 0.86, for work burnout was 0.87 and for client burnout 0.85. The inter-item correlation ranged from 0.37-0.67.

Results

To seek the causes of stress in doctors, the researcher has asked an open ended question before going through the standardized questionnaire of stress. The responses made by both groups of doctors were categorized as causes of stress related to work place and family. These were presented in Tables 14.1 and 14.2 respectively. Table 14.1 demonstrated that four

Table 14.1: Causes of stress produced by work as mentioned by doctors

Doctor Groups	*Causes*
General Practitioners (Not Frequently exposed to Emergency duties)	1. Poor Working Conditions 2. Work Overload 3. Patient Overload 4. Malfunctioning Health Care systems 5. Incomes less than their expectations 6. Lack of patient cooperation 7. Lack of Knowledge of patients is frustrating 8. Poor social recognition and prestige as compared to specialized doctors
Specialized Doctors (Frequently involved in Emergency and Critical Care)	1. Poor working conditions 2. Work Overload 3. Patient Overload 4. Malfunctioning Health Care Systems 5. Untimely Emergency Calls 6. Neglect by paramedical staff 7. Poor assistant staff to post-operative care of patients 8. Myths and misconceptions of patients regarding surgery 9. Poor adherence of patients

causes of work stress were common in two groups of doctors, i.e. poor working conditions, work overload, patient overload and malfunctioning health care system. However, the general practitioners had also emphasized that sometimes patients do not cooperate in the treatment process and it is frustrating. Apart from this in comparison to specialized doctors they earn less and have poor social recognition and prestige.

The specialized doctors are frequently engaged in emergency services, therefore, untimely emergency calls sometimes produces stress to them as they have to cut their family time for their profession. Other causes of stress as delineated by these doctors are related to surgery and paramedical staff. The doctors felt that many a time's unskilled paramedical staff and unsatisfactory post-operative care spoil all their efforts of doing good surgical procedure and giving relief to patients. From patient's point of view, the doctors said that there are many myths and misconceptions regarding surgery are prevailing in society and they hinder in recovery process and this is stressful for doctors.

Table 14.2: Causes of Stress produced by family

Doctor Groups	*Causes*
General Practitioners (Not Frequently exposed to Emergency duties)	1. Time Pressure 2. Unhealthy life style 3. Little time to spend with family 4. Education of children as not good schools at interior places
Specialized Doctors (Frequently involved in emergency and Critical Care)	1. Time Pressure 2. Unhealthy life style 3. Little time to spend with family

The three family related causes, i.e. time pressure, unhealthy life style and little leisure time to spend with family was voiced by both groups of doctors. The general practitioners were generally doing medical practices at the places far away from the district headquarters, where schooling for children is not up to their expectation. Therefore, they established their families at headquarters and daily commute to their work place to home and *vice versa*.

Stress-Burnout Relationship

The mean, S.D. and F-ratio of stress and burnout score in two groups, i.e. general practitioners and specialized groups have been presented in Table 14.3.

Table 14.3: Mean, S.D. of Stress and Burnout as a function of Profession Specialization

Variables	General Practitioners		Specialized Doctors		F
	Mean	S.D.	Mean	S.D	
Stress	62.83	7.02	55.97	9.12	35.74**
Burnout	48.57	7.17	41.47	8.25	42.42**

Note: P < .01** P < .05 *

The results showed that the F-ratio for the main effect of stress was significant. The stress level of general practitioners (M = 62.83) was significantly higher than mean stress of specialized group (M = 55.97). Similarly, the F-ratio for burnout was also found significant. The mean table indicated that mean burnout for general practitioners group (M =48.57) was higher, than the mean of specialized doctors group (M = 41.47). These findings display that general practitioners have more stress and burnout than their specialized counterparts (Table 14.3).

The findings are in consonance with the earlier researches that stress and burnout are significantly and highly correlated. This section of results had also made it clear that general practitioners group of doctors have more stress and related burnout than the group of doctors having post-graduate degrees in specialized areas.

Discussion

Causes of Stress in Doctors

The job demands and job stress is higher in the medical professionals working at the upper level of medical organizations hierarchy (both General practitioners and specialized) in comparison to other medical personals like nurses, technicians, ward boys and paramedical staffs. In an answer to the question "Why are doctors so unhappy?" Smith (2001) concluded that the most obvious case of doctors' unhappiness is that they feel over worked and under supported. The fundamentals of good health (i.e. healthy diet, regular exercise, adequate rest and sleep, sufficient recreation, social interaction, and meaningful involvement in one's family and community) are well-known to all practitioners, despite this they frequently trapped in stress and burnout.

In this study, poor working conditions, work overload and above all malfunctioning health care system, the causes of stress related to work environment as mentioned by doctors in interview schedule (Table 14.1). Especially in the case of specialized doctors, one of the major reasons of stress was untimely emergency calls and neglect by paramedical and assistant staff to post operative care of patients (Table 14.1). Doctors spend a great deal of their working time with patients who desperately need help. When patients show gratification after recovery, it can be rewarding. However, as patients become more demanding doctors are more regularly confronted with lack of reciprocity. Along with this the doctors in emergency care have always had little time to spend with family and children (Table 14.2). As the findings of the present investigation are clearly indicating that burnout was significantly more in general practitioners (MBBS) than in specialized doctors (MS/MD) group of participants. Work overload, job demands, work pressure, emotional demands were the factors which most significantly predict burnout (Cam, 2001; Bakker, Demerouti and Verbeke, 2004). Other researchers have also found a strong relationship between work overload and burnout (Brewer and Shapard, 2004). The overload can be physical or emotional and no matter which one of them it is, if the overload exceeds a person's ability to cope with it, we call it stress. Both workload and time pressure have been significantly connected to burnout.

Stress-Burnout Relationship

Burnout is a combination of three types of exhaustion such as physical, mental and emotional exhaustion that leads to employee turnover and low job satisfaction (Weisberg, 1994). The current study undertakes the same concept but with few adjustments. This study is based on examining the relationship of burnout (i.e. work burnout, personal burnout and client burnout) among general practitioners and specialized doctors with work life balance, psychological immunity with well-being. This study found a high degree of stress and burnout among general physicians. The lack of association between stress and burnout with any demographic factors, including age, sex, practice experience, or type of remuneration, suggests that all medical practitioners are vulnerable. Burnout might not be due to demographic factors, but could be due to practice or personal issues. Previous studies have also shown no association between demographic characteristics and burnout or work satisfaction (Zuger, 2004; Bovier and Perneger, 2003). Stress and burnout experienced by specialists in their work environment have been shown to have an impact on their mental and physical health (Spurgeon and Harrington, 1989). Employees with excessive workload would experience negative emotions, fatigue and tension (Jones *et al.*, 2010; Peiro *et al.*, 2001; Fu and Shaffer, 2001). Such feelings would then lead to an increase in the intensity of emotional exhaustion. Firth-Cozens (1998, 2003) had attributed the role overload of physicians in his study to the increase in the number of outpatients to be attended each day and the increase in the number of patients in the ward. The considerably high level of role overload experienced by the physicians in this present study could be due to similar reasons. In the present investigation the doctors of both groups had mentioned work and patient overload as a major cause of stress which leads to burnout.

Doctors being on integral part of the society provide health care services to the community. Ahmed (2010) reported that in Pakistan there is only one doctor available to 1212 persons to get health care facilities (Economic Survey of Pakistan, 2008-09). This ascertains that burnout affects on their job satisfaction, work life balance, work life conflict, and turnover intentions. This study provides the insight for the doctors to manage their burnout level by availing maximum work life balance facilities and to maximum the job satisfaction is a developing country like Pakistan. The situation in India is not very different from that of Pakistan. The doctor patient ratio is very poor here also and condition in rural areas is worse than cities.

Generally, the studies had indicated that the doctors with specialization report more stress and burnout than the doctors having only bachelor's degree in medicine and not frequently involved in emergency care (Goldberg *et al.*, 1996). The doctor's who perceive high level of job related stress and are in emergency branches are having more burnout and stress. The major correlates of burnout were identified as negative perception of self, negative practice habits and attitudes, unhealthy life styles, lack of job involvement, dissatisfaction with career, high level of alcohol consumption, intent to leave practice within 10 years and lower level of exercise (Goldberg *et al.*, 1996) and emotional maturity was the most significant protective factors against burnout along with adjustment capabilities, sense of physical well-being (Chakraborty, Chatterjee and Chaudhary, 2012). The others associated factors which inter-section the level of stress and burnout were family problem, time pressure, unhealthy life styles and over work load. Emergency medical services provided outside the hospital emergency room setting are often delivered in a hostile world where darkness, adverse weather conditions, difficult terrain, and unpredictable dangers magnify the pressure (Linton,

Kommor, and Webb, 1993; Miller, 1995). Added to these environmental stressors is the constant pressure for practitioners to perform competently.

However, in the present investigation the results are contradictory to some of the earlier research findings. Doctors in general practice have more stress and burnout than there more specialized counterparts who frequently involved in emergency and critical care. The reasons for this as given by general practitioners were related to both work and family. The work related causes were poor working conditions, work and patient overload and over all malfunctioning health care system. The general practitioners were mostly practicing in the rural areas of the region both in government hospitals and in private setup; they are not satisfied with their prestige and income. Besides this they have tremendous patients overload with least facilities both at infrastructure level and of staff and paramedical help. The patients of the rural background having their own belief system also causes stress as many a times they are not being able to understand the treatment process and therefore, do not adhere and cooperate. All these factors are major sources of stress and over a period of time, these stressors have made a cumulative impact and the doctors feel burnout.

Nevertheless, these findings are in consonance with the earlier researches that stress and burnout are significantly and highly correlated. The results had also made it clear that in both general practitioners and the specialized doctors group the stress and burnout had a strong, significant and positive correlation (Table 14.3) (Steijn, 2004; Noor and Moad, 2008). Stress was not only correlated with total burnout but also with all the three aspects of burnout, i.e. personal, work and client burnout in both groups. Noor and Moad (2008) revealed that the relationship between stress, one of the causes of burnout, work life conflict and stress have a significant positive relationship with turnover intentions.

This significant finding is worth to mention that the general practitioners with high stress are especially at risk of burnout. This is alarming as the consequences of doctors' burnout are serious, not only because it reflects personal suffering but also because burnout threatens the quality of care doctors are expected to deliver. General practitioners, physicians working in the public sector, those who have more shifts, and have fewer vacations per year, seem to be at high risk of burnout (Ozyurt, Hayran, and Sur, 2010). These findings are similar to the results of other studies. For example, in a Finnish study, the highest burnout scores were noted in general practitioners and non-specialists working in health centres. This was attributed to heavy patient loads, long hours, and problems of professional identity (Olkinuora, Asp, Juntunen *et al.*, 1990). However, because medical specialties differ widely in their job characteristics in ways that appear to affect the relative prevalence of burnout, it is difficult to reach universal conclusions.

References

Ahmad, A. (2010). Work-Family Conflict among Junior Physicians: Its Mediating Role in the Relationship between Role Overload and Emotional Exhaustion. *Journal of Social Sciences,* 6(2), 265-271.

Al-Aameri, A.S. (2000). Job satisfaction and organizational commitment for nurses. *Saudi Medical Journal*, 21(6): 531-535.

Allegra, C.J.; Hall, R. and Yothers, G. (2005). Prevalence of burnout in the U.S. oncology community: Results of a 2003 survey. *Journal of Oncology Practice*, 1: 140-147.

Alphonsa, A.K. (2011). A study on stress among health care professionals in Father Muller Medical hospital. A dissertation submitted to Rajiv Gandhi University of Health Sciences, Bangalore, Karnataka.

Al-Omar, B.A. (2003). Sources of work stress among hospital staff at the Saudi MOH, *JAKU: Economics and Administration*, Vol. 17(1), 3-16.

Anderson, S. Jr.; Gabbe, S.G.; and Christensen, J.F., (2002). Mid-career burnout in Generalist and Specialist physicians, *JAMA*, 288(12), 1447-1450.

Appleton, K.; House, A.; and Dowell, A. (1998). A survey of job satisfaction, sources of stress and psychological symptoms among general practitioners in Leeds. *British Journal of General Practice*, 48, 1059-1063.

Bailie, R.; Sibthorpe, B.; Douglas, B.; Broom, D., Attewell, R., and McGuiness, C. (1998). Mixed feelings: Satisfaction and disillusionment among Australian GPs. *Family Practice,* 15: 58-66.

Bakker, A.B., Demerouti, E. and Verbeke, W. (2004). Using the job demands-resources model to predict burnout and performance. *Human Resource Management*, Vol. 43(1), 83-104.

Bergman, B.; Ahmad F. and Stewart, D.F. (2008). Work family balance, stress and salivary cortisol in men. and women academic physicians. *International Journal of Behavioural Medicine,* 15(1), 54-61.

Bhugra, D.; Bhui, K.S. and Gupta, K.R. (2008). Burnout among doctors and dentists in North India. *International Journal of Culture and Mental Health,* Vol. 1(1), 24-29.

Bovier, P., and Perneger, T. (2003). Predictors of work satisfaction among physicians. *European Journal of Public Health,* 13(1): 81–87.

Borritz, M. (1999). The Copenhagen Burnout Inventory: A new tool for the assessment of burnout. *Work and Stress: An International Journal of Work, Health and Organizations*, Volume 19, Issue 3, 192-207.

Brewer, E.W., Shapard, L., (2004). Employee burnout: A meta analysis of the relationship between age or years of experience. *Human Resource Development Review*, 3, 102-123.

Burdi, M.D. and Baker, L.C. (1998). *Physicians' perceptions of autonomy and satisfaction in California.* Health Aff (Millwood), 18: 134-145.

Calnan, M.; Wainwright, D.; Forsythe, M.; Wall, B., and Almond, S. (2001). Mental health and stress in the workplace: the case of general practice in the UK. *Social Science Medicine,* 52: 499-507.

Cam, O. (2001). The burnout in nursing academicians. *International Journal of Nursing Studies*, Vol. 38 (1), 201-207.

Chakraborty, R.; Chatterjee, A.; and Chaudhary, S. (2012). Internal predictors of burnout in psychiatric nurses: An Indian study. *Industrial Psychiatry Journal,* 21(2): 119-124.

Cohen, J. (1988). *Statistical power analysis for the behavioural sciences* (2nd ed.). Hillsdale, NJ: Lawrence Erlbaum.

Cole, T.R. and Carlin, N. (2009). The suffering of physicians. *Lancet.* October 24, 374 (9699): 1414-15.

Crane. M. (1998). Why burned-out doctors get sued more often. *Med Econ.,* 75:210-218.

Demerouti, E.; Bakker, A.B.; Nachreiner, F. and Schaufeli, W.B. (2001). The job demands resources model of burnout. *Journal of Applied Psychology,* 86, 499-512.

Dowell, A.C.; Hamilton, S.; McLeod, D.K. (2000). Job satisfaction, psychological morbidity and job stress among New Zealand general practitioners. *New Zealand Medical Journal*, 113: 269-272.

Dowell, A.C.; Coster, G.; and Maffey, C. (2002). Morale in general practice: crisis and solutions. *New Zealand Medical Journal,* 115(1158): U102.

Elit, L.; Trim, K.; Mand-Bains, I.G.; Sussman, J. and Grunfeld, E. (2004). Job Satisfaction, stress and burnout among Canadian gynaecologic oncologists, *Gynaecologic Oncologist*, 94, 134-139.

Firth-Cozens, Jenny (2003). Doctors, their well-being, and their stress. *BMJ.* March 29, 2003; 326(7391): 670-671.

Firth-Cozens, Jenny and Moss, Fiona. (1998). Hours, sleep, teamwork, and stress: Sleep and teamwork matter as much as hours in reducing doctors' stress. *British Medical Journal,* 317 (14 November): 1335-1336.

Freudenberger, H.J. (1974). Staff burnout. *Journal of Social Issues,* 30(1).

Fu, C.K. and Shaffer, M.A. (2001). The tug of work and family: Direct and indirect domain-specific determinants of work family conflict. *Personal Review*, Vol. 30(5), 502-522.

Gabbard, G.O. (1985). The role of compulsiveness in the normal physician, *JAMA*; 254(20): 2926-9.

Gianakos, I. (2000). "Gender Roles and Coping with work stress", *Sex Roles: A Journal of Research* (June): 1-13. http://www.findarticles.com/cf_0/m2294/2000_June/66011972/print.jhtml in 12/12/1420h.

Gil-Monte, P.R.; Peiró, J.M.; and Valcárcel, P. (1998). A model of burnout process development: an alternative from appraisal models of stress. *Comportamen to Organizacional e gestao,* 4(1), 165-179.

Goldberg, R.; Boss, R.W.; Chan, L.; Goldberg, J.; Mallon, W.K.; Morazadeh, D.; Goodman, E.A. and Mclonkie, M.L. (1996). Burnout and its correlates in emergency physicians: Four years experience with a wellness booth. *Academy of Emergency Medicine,* 3 (12), 1156-64.

Huby, G.; Gerry, M.; McKinstry, B.; Porter, M.; Shaw, J.; and Wrate, R., (2002). Morale among general practitioners: Qualitative study exploring relations between partnership arrangements, personal style, and workload. *British Medical Journal,* 325(7356): 140-144.

Jackson, S.E.; Schwab, R.L.; and Schuler, R.S. (1986). Toward an understanding of the burnout phenomenon. *Journal of Applied Psychology,* 71(4), 630-640.

Jamal, M. (2008). Burnout among Employees of a Multinational Corporation in Malasia and Pakistan: An Empirical Investigation, *International Management Review,* 4(i), 60-70.

Jones, A.; C.S. Norman and B. Wier, (2010). Healthy lifestyle as a coping mechanism for role stress in public accounting. *Behaviour Research Account.,* 22: 21-41. DOI: 10.2308/bria.2010.22.1.21.

Judge, T.A. (2000) Promote job satisfaction through mental challenge. In E.A. Lacke (Ed.) *Handbook of Principles of Organizational Behaviour*, pp. 75-89. Oxford, England: Black Well.

Kirwan, M.F.; and Armstrong, D. (1995). Investigation of burnout in a sample of British general practitioners. *British Journal General Practice,* 45: 259-260.

Khudsen, H.K.; Ducharme, L.J. and Romen, P.M. (2006). Counselor emotional exhaustion and turnover intentions, in therapeutic communities, *Journal of Substance Abuse, Treatment*, 31, 73-180.

Leiter, M.P.; Frank, E.; and Matheson, T.J. (2009). Demands, values and burnout. *Canadian Family Physician*, 55, 1224-25.

Leiter, M.P.; Harvie, P.; and Frizzell, C. (1998). The correspondence of patient satisfaction and nurse burnout. *Social Science Medicine,* 47(10): 1611-17.

Linton, J.C.; Kommor, M.J.; and Webb, C.H. (1993). Helping the helpers: The development of a critical incident stress management team through university/community cooperation. *Annals of Emergency Medicine*, 22, 663-668.

Linzer, M.; Konrad, T.R.; Douglas, J.; *et al.* (2002). Managed care, time pressure, and physician job satisfaction. *Journal of General Internal Medicine,* 15:441-450.

Mateen, F.J.; and Dorji, C. (2009). Health-care worker burnout and the mental health imperative. *Lancet,* 22; 374(9690): 595-97.

Miller, L. (1995). Tough guys: Psychotherapeutic strategies with law enforcement and emergency services personnel. *Psychotherapy*, 32(4), 592-600.

Mirvis, D.M.; Graney, M.J.; and Kilpatrick, A.O. (1999). Burnout among leaders of the Department of Veterans Affairs medical centers: contributing factors as determined by a longitudinal study. *J Health Hum Serv Adm* 21(3): 390-412.

McManus, I.C.; Keeling, A. and Paice, E. (2004). Burnout and doctors' attitude to work and determined by personality and learning style: A twelve years longitudinal study of U.K. medical graduates. *BMC Medicine,* 1186-1741-7015-2-29.

Newman, J. and Beehr, T. (1979). Personal and organizational strategies for Handling stress. A Review of Research and Opinion ? *Personnel Psychology,* spring: 1-44.

Noor, S. and Moad, N. (2008). Examining the Relationship between work life conflict, stress and Turnover Intentions among Marketing Executives in Pakistan. *International Journal of Business and Management,* 3(2), 93-102.

Olkinuora, M.; Asp, S.; Juntunen, J., *et al. (1990).* Stress symptoms, burnout and suicidal thoughts in Finnish physicians. *Social Psychiatry Epidemiology,* 25:81-86.

Ozyurt, A.; Hayran, O. and Sur, A. (2010). Predictors of burnout and job satisfaction among Turkish physicians, *QJM: An International Journal of Medicine,* Vol. 99 (3), 161-169.

Paine, W.S. (1982). *Job stress and burnout: Research, theory and intervention.* London: Sage Publications.

Peiró, J.M.; González-Romá, V.; Tordera, N.; and Mañas, M.A. (2001). Does role stress predict burnout over time among health care professionals? *Psychology and Health,* Volume 16, Issue 5, 511-525.

Piko, B.F. (2006). Burnout, role conflict, job satisfaction and psychosocial health among Hungarian health care staff: A questionnaire survey. *International Journal of Nursing Studies,* doi:10.1016/j.ijnurstu.2005.05.00.

Ray, E.B. and K.I. Miller (1994). Social support, home/work stress and burnout: Who can help? *Journal of Applied Behaviour Science,* 30: 357-373.

Shanafelt, Tait D.; Balch, Charles, M., Bechamps, Gerald J., Russell, Thomas, Dyrbye, Lotte, Satele, Daniel, Collicott, Paul, Novotny, Paul, J., Sloan, Jeff, Freischlag, Julie, A. (2009). Burnout and Career Satisfaction Among American Surgeons. *Annals of Surgery,* Vol. 205(3), 461-473.

Sanders, G.S.; Suls, J.; Maslach, C.; and Jackson, S.E. (1982). Burnout in health professions: A social psychological analysis. *In:* Sanders, G.S., Suls, J., (ed). *Social Psychology of Health and Illness.* 3rd eds. Hillsdale NJ: Lawrence Erlbaum, pp. 227-51.

Schaufeli, W.B.; and Bakker, A.B. (2004). Job demands, job resources and their relationship with burnout and engagement: a multi-sample study. *Journal of Organizational Behaviour,* 25(3): 293-315.

Sibbald, B.; Bojke, C.; and Gravelle, H. (2003). National survey of job satisfaction and retirement intentions among general practitioners in England. *British Medical Journal,* 326: 22-25.

Smith, R. (2001). Why are doctors so unhappy? *British Medical Journal,* 322:1073-1074.

Spickard, A.; Gabbe, S.; Christensen J. (2002). Mid-career burnout in generalist and specialist physicians. *JAMA*, 288:1447-1450.

Spurgeon, A.; and Harrington, J.M. (1989). Work performance and health of junior hospital doctors: A review of the literature. *Work and Stress,* 3, 117-128.

Steijn, B. (2004). Human Resources Management and Job satisfaction in the Dutch Public Sector. *Review of Public Personal Administration*, 24(4), 291-303.

Velentine, Sean, Greller, Martin, M., and Richtermeyer, Sandra, B. (2006). Employee job response as a function of ethical context and perceived organization support. *Journal of Business Research*, 59, 582-88.

Van Dierendonck, D., Schaufeli, W., and Sixma, H. (1994). Burnout among general practitioners: A perspective from equity theory. *Journal of Social and Clinical Psychology,* 13(1): 86-100.

Weisberg, J. (1994). Measuring workers burnout and intention to leave, *International Journal of Manpower*, 15 (1), 4-14.

Williams, E.S.; Konrad, T.R.; Scheckler, D.P. (2001). Understanding physicians' intentions to withdraw from practice: the role of job satisfaction, job stress, mental and physical health. *Health Care Management Review,* 26, 7-19.

Xianyu, Y. and Lambert, V.A. (2006), Investigation of the relationships among workplace stressors, ways of coping, and the mental health of Chinese head nurses. *Nursing and Health Sciences*, 8: 147-155. doi: 10.1111/j.1442-2018.2006.00281.x

Zhu, W., Wang, Z.M., Wang, Z.M., Lan, Y.Z., and Wu, S.Y. (2006). Occupational stress and job burnout in doctors. *SichuanDa Xue XueBao Yi Xue Ban,* 37 (2), 281-308.

Zuger, A. (2004). Dissatisfaction with medical practice. *New England Journal of Medicine*; 350(1): 69-75.

15

Environmental Toxins

A Threat to Mental Health

Jyotsana Shukla

There is evidence regarding mental health outcomes of toxic exposure for humans, the role of environmental toxins in suppressing the healthy development of the brain and nervous system and how certain environmental pollutants could be undermining the health conditions of those who already have a learning, developmental or behavioural disorder? In a developing country like ours where we are already pressed with various social problems and lack of health infrastructure, exposure to toxic chemicals and their harmful consequences on mental health would be an additional burden.

Behavioural Toxicology is a well-known area of scientific inquiry. It recognizes the fact that the adverse health impact of environmental chemicals should also be seen from the perspective of how people feel and behave, not just by the number of deaths and by the extent of tissue damage.

The mental health impacts of toxins cover a wide spectrum of mental illnesses, such as, neurotoxicity, acute stress, combined neurotoxic injury, pre-existing mental illness made worse by neurotoxicity and/or acute stress, mass hysteria (no chemical is present but mass panic occurs).

Evidence has shown association between toxic exposures and mental illnesses such as Attention Deficit and Hyperactivity Disorders (ADHD), Cognitive disability/Intellectual disability/Developmental delays, Psychomotor delays/decreased coordination, Behavioural dsiorders, psychiatric disorders. A variety of toxins such as ethanol, lead, mercury, PCBs (Polychlorinated Biphenyl), BPA (Bisphenol A.), tobacco, smoke, ethanol, carbon monoxide, multiple pesticides, solvents, manganese, nicotine, solvents, tobacco smoke, arsenic, cadmium, fluoride, PBDEs

(Polybrominated Diphenyl Ethers), multiple pesticides, smoke, nicotine, carbon disulphide, Acrylamide,, aluminum, manganese, methyl bromide, styrene, toluene, have been implicated individually and in groups in the etiology of these disorders to varied degrees.

Toxins are also one of the physical causes of depression. There have been theories of schizophrenia based on the toxic effects of the drug, phencyclidine (PCP), and a few other experimental chemicals. Nevertheless, toxicological theories of mental illness are not usually explored.

In 2008, an endocrine disruption theory of schizophrenia based on the effects of BPA (Brown, 2008) was proposed. The theory demonstrated that BPA causes abnormalities in animals also observed in schizophrenia. Studies have found an association between prenatal lead exposure and schizophrenia (Opler *et al.*, 2004).

A growing body of peer-reviewed scientific research reveals that for the most vulnerable populations, exposure to even minute doses of neuro-toxic chemicals can lead to learning and developmental disabilities. It is believed that by minimizing exposure to neuro-toxic chemicals we may mitigate the severity of the condition and improve the quality of life of those who are already suffering from learning or developmental disabilities.

Toxicity from chronic low-level exposure affects in a much more insidious manner. Chronic low-level exposure has been found to lead to such wide ranging mental health problems such as neuropsychiatric disturbances, e.g. aggressive behaviour, memory loss, depression, irritability, and learning deficits.

Although efforts are being made to contain the release of toxins and heavy metals into the environment, we are far from resolving the challenge. In developing countries like India, and even in the United States, thousands of tonnes of toxic industrial wastes, including heavy metals, are dumped into the environment every year.

Scientists believe that by implementing strong health-based policies emphasizing safer alternatives, we could eliminate these exposures to substances that we know can have these impacts. In addition, we need to conduct studies on other environmental contaminants of concern for which we do not yet have sufficient safety data relating to their physical and mental health impact.

Researchers have suggested that there is a need to read and monitor the mainstream toxicological, environmental and occupational-medicine literature and to reinterpret the genetic and viral theories of mental illness using toxicological mechanisms to explain them. It has been suggested by scientists that there is a need to encourage collaborations and joint meetings between psychology and scientific disciplines that study the natural and synthetic environments as sources of disease (environmental medicine, toxicology).

Disciplines like toxicology, environmental sciences, and occupational medicine—study toxicological causes of diseases including mental diseases, hence it is pleaded that psychological research needs to be included in environmental and occupational medicine, and toxicology in particular.

As reported in the current literature on the subject, the financial and emotional costs of mental health impacts of toxic chemicals have already reached alarming levels for affected. Every possible measure needs to be taken to prevent and treat the growing health problems. In some instances, by reducing exposure to harmful substances from our environment—such as lead—billions of dollars have been saved and there has been an increase in the quality of life of millions of individuals, families and their communities.

Psychology can provide help to deal with many of the rising issues and challenges in environmental health. These mental health outcomes pose a serious challenge to those who are working to improve the public health. Preventive policy imperatives through which governments and corporations can deal with the mental health challenges from toxic exposures are the need of the hour.

There is a need to bring about fundamental changes in the regulatory laws regarding how we develop and produce chemicals, so that the health of current and future generations is not compromised. Researchers hope that reducing exposures to toxic chemicals will result in a healthier population and will also lead to positive occupational health outcomes, and a reduction in health care costs to governments and employers.

The mounting scientific evidence indicates that we need to reduce our exposure to toxic chemicals and develop safer alternative to these chemicals, otherwise ever increasing costs of mental health care and developmental disabilities will only increase further.

Policy alternatives for governments and corporations to protect the health of their workers and the general population need to be explored so that everyone may realize their full potential in a safe and healthy environment.

References

Brown, J.S. (2008). Toxicological Theories of Mental Illness: A Clash of Paradigms and Call for Reunification, *The NADD Bulletin*, Volume 11, Number 5, September/October 2008, pp. 97-100.

Brown, J.S. Jr. (2002). Environmental and chemical toxins and psychiatric illness, Washington, D.C. *American Psychiatric Publishing*.

Brown, J.S. Jr. (2007). Psychiatric issues in toxic exposure. *Psychiatric Clinics of North America*, 30, 837-54.

Brown, J.S., Jr. (2008). Effects of bisphenol—A and other endocrine disruptors compared with abnormalities of schizophrenia: An endocrine-disruption theory of schizophrenia. *Schizophrenia Bulletin*, [Epub ahead of print].

Crow, T.J. (2008). The emperors of the schizophrenia polygene have no clothes. *Psychological Medicine*, [Epub ahead of print].

Filidei, M.D. (2002). Toxic Metals and Mental Health, http://www.alternativementalhealth.com/articles/toxicmetals.htmaccesed 02-05-2013.

Havenaar, J.M. (1997). Psychological Factors Affecting Health after Toxicological Disasters, *Clinical Psychology Review*, Vol. 17, No. 4, pp. 359-374.

Herbstman, J.B.; Sjodin, A.; Jones, R.; Kurzon, M.; Lederman, S.A.; Rauh, V.A.; Needham, L.L.; Wang, R.; Perera, F.P. (2008). Prenatal Exposure to PBDEs and Neurodevelopment, *Environmental Health Perspectives* doi: 10.1289/ehp.0901340.

Koch, T. (2005). Cartographies of disease. Maps, mapping, and medicine. Redlands, CA: ESRI Press.

Opler, M.G., Brown, A.S., Graziano, J., Desai, M., Zheng, W., Schaefer, C., Factor-Litvak, P., and Susser, E.S. (2004). Prenatal lead exposure, delta-aminolevulinic acid, and schizophrenia. *Environmental Health Perspectives*, 112, 548-552.

Opportunity and Challenge for Psychology. *American Psychologist*, November, 1174-1187

Sinclair, J. (2010). How Exposure to Toxins Can Cause Depression, Anxiety and Other Mental Health Illnesses, http://www.breakingfreefromdepression.com/evidence-zinc-deficiency-in-depression/comment-page-1/-comment-1136 accesed, 02-05-2013

Sinclair, J. (2011). More Evidence Showing Zinc deficiency is involved in Depression, http://www.breakingfreefromdepression.com/evidence-zinc-deficiency-in-depression/comment-page-1/-comment-1136.

Sullivan, P.F., Lin, D., Tzeng, J.Y., van den, O.E., Perkins, D., Stroup, T.S., Wagner, M., Lee, S., Wright, F.A., Zou, F., Liu, W., Downing, A.M., Lieberman, J., and Close, S.L. (2008). Genomewide association for schizophrenia in the CATIE study: results of stage 1. *Molecular Psychiatry*, 13:570-84.

The Learning and Developmental Disabilities Initiative (2010), Mind Disrupted Report, available at www.minddisrupted.org

Weiss, B. (1983). Behavioural Toxicology and Environmental-Health Science.

16

Mental Health and Meditation at the Individual Level

Akbar Husain

Mental health refers to the development, preservation, prevention and treatment and enhancement of total personality in all its varied aspects. It deals with individuals, groups and social institutions as interdependent systems. According to the dual factor theory of mental health, both negative and positive aspects need to be considered together and not separately. While one deals with mental disorders, their prevention, diagnosis prognosis and treatment, the other deals with the positive aspects like sense of well-being, satisfaction in all spheres of life, adjustment, realization of one's full potential including creativity and originality, looking forward to get support from others and later providing support to all others when and wherever required—according to ones' abilities.

Mental health is not a mere absence of mental illness or mental ill health. It is definitely much more than that, various health services like mental hospitals, government and private psychiatric nursing homes, psychiatric illness, child guidance centres, mental retardation homes, etc. deal more with the negative mental health while ignoring to a great extent, the positive aspects of the individual mental health. Mental health is an important dimension of holistic health. According to Charandas (1986), mental health is the adjustment of human being to the world and to each other with maximum of effectiveness and happiness.

On the WHO Website as of October 2011, mental health is defined as "a state of well-being in which every individual realizes his or her potential, can cope with the normal stresses of life, can work productively and fruitfully, and is able to make a contribution to her or his community."

Considering the field of 'Positive Psychology', mental health is found to be positively related to various positive capacities such as resilience

(Nygren, Alex, Jonsen, Gustafson, Norberg, and Lundman, 200... 2010), life satisfaction and happiness (Bray and Gunnell, 2006), ... (Gestel-Timmermans, Boggard, Brouwers, Herth, and Nieuwenhuize... 2010), humour (Miller, 2003), emotional intelligence and self-efficacy (Gupta and Kumar, 2010).

In the course of our daily lives we face a lot of stress at physical, social, occupational, and mental levels. We should get rid of them through meditation. Many of us do the meditation to cleanse the mind so that mind get better and there is a general feeling of mental well-being. Meditation brings greater benefits to the meditator. Once the mind gets cleansed by such a system it also affects the thought process. Meditation brings calmness and rejuvenates both mind and soul.

Constituents of Positive Mental Health

Positive mental health is not a unitary concept. It consists of different, somewhat interdependent factors. A mentally healthy person may have one or more of these factors, in varied levels.

1. Creative use of leisure
2. Achievement value
3. Internal locus of control
4. Ego-strength
5. Hardiness
6. Psychological well-being
7. Hope
8. Social support
9. Quality of life
10. Mental efficiency
11. Self-help
12. Job satisfaction
13. Adjustment in most, if not all situations.
14. Always ready to learn and readjust.

Husain and Khan (2013) proposed a model to define the concept of mental health and consider it as both multidimensional and value-laden. They include Meaning in Life, Emotional Stability, Nurturance, Temperament, Adjustment, Life Satisfaction under the MENTAL and Hope, Environment, Altruism, Lifestyle, Tension and Hardiness under the HEALTH dimensions.

Who is Mentally Healthy?

If one thinks of a dimensional approach to the mental health, it could be like mentally ill to normal to mentally healthy. Here mentally healthy would be a deviant person from the normal in the positive direction while a mentally ill person would be a deviant person from the normal towards the negative direction. Thus, there would be a qualitative difference in the characteristics of the person at the poles, with little or no overlap between the two.

A better approach to understand the concept of mental health is the Dual factor theory. Verma, Nehru and Puri (1998) proposed a dual theory of mental health. This theory regards mental health as an absence of mental illness and a presence of certain factors of positive mental health. The positive mental health factors include the following sense of well-being, satisfaction, hope, adjustment, ego-strength, super-ego, creativity, ability to enjoy, happiness, honour, quality of life, self-realization, social support, etc. Here, the two sides can have differences on many (not necessarily) characteristics. For example, a mentally ill may be satisfied in his job but not very creative, not very productive or, original. He may even be normal with regard to a few characteristics, whereas mentally healthy would be one with lots of (if not all) the characteristics described below:

1. A mentally healthy individual is one who is usually satisfied in most situations. Even if he is not very satisfied in some situation, he can still take things in the stride and be creative, productive, happy, and well-adjusted.
2. A mentally healthy individual is mostly optimistic never giving up hope even in a most trying situation. He would still be stress-free and tolerate any amount of frustration to keep on trying his level best to cope with the situation and would generally be more resilient.
3. A mentally healthy individual would always look for original, creative solutions for his as well as others' problems.
4. A mentally healthy individual would welcome genuine help from others as well as be ready to help others. He would be at the centre of any Self Help Group and contribute to the welfare of self, family and of the society at large.
5. A mentally healthy individual is one who would be able to enjoy things in life, take pleasure even in ordinary things and share it with others around him.
6. A mentally healthy individual is one who is able to see the positive things even in a difficult situation, like recognizing real (true) friendship even in the face of calamities and seeing the true face of people deserting him in times of adversity.

7. A mentally healthy individual is one who is always able to remain self-confident and infuse confidence even in distressed/depressed individuals. Others seek reassurance from him and feel relaxed and at ease in his presence, by mere talking to him.
8. A mentally healthy individual is always relaxed, smiling, reassured, stress-free and able to induce the same feelings and attitudes in others.
9. A mentally healthy individual is one who has constructive habits and leisure time activities. He makes creative use of leisure.
10. A mentally healthy individual is able to see hope even if put to a disadvantage and handicap.

How can One Achieve Positive Mental Health?

Positive mental health is an attitude, a way of life, nurturing of competencies to deal with the exigencies of everyday life. This competence prepares an individual to learn the skills of 'how' and 'when' to do things. Achievement of these leads to happiness and success and they serve as a protective mechanism. Promotion and enhancement of competence, socially and psychologically would require one to practice the skills necessary for social functioning, mental health and well-being. Most humane and cost-effective way to protect and enhance psychological well-being is through prevention. This can be done by life skill training which should occur at a young age and should be taught to enhance coping with life stresses and pressures, failure of which may give rise to negative health behaviours and social problems.

One can believe in good things in life as expressed by our elders/ wise men/poets/philosophers, etc. A few examples are as follows:

1. God is in the heaven.
2. Everything is right with the world.
3. Grow old with me; the best is yet to be.
4. There is always sunshine/light after the darkest night.
5. Barking dogs seldom bite.
6. Our sweetest songs are those that tell of saddest thoughts.
7. Praise cannot harm you don't inhale it.
8. Old order chargeth, lest one good order should corrupt the world.
9. The greatest punishment of a liar is that he cannot believe others.
10. A friend in need is friend indeed.
11. Love is divine, Love is immortal.

12. Practice what you preach.
13. Love is God, God is love.
14. Love me; love my creatures.
15. Do not ask what the nation can do for you, ask what you can do for the nation.
16. Than God that I am not God, I did not create this world. I am not responsible for it. I don't have to explain anything.
17. Old is gold.
18. Health is wealth.
19. A thing of beauty is joy for ever.
20. The brave dies once, the coward dies many times.
21. Live in the living present, future will take care of itself.
22. Poetry is what was oft thought but never so well expressed.
23. Genius is one per cent inspiration but ninety-nine per cent perspiration.
24. Insight can best be described as an "Aha" experience.
25. Brave write history that cowards can only wonder.
26. There are always greater horizons to be reached/won.
27. Change what you can, tolerate and accept what you cannot change and have wisdom to know the difference the two have.
28. In the end we do get what we deserve.
29. Hope for the best but be prepared for the worst.
30. Those who refuse to go beyond the facts, rarely go as far as facts.
31. God helps those who help themselves.
32. Losing faith in younger generation is a sign of old age.
33. Life is immortal, soul never dies, only form changes.
34. God loves you. He has created this world for you.
35. It is better to have loved and lost than ever to have loved at all.
36. There is always life after death.
37. There is unity in diversity.
38. Live and let live.
39. Life is precious; make the best use of it.
40. Happiness increases by sharing it with others.
41. What cannot be cured must be endured.
42. Meditate on God.

There are numerous scales to measure positive mental health being used in different languages throughout the world but the basic concept remains more or less the same. The way mental health is defined and conceptualized will affect how it is measured.

A common question that is posed by people is how to equip oneself to face the challenges of life and maintain positive health. I am suggesting the following tips to deal with the stresses of daily life and maintain positive mental health.

Talk about your feelings	Promote joy and hope
Keep active	Eat well
Sleep well	Express Positive Emotions
Keep in touch with loved ones	Do mindfulness meditation
Acquire the knowledge	Get professional help
Look beyond drug therapies	Time management
Hold that thought	Cultivate universal compassion
Let there be light	Apologize with sincerity and remorse
Improve your coping skills	Set realistic goals
Keep an eye on personal stress	Three good things
Love for all living creatures	Be calm in mind, speech, and action
Find a hobby	Do Good to others
Rely on self-help	Open your ears to music.
Develop inner strength	Attain eternal peace
Cultivate spiritual virtues	Resolved misunderstanding
Gain serenity	Enhancing communication skill

Meditation and Mental Health

Meditation is a spiritual exercise in which a person discover the essence of his or her being, or the deepest meaning by which people live. To me meditation is the process for the development of inner peace and attains mental health.

Meditation has been practiced within religious traditions since ancient times. Today mindfulness-based meditative practices have become popular within the Western medical and psychological community, mainly due to the observable and positive impact on patients suffering from stress-related health conditions (Ospina and Bond, 2007).

There has been a dramatic increase in the past 20 years or so of studies on the impact of meditation upon one's health. There are various potential positive effects such as brain activity during meditation, brain waves during meditation, meditation and perception, sleep need, and elevation of positive emotions and outcomes, and positive behaviour have been noted in the previous studies. These researches are based on various styles of meditative techniques: Insight meditation, *Kundalini yoga* meditation, Integrative body-mind training, Zazen, Theoria, Non-referential compassion meditation, Mental Silence, Transcendental Meditation, and Tasbih meditation. Relaxation and different meditation techniques including biofeedback, shavasana, transcendental meditation, *vipasana*, *sudarshan kriyas*, devotional songs, etc. are of immense use in maintaining positive mental health.

In the face of stressful and conflict situations, humans fight, flight, or simply freeze. Meditation is spiritual exercise which saps our mental energy and life force. Meditation is a spiritual exercise which develops great strength among individuals in mind, heart, spirit. It nourishes and refreshes one's mind. Meditation keeps our mind active and clear. We need to practice meditation to improve our mental health. Though meditation is a purely mental in nature, it gives rise to heal mental suffering.

Yogic traditions have suggested various processes of doing meditation. Becoming silent is the true heart of meditation. During the process of meditation complete silence is observed. Meditation is assumed to control our senses and connect us to the Supreme. *Japa* or Chanting of *mantra* '*Aum*' activates the mind and consequently we feel mentally healthy. *Aum* is the active word of God.

It is of paramount importance that one should devote at least 15 minutes everyday to do meditation, preferably early in the morning. Through the practice of either concentrative or mindfulness meditation, one can eliminate the bad thoughts by creating positive thoughts. For example, thoughts of hatred and anger can be controlled by generating thoughts of forgiveness, mercy, and non-violence; thoughts of pride and arrogance can be eradicated through inculcating thoughts of humility and a down-to-earth attitude; greed and possessiveness can be dispelled by pursuit of magnanimity and contentment; jealousy and meanness can be replaced with thoughts of love and generosity.

We may differ variously by religion or caste, but we all agree with the value of having a peaceful mind. In our modern age of ever-increasing complexity, greater importance should be given to mental health, and to reach peace of mind, certain self-disciplines are to be practiced. Whenever we meditate, we have mental clarity, spiritual alertness, and Divine awakening within us, and at that moment the mind is pure and silent.

Conclusion

Mental health is still much debated concept with no universally accepted definition because it is multidimensional and value laden (Friedli, 2004; Herron and Trent, 2000).

A thought over the suggestions given by the author can help an individual to adopt any or many of these to achieve positive mental health. Think positively and feel positively should be the motto of every individual.

Meditation is the essence of spiritual life. It is our mental attitude which brings in thoughts and shows us the positive outlook of life. Lots of patience is required to perform meditation. So everyone of us should do meditation to maintain a positive attitude towards life. Performing meditation during stressful times in our life will make a big difference. To keep the mind strong, meditation is a duty.

References

Bray, I., and Gunnell, D. (2006). Suicide rates, life satisfaction, and happiness as markers for population mental health. *Social Psychiatry and Psychiatric Epidemiology,* 41, 333-337.

Charandas, N. (1986). Mental health and the community. *Indian Journal of Community Guidance and Service,* 3(2), 25-27.

Friedli, L. (2004). *Mental health improvement 'concepts and definitions': Briefing paper for the National Advisory Group.* Edinburgh, Scottish Executive.

Gestel-Timmermans, H., Boggard, J., Brouwers, E., Herth, K., and Nieuwenhuizen, C. (2010). Hope as a determinant of mental health recovery: A psychometric of the Hert Hope Index-Dutch version. *Scandinavian Journal of Caring Science,* 24, 67-74.

Gupta, G., and Kumar, S. (2010). Mental health in relation to emotional intelligence and self-efficacy among college students. *Journal of the Indian Academy of Applied Psychology,* 36(1), 61-67.

Herron, S., and Trent, D.R. (2000). Mental health: A secondary concept to mental health illness. *International Journal of Mental Health Promotion,* 2, 29-38.

Husain, A. and Khan, S. (2013). Mental Health: A New Interpretation. In D. Hooda and N.R. Sharma (Eds.) *Mental Health: Risk and Resources* (1-19). New Delhi: Global Vision Publishing House.

Miller, D.M. (2003). *The Correlation between Sense of Humour and Mental Health.* Unpublished Ph.D thesis. Missouri Western State University, United States.

Nygren, B., Alex, L., Jonsen, E., Gustafson, Y., Norberg, A., and Lundman, B. (2005). Resilience, sense of coherence, purpose in life, and self-transcendence, in relation to perceived physical and mental health among the oldest old. *Aging and Mental Health,* 9(4), 354-362.

Ospina, M., and Bond, T. (2007). "Meditation practices for health: State of the Research. Evidence Report/Technology Assessment No. 155" (e-text). *Agency for Healthcare Research and Quality.*

Verma, S.K., Nehru, A., and Puri, A. (1998). Quality and quantity of mental health. *Journal of the Indian Academy of Applied Psychology*, 24, 59-62.

Wells, M. (2010). Resilience in older adults living in rural suburban and urban areas. *Online Journal of Rural Nursing and Health Care,* 10(2), 45-54.

World Health Organization (2011). *Defining the Concept of Mental Health.*

17

Organizational Effectiveness a Precursor to Organizational Health

Tanu Shukla

Introduction

Organizations are usually identified as instrument of purpose and are seen as synchronized by objectives and ends. Explaining variation in performance or effectiveness is indeed an enduring theme in the field of the organizational study. The concept of organizational effectiveness has accomplished vital attention in recent years. Social scientists from numerous disciplines have been focusing their writings on the question of what is required for good organizational health. There has been a constant demand upon educational organizations to improve performance, so to grow to be more effective and efficient. These developments have consequences for the practice of educational management; hence, effective management should be central to the professional development and for the overall proficient organization. Organizations are not closed system; they surely have inputs from the environment that they exchange for a portion of their outputs. Organizations are social actors responsible for ethical and unethical behaviours, Clinard and Yeagner (1998).

The concepts of effectiveness, efficiency and excellence of organizations are such issues that have provoked the writings of economists, organization theorists, management philosophers and psychologists. Yet, organizational effectiveness remains a complex and difficult problem for both theorists and researchers as well as for practitioners. Since organization and management science emerged in the early 1900s in conjunction with the industrial revolution, an evolution has occurred in concepts about the nature and function of organizations and the criteria for organizational effectiveness. A wide range of organizational characteristics, i.e. structures, compositions, behaviour and output has been proposed and applied as criteria of organizational effectiveness, Mahoney (1997). By this means, organizational effectiveness can be taken up as a composite construct that depends on multiple factors and their interactions.

Social scientists from numerous disciplines have been focusing their writings on the question of what makes for an effective organization. Organizations look for ascertaining correspondence between the social values connected with their suitable behaviour in the social system. The term is not new fangled; it has its inclusion in Beckhard's (1969) well-known definition in organizational development. Indeed, researchers have been working to define its characteristics, precursors and determinants of OE from many years, Cameron and Whetton (1981). Many early studies concentrated on quantitative and objective measures on outcomes of what constitutes of an effective organization. Now, the shift is as such that the term refers to the individual's involvement and satisfaction with as well as enthusiasm for work (Harter, Schmidt and Hayes, 2002). The concepts of organizational effectiveness are the basis of theories of management and organization behaviour and there is relatively less consensus about this concept.

If organizational values are well defined and clarified then this will be of great help in decision-making and prioritizing the expectations to be fulfilled. Well defined and accepted values can guide an organization to the right path in the right manner with collective consciousness. Dennison (1995) argued that effectiveness is one of the most pervasive yet delineated constructs in the study of organizations. As organizational values are aggregate manifestations of individual values, so, no organizational strategy for excellence can be implemented unless they have the values for doing so along with the knowledge, skills and attitudes. Thus, selection of appropriate basis for assessing organizational effectiveness presents a challenge for researchers.

Models of Organizational Effectiveness

A variety of approaches to the definition of Organizational Effectiveness (OE) appears in literature. The different approaches have emerged from different conceptualizations of the meaning of an organization. The conceptualization of different types of organization leads the change in definitions and approaches to organizational effectiveness. Few of the most appearing approaches in the literature are discussed here. The traditionalist way to study effectively is "goal approach". Its distinguishing characteristic is that it defines effectiveness in terms of the degree of goal-achievement. According to this approach, the greater, the degree to which an organization achieves its goals, the superior its effectiveness. As effectiveness is defined with respect to the degree of goal-achievement, the definition of "goal" becomes crucial. Etzioni (1964) asserts that organizational goal is a desired state of affairs which the organization attempts to realize. Those who describe effectiveness in terms of the degree of goal-achievement typically equate "goal", "objective", "purpose", "mission", "aim", and "task", Campbell (1977), Scott (1995) and Price (1972). Within the purview of goal accomplishment model, Interactive system model attempts to relate individual subsystem performance to organizational goal achievement.

The goal approach to the study of effectiveness has been criticized by those who use the "system resource approach". This approach defines effectiveness, not with respect to the degree of goal-achievement, but in terms of the skill of the organization to make use of its milieu in the attainment of limited and valued resources. As a criticism, System Resource Model was proposed by Yutchtman and Seashore (1967) evaluates the organizational effectiveness in terms of its ability to compete for and to gain scores and value resources over a period of time. They held that the goal approach does not give adequate consideration to the conceptual problems of the relation between the organization and its environment. As per this approach, the effective organization is capable of exploiting its environment and acquiring the optimum amount of resource for its operation. The model actually evaluates effectiveness in terms of the input, the output feedback cycle of the organization.

Strategic Constituency Model also called participant satisfaction model which suggests that OE is attained whenever an organization distinguishes among its strategic groups and satisfies their demands or it may be described as the extent to which all organizations' strategic constituencies are at least minimally satisfied or reduces the regret of these major strategic constituencies, Keeley (1978). It also has an extension as Ecological Model, Keeley (1978) and Miles (1980). Effectiveness, as per this, is described as the degree to which the needs and expectations of strategic constituencies are met by the organization. This approach may be defined as a summary measure for an organization or a series of different scores from a variety of constituencies. The interrelations among contingent multiple models of OE and the situational nature of OE allows the definition of OE to reflect 'user' values not 'expert' values. In the sector of higher education, contradictory findings exemplify OE due to the distinctive organizational characteristics of institutions that differ in their domain effectiveness. Cummings (1980) states that relationships among institutional variables are very vague and complex. Also, relationships are likely to change with different outlines of effectiveness across domains.

Each of these approaches, bears certain advantages as a research and theoretical tool, but each also has weaknesses, Cameron (1986). As these models are analytically independent, uniform approach cannot be appropriate in all circumstances. The problem that appears in determining which model is appropriate in assessing effectiveness is difficult to choose. Organizations generally operate in multiple domains, but few organizations maximize effectiveness in all domains, Cyert (1963), Pennings and Goodman (1977) and Steers (1977). In short, it can be stated that because each of the four major approaches to organizational effectiveness emphasizes a limited domain set and so the complexities are inherent in each organization. Thus, not only models of effectiveness are needed for different types of organizations, but that appropriate model may differ even in organizational subunits.

Based on various variables, Steers outlined a process model for analyzing effectiveness, which has a major influence on environmental characteristics, employee characteristics, and organizational characteristics. Describing required resources and sustaining a harmonious relationship with the environment is essential to the application of the model. Steers concluded that OE is best understood as a continuous process rather than end state and this process is of a dependent nature. Argyris (1985), Bennis (1966) and Likert (1967) symbolizes this model in their explorations and according to them, effectiveness is equated with internal organizational health, efficiency, internal processes and procedures.

An effective organization, as per this model, is the one with a high degree of match and congruence between its internal environment and its external environment. In an educational setting, it is always advisable to take this approach for understanding the organization. Rather than requiring inferences from outcomes to performance characteristics, it assesses performance values. Process measures are based on the assumption that it is known what activities are required to ensure effectiveness, Suchman (1967). Also, it is imperative to observe that this indicator represents an assessment of input or energy regardless of output.

The process model emphasizes more on the series of activity that may lead to the effectiveness of the organization. In other words, it does not view the organizational effectiveness in the disjointed efficacy of the outcomes, rather necessitates involvement of the stakeholders in the organizational processes. The process model assumes vital substance in the context of higher education where an outcome is often not readily measurable and requires considerable time to realize result of any activity. The process model is largely seen as human resources perspective with their focus on the relationships between internal characteristics of functional organizational subunits.

Organizational Effectiveness, in the present study, refers to the degree to which educational means or processes result in making an organization, an effective organization. The objectives of the study lays emphasis on reviewing the existing literature that deals about the organizational effectiveness for flourishing organizational health and to find out the contribution of each of the facets of organizational effectiveness that helps in explaining the concerned variable.

Methodology

The study is descriptive in nature. A crucial limitation recognized by the investigator through review of literature reveals that most of the studies were frequently explored merely on a theoretical basis. Hence, the present study attempts to view the factor of organizational effectiveness in a more understandable way by field inquisition. The data base of the present study involves sample of 198 (75%) teachers out of the total population of all the teachers, i.e. 264 from one of the state universities of Uttar Pradesh. The selection of teachers was made by using a stratified random sampling technique. The university constitutes diverse area of knowledge and discipline spread through different academic faculties. Hence, multiple reasons stimulated the researcher to take it as sample for the study.

Here, the emphasis has been placed on behavioural aspects of effectiveness. In the tool, OE has been defined in terms of teachers' perceptions of organizational structure and system, congenial organizational climate, interpersonal harmony and cooperation, efficient leadership, higher morale and job satisfaction, organizational procedure and functioning such as decision-making, implementation of policies, planning human relations, adopting innovations and making certain high standards of teaching-learning. Organizational effectiveness scale contains forty short descriptive statements.

Factor analysis was exercised to identify the factors contributing in the OE as a main variable. Principal component method was used to extract various components that are exercised in the following analysis. This calculates approximately how much of the variability is due to frequent factors i.e. communality. It has also been explained by Eigenvalues, using scree plots, as how much the variance in all the variables is explicated by a particular factor.

Background Literature

Organizational Effectiveness (OE) may be defined as situation specific, multidimensional construct that is useful for evaluation of largely performance of an organization. Units of every subsector in the larger framework of an organization differ, so units to judge the effectiveness would also be probably different that together makes complexity in assessment of OE. A rising knowledge about the effectiveness in organizations is developed, but modest researches have been done on organizational effectiveness in higher education milieu. Few of the studies have been carried out highlighting the dimensions of effectiveness of higher education. Measures of OE are meant to denote the parameters as the dependent variable. The review expresses the miscellaneous meanings of construct, here, the literature specifically discusses in a higher education context along with studies conducted in allied areas.

The well-known contributor, Cameron (1978) is the most illustrious in the current context; he has made an enormous input in higher education system. He identified nine famous effectiveness dimensions, selected the criteria, constituencies, and institutions and has chosen a sound methodology for his study. The nine dimensions that he has described are students' educational satisfaction, their academic, personal and professional development, faculty job satisfaction, professional development of teachers, resource acquisition, system clarity and organizational health. Soon after, in his exploration, he further elaborated that unstable environmental conditions have revealed a strong impact on the effectiveness of academic institutes. Cameron (1986) demonstrates why organizational effectiveness studies are crucial in certain types of organizations. The results of this study of twenty-nine organizations indicate that certain managerial strategies are strongly associated with high static scores and with improving effectiveness over time. Managerial strategies, in fact, were found to be more important than structure, demographics, finances, and other factors. Proactive strategies and those with an external emphasis are more successful than internal and reactive strategies. Managerial strategies that are multifaceted are more likely to lead to effectiveness than monolithic strategies. The independent and conditional effects of organizational culture type and level of mission agreement on the organizational effectiveness of colleges and universities is described by also, Sisman (1996) provided features of an effective institute in terms of useful and capable management, students, teachers, strong culture, parental involvement, etc. Sisman (1996) described as management of an academic institute is regarded to be vital dimensions in students' and faculty's perception. Moreover, Chenhall (2006) pointed out that employees are the key skill of any organization and they should be motivated depending upon the changeable perspective of the organization in which it operates. Likewise, Cheng and Wong (1996) conducted a research in Asian institutions that have sketched few effectiveness dimensions as; support of internal and external environment and professionalizing of teaching staff.

The study of Davadoss and Muth (1984) found that power behaviours variously affect one's sense of job involvement and overall effectiveness of one's college, focusing on theoretical and empirical relations among power variables, faculty job involvement, and college organizational effectiveness. In particular, the influence was found to be positively related to the involvement and to effectiveness, while coercion was found to be negatively related to effectiveness but not related to involvement. The findings suggest that empirical integration of divergent normative theories is useful for understanding how academic administrators might behave to improve the performance of their institutions and provide support for earlier studies which have used the empirical model. Likewise, the correlation between managerial leadership style and individual factors with organizational effectiveness was investigated by Verma (2001). Ninety-two higher and middle level managers from private corporations were administered a leadership style scale. Variables of organizations, education and length of the experiment did not show any significant relation with organizational effectiveness at higher level. It was not considered to be the ideological reason, but what else could do to improve organizational effectiveness.

Many other researchers have witnessed that organizational effectiveness has multiple dimensions and all the underlying indicators should be considered while measuring it, Cameron (1978). Most of the underlying indicators have been discussed earlier. The effectiveness indicators that are present in more or less in each study area as students' development, effective management and leadership of academic organizations, faculty satisfaction, quality of teaching, university culture, environmental impact, parental involvement, acquisition of resources and their efficient use. Cameron (1978) has described that not a single model can be used to measure organizational effectiveness, as it is multidimensional field, so one has to measure all the underlying variables to measure it. Further, the contextual factor should be considered before selecting any organizational effectiveness criteria. As context varies across countries and even within countries, so if one factor proves to be successful at one part of the world may prove to be futile with another.

The other approach of goal model is the System Resource Model or the Natural System Approach that explains how an organization interacts with its surroundings, including its internal, external environment and how successful an organization exploits resources from its environment, Yuchtman and Seashore (1967). Here, the focus shifts from output to input Cameron (1980). So resources acquirement is regarded as the chief condition than the achievements of goals, hence, an organization is effective if it has the ability to acquire valued resources from its environment for its gratifying a range of system requirements. Another model of OE is an Internal Process Model that functions on the assumption that if processes are effective, the goals will be met effectively. As per this, an effective organization is featured by absence of internal stress, smooth internal functioning, trust, benevolence, high integration of members into the system, smooth information flows vertically as well as horizontally. It will be more effective when the organization possesses a greater degree of these characteristics, Cameron (1980).

As per Internal Organizational Process, effectiveness is equated with internal organizational health, efficiency, internal processes and procedures. Argyris (1964), Bennis (1966) and Likert (1967) symbolize this model in their explorations. Steers and Richard (1977) have illustrated that organizational effectiveness should be measured in terms of processes carried out in an organization than ultimate results outcomes. According to them, the approach is applicable to all types of organizations.

The study conducted by Webb (2001) identifies organizational characteristics which act as determinants of effectiveness of voluntary educational organizations. The findings differ distinctly from earlier studies of organizational effectiveness and indicate that organization development in such organizations needs to undergo rethinking. The study conducted by Cameron (1978) examines the obstacles to the assessment of organizational effectiveness in higher education in the paper. Some of those are discussed, namely criteria problems and the unique organizational attributes of colleges and universities, and criteria choices addressing these issues are outlined. Criteria were generated from dominant coalition members in six institutions, and tested, and evidence was found for certain patterns of effectiveness across the nine dimensions nine dimensions of organizational effectiveness were derived.

The role of organizational context in predicting service effectiveness was discovered by Yoo and Brooks (2006). The study found the trend of expanding knowledge of intervention effects in social work and other disciplines in the human services. A total of 3,883 children and 13 networks of organizations comprised the study sample. To determine whether the organizational context explains intervention effects, a multilevel model of a hypothesized relationship between organizational variables, child characteristics, and child outcomes was tested. The results indicate that children's outcome (measured as out-of-home placement) varies across networks, and this variance is largely explained by workplace conditions. The study suggests that organizational characteristics are potentially strong determinants of service effectiveness Cameron and Ettington (1988).

The investigation of Osburn and Hunt (1974) found that environmental complexity is based on a unique conceptual view of organizational environments which distinguishes among broad factors facing many organizations, conditions unique to a system, and inter organizational characteristics. Environmental complexity is viewed as the interaction between environmental risks, dependency, and inters organizational relationships. Research questions concerning complexity in the task environment are investigated in 26 small, rigidly structured social service organizations in a populous mid-western state. Results show that neither complexity nor risk is associated with organizational effectiveness. Both task environments dependency and inter-organizational interaction alone and in combination are positively and significantly correlated with effectiveness.

A theoretical framework designed by Gornitzka (1999) for a comparative research project on organizational change in higher education is presented. The main focus is on how organizational change in universities and colleges is affected by governmental policies and programmes. The framework is based upon two major theoretical perspectives, resource dependency and neo-institutionalism. It is argued that for examining changes in universities and colleges both the relationship between these organizations and the government, as well as their internal dynamics is of importance. The article suggests that these models offer a meaningful insight into how and why governmental steering approaches have been changed over time. The paper of Fey and Denison (2003) examines the link between organizational culture and effectiveness for foreign-owned firms operating in Russia. Beginning with a model of organizational culture developed in the United States, the paper presents a multi-method analysis of culture and effectiveness in a transition economy. We argue that effectiveness in Russia relies more on adaptability and flexibility than it does in the United States. The authors explore these ideas using survey data on 179 foreign-owned firms operating in Russia and compare the results to those obtained from firms in the United States then present four case studies designed to ground the results in the Russian context.

Most studies of organizational performance define performance as a dependent variable and seek to identify variables that produce variations in performance. March and Sutton (1997) specifies organizational performance in this way typically devote little attention to the complications of using such a formulation to characterize the causal structure of performance phenomena. The authors conclude by considering a few virtues and hazards of such a solution to dilemmas involving compelling contradictory imperatives and the generality of the issues involved. In the study of organizational effectiveness of training, Nordhaug (1992) presented an analytical framework aimed at the study of aggregation of individual outcomes from personnel training into organizational effectiveness of the first and second order. The focus is set on possible inter linkages between outcomes at the level of employees and the level of firms. Results revealed that usefulness of how concrete individual aggregate and later transformed into organizational resources as well as dysfunctional effects.

The application of a theory of partial system and its implications for organizational effectiveness was examined by Klien (1992). Quasi system ineffective oriented to compliance with standards rather than exchange with the environment. The minimally effective pseudo system includes one, self involved incestuous process representing interaction confirmed largely to participants due to limited energy inputs and second, self-justifying cannibalistic processes representing interaction with a subset of environment restricted to a degree that participants fail to recognize due to limited information input. Results indicated that an organization represents a system and achieved effectiveness not by definition but through developing an active and continuous process of self-evaluation and redemption and when needed.

Denison and Mishra (1995) explored case studies and surveyed data the relationship between organizational culture and effectiveness. The results provide evidence for the existence of four cultural traits—involvement, consistency, adaptability, and mission—and indicate that these characteristics are positively related to perceptions of performance as well as objective measures such as return on assets and sales growth. Organizational culture is found to be measured and to be related to important organizational outcomes. Similarly, the relationship between work related values perceives organizational support, organizational effectiveness and coping in 45 executives representing different departments of TISCO in India was assessed by Mishra (1992). No significant relationship was found any all the variables for executives. However, in both groups, the relations between coping and organizational effectiveness was significant. The coping styles of no executives were contingent on their perception of physical well-being.

Campbell (1977) reviewed the organizational effectiveness literature, suggesting "how criterion measures of organizational effectiveness should be developed so that they can be used to compare organizations, evaluate the effects of organizational development efforts and determine what characteristics of organizations are significantly associated with organizational effectiveness as a basic construct." Organizations were seen to be presented in terms of two general models, popularly labelled "goal-centred" and "natural system". Campbell also presented taxonomy of the various criteria as being used in the literature, to account for "all variables that have been proposed seriously as indices of organizational effectiveness". Campbell went on to suggest a relative lack of value in "objective" inquiry, arguing that the development of organization-specific models based on clear, explicit assumptions would be generally more promising. Organizational effectiveness, then, would be the degree to which the organization's 'end' objectives are accomplished subject to certain constraints.

The psycho-social assumptions underlying dominant modes of management in Irish work were investigated by McCarthy (1996), the model stresses the need to build systems of work which fuse individuals and group orientations in order to facilitate the evolution of Irish work systems and demand a new set of organizational behaviour, i.e. trust, empowerment, personal accountability and teamwork. This model reflects the potential of male female workers and to allow for creation and innovation in information, environment in the future. Management diversity was analyzed by Amason (1997) and noted that social traps are situations where decision problems involve conflicts between individuals and long term consequences implying that management of diversity is created by workplace diversity.

Three areas of Organizational Effectiveness (OE)—one definition, second criteria and third evaluation—were reviewed by Gbadamosi (1999). Several alternative definitions, viewpoints are examined and concluded that there is no single definition that is universally accepted. Common approaches in literature are compared in relation to goal attainment, second system strategic constituencies and third competing values. Several criteria for organizational effectiveness are listed that indicates lack of consensus. Identified measurement problems included constructing validity, criterion stability and time perception. It was concluded that there seems to be an agreement on the need to use multiple criteria for measurement of organizational effectiveness and disagreement may actually benefit to the growing literature on the concept of organizational effectiveness.

A variety of predictors, as they related to survival of small business and their perceived success, was assessed by Goldenberg (1999). It showed organizational capacities transforms vision into productive activity using resources of an organization act through a productive empowerment and develops commitment, cohesiveness and consciousness towards enhancing development capacities.

The studies related to work groups were examined by Sundstrom (2000) and their legacy, related empirical researches of work group's effectiveness conducted in the work setting in last twenty years addressed four questions: (a) What have field researchers identified in operationally defining work groups? (b) What have research strategies been used? (c) What have criteria of work groups' effectiveness the field researchers measured using what sources of data? and (d) What have variables researchers sought to list with measures of work group effectiveness?

The study of Yoo and Brooks (2005) examines the role of organizational context in predicting service effectiveness. It highlights methods for studying this phenomenon for expanding knowledge of intervention effects in social work and other disciplines in the human services. A total of 3,883 children and 13 networks of organizations comprised the study sample. To determine whether the organizational context explains intervention effects, a multilevel model of a hypothesized relationship between organizational variables, child characteristics, and child outcomes was tested. The results indicate that child outcome (measured as out-of-home placement) varies across networks, and this variance is largely explained by workplace conditions. Specifically, organizations that are characterized by their respective workers as have occurrences of out-of-home placement for children who participated in a family preservation programme. This study suggests that organizational characteristics are potentially strong determinants of service effectiveness.

The significance of virtuousness in organizations has recently been acknowledged in the organizational sciences, but research remains inadequate. Cameron (2004) defines virtuousness and connects it to scholarly literature in organizational science. An empirical study is described in which the relationships between virtuousness and performance in 18 organizations are empirically examined. Significant relationships between virtuousness and both perceived and objective measures of organizational performance were found. The findings are explained in terms of the two major functions played by virtuousness in organizations: an amplifying function that creates self-reinforcing positive spirals, and a buffering function that strengthens and protects organizations from traumas such as downsizing.

Theoretical views of the relationship between poor performance and subsequent organizational action has been discussed by Ketchen (1999). The behavioural theory of the firm posits that poor performing organizations will make strategic changes in, for example, the products and services they offer. In contrast, the threat-rigidity perspective predicts rather conservative responses; poor performers are expected to rely on previous actions to reverse their poor outcomes. These were examined by competing predictions using data from a regional sample of hospitals. The results offer support for the behavioural theory of the firm and no support for threat-rigidity. We derive several implications of these findings in an effort to guide future research. The article of Nobbie (2003) presents an empirical study of the relationships between implementation of the policy governance model in non profit organizations, board performance, and organizational effectiveness. An implementation measure of the policy governance model was created to investigate these relationships. Data were gathered from three samples: organizations that have implemented policy governance, a matched sample of randomly selected non-profit organizations, and non-profit organizations that had received board development from the National Centre for Non-profit Boards. The analysis yielded several positive, significant relationships between the extent of implementation of policy governance board behaviours, perceptions of improvement in board performance following implementation of policy governance, and some aspects of organizational effectiveness.

Cameron (1986) demonstrates why organizational effectiveness studies are crucial in certain types of organizations. The results of this study of twenty-nine organizations indicate that certain managerial strategies are strongly associated with high static scores and with improving effectiveness over time. Managerial strategies, in fact, were found to be more important than structure, demographics, finances, and other factors. Proactive strategies and those with an external emphasis are more successful than internal and reactive strategies. Managerial strategies that are multifaceted are more likely to lead to effectiveness than monolithic strategies. The independent and conditional effects of organizational culture type and level of mission agreement on the organizational effectiveness of colleges and universities is described by Fjortoft and Smart (2002) while significant differences are found for both culture type and mission agreement, there are important conditional effects on two of the effectiveness measures.

Clark, Lotto and Astuto (1984) have known features of an effective academic institute as students' acquisition of important skills, students' success and development, learning targets, strong culture, and prominent academic leadership. Similarly, Hoy and Ferguson (1985) have described the indicators of effectiveness as students' success, effective management of teachers, institution's satisfaction and the way in which academic leaders cope with the environment, are those dimensions that should be considered while measuring organizational effectiveness. Gun and Holdaway (1986) have portrayed effectiveness indicator as teachers and students' satisfaction, academic development, parents' satisfaction, grooming of students as a responsible citizen, employment of expert staff and finally preparing students for moving into markets and getting good jobs, as building up their professional carriers.

The verdict of the paper by Mahoney and Weitzel (2006) is interpreted within the framework of a hierarchical model of criteria of effectiveness. Measurable organizational characteristics serve as operators, short-run substitutes for the more subjective, long-run ultimate criterion of organizational effectiveness. The paper by Price (1972) reviews the goal approach and the system resource approach to the study of organizational effectiveness. The goal approach is defended with respect to the criticisms made by the users of the system resource approach. Next, it is criticized for its failure to develop general measures of effectiveness. The system resource approach is then criticized as optimization is not measured, few general measures are used and the basic rule of mutual exclusiveness is seriously violated.

Cunningham (1977) presented seven alternative approaches for assessing organizational effectiveness as rational goal, system resource, managerial process, organizational development, bargaining, structural functional and functional. A paradigm is proposed by Gregory, Gaertner and Ramnarayan (1983), regarding effectiveness as the ability of an organization to account successfully for its outputs and operations to its various internal and external constituencies. This framework can be used to assess effectiveness by examining organizational outputs and processes in a critical and holistic way. A review of the existing literatures on organizational effectiveness and a case example, are used to develop the proposed framework.

A research approach is proposed by Lewin and Minton (1986) as well as considered the problems of organizational effectiveness utilizing a strategy of organizational effectiveness, which could lead to an inductive, applied, empirically-based theory of contingent organization design. The role of organizational context in predicting service effectiveness was discovered by Yoo and Brooks (2006). The study found the trend of expanding knowledge of intervention effects in social work and other disciplines in the human services. A total of 3,883 children and 13 networks of organizations comprised the study sample. To determine whether the organizational context explains intervention effects, a multilevel model of a hypothesized relationship between organizational variables, child characteristics, and child outcomes was tested. The results indicate that children's outcome (measured as out-of-home placement) varies across networks, and this variance is largely explained by workplace conditions. The study suggests that organizational characteristics are potentially strong determinants of service effectiveness.

Analysis using Factor Analysis

The definitional peripheries of OE have been clearly stated and thus, here, researcher has referred to process oriented model. An effective organization, as per process oriented model, is the one with a high degree of match and congruence between its internal environment and its external environment. In an educational setting, it is always advisable to take this approach for understanding the notion of OE. Here, researcher in the present study has viewed the study from a process oriented approach where focus is on quality rather than quantity of activities carried on by the organization. Rather than requiring inferences from outcomes to performance characteristics, it assesses performance values. Process measures are based on the assumption that it is known what activities are required to ensure effectiveness, Suchman (1967). Also, it is imperative to observe that this indicator represents an assessment of input or energy regardless of output.

Factor analysis was employed and it was observed that exclusively the dimension as Congenial Climate was identified as a factor having eigen-value greater than one (shown in the Table 17.1 and Fig. 17.1 mentioned below). Interpersonal Harmony contributes fifteen per cent of the variance. Dynamism and adaptability explained fourteen per cent of

Table 17.1: Organizational Procedure

Component	*Total Variance Explained*					
	Initial Eigenvalues			*Extraction Sums of Squared Loadings*		
	Total	*% of Variance*	*Cumulative %*	*Total*	*% of Variance*	*Cumulative %*
1. Congenial climate	3.111	51.843	51.843	3.111	51.843	51.843
2. Harmony	.950	15.841	67.684			
3. Dynamism and adaptability	.804	13.406	81.090			
4. Commitment	.450	7.498	88.589			
5. Organizational Procedure	.363	6.053	94.642			
6. Organizational structure	.321	5.358	100.000			

Extraction Method: Principal Component Analysis

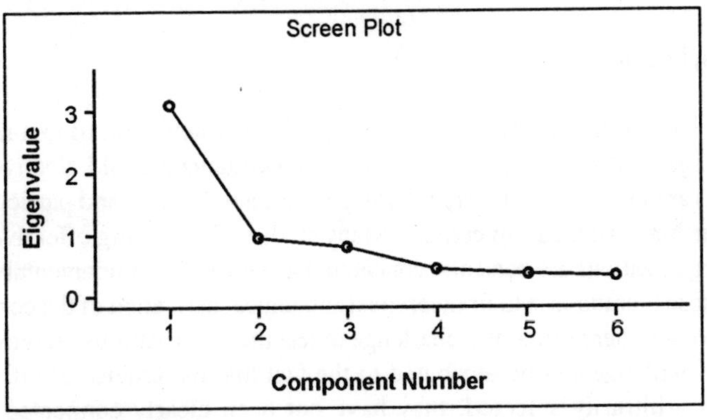

Fig. 17.1: Eigen-value

the total variance. Commitment explained eight per cent of total variance. The dimension like Organizational Procedure and Efficiency explained six per cent and five per cent respectively of total variance in Organizational Effectiveness (OE).

The analysis shows that teachers' perceived congenial climate as a main contributor of organizational effectiveness. It is presumed that organizations are created on the basis that more can be achieved by employees working in harmony and towards a stated purpose than by individuals acting alone. It is revealed in various literatures that the execution of responsible judgment is the spirit of professional actions. The act of caring of committed teachers to help every student to defend and endorse the interests, well-being of students and make every endeaour to guard students are vital features of promising action of teachers. The teacher should support collegiality amongst colleagues by regarding their professional standing and views. When teachers are prepared to offer advice and assistance, particularly to those beginning their career in teaching, it is a step for effective organization and also a crucial factor towards human relations. It is quite logical to believe that commitment of a teacher results in better efforts on learning, teaching conditions which is definitely an important measure of organizational effectiveness. Specifically, teachers with dynamism and ability to adapt to the environment invites a higher level of success and had higher expectations for integrity towards their services. These findings may have practical implications for administrators who have a positive attitude towards efficient and competent university. Organizational structure and procedure are product driven variables and hence teachers' perceived it as less effective as compared to the other variables.

Conclusion

The idea of organizational effectiveness is the foundation of theories of management and organization. Studies on Organizational Effectiveness (OE) are fairly limited, generally in educational contexts and particularly in the higher education context. Many studies, for viewing effectiveness in organizations are basically conceptual in nature. The fundamental merit of those literatures is their theoretical and logical derivation of the concept. However, there remains a challenge to test these derivations empirically. The challenge can be attributed to the fact that the criteria of OE have been arbitrarily selected, they have not been clearly connected with organizational performance and the chief factors that predict effectiveness have not been fairly articulated.

Less in empirical studies makes the area of organizational effectiveness fertile to examine. It can be mentioned by reviewing the related literature on Organizational Effectiveness that different kinds of organization have different criterion to assess organizational effectiveness. For example, business organizations are likely to find production efficiency, whereas academic organizations are more expected to emphasize reliability, cooperation and professional competence in determining effectiveness. For the assessment of organizational effectiveness of educational organizations, there are distinct measures, but quite a few have contributed on this particular domain. Few of the important researchers as Cameron and Callahan investigated the concept of organizational effectiveness in higher education, but the limitations were discovered in the contributions related to higher education and not much escalating dimension could be settled in relation to organizational effectiveness of higher education. Theoretical contributions in OE are essentially needed that could be helpful in making generalizations to other types of similar organizations.

Different literature suggests a number of criteria for evaluating effectiveness; broadly two criteria can be classified as external criteria and internal criteria. External criteria include adaptiveness, bargaining position for resources, the ability of organization to perceive reality and the achievement of organization. Internal criteria include morale, turnover as a measure, stability, stress and most importantly employee opinions. Researchers are not much willing to accept random criteria of effectiveness so intense struggle is identified in the settlement of indicators of organizational performance. Thus, it can be asserted that Organizational Effectiveness is a very crucial concept to study and there has been relatively less consensus about the concept. Although the organizational effectiveness has been well studied concept, but it has not been dealt effectively in the context of the education system. Researcher admits that it is difficult to define organizational effectiveness in an absolute sense as there are various perspectives on this concept, remaining flexible in interpretation. The review indicates that the domains of organizational effectiveness need to undergo rethinking, especially at the higher education system. Researcher unfolds that most studies had been conducted in industrial and business level, but definitely there is enormous requirement of research for this concept in the educational sector.

The inherent problem to define the organizational effectiveness is the serious concern for its measurement. There is a solemn need to reorient research on organization effectiveness by growing a research approach to develop pertinent indicators of it, exclusively at higher educational institutions. Among many, two of the critical education's challenges are quality and effectiveness, yet the features of quality and criterion to assess effectiveness are not simply recognized and universally straight. The background nature, constituent perspectives, institutional policies, characteristics and culture make it complicated to articulate common operational definitions of quality and effectiveness. It is indeed very intricate since the troubles lie inherent in defining the construct. Organizational researchers hardly ever presented any systematic data regarding the validity and reliability of their measures, leading to the dilemma in establishing a sole cumulative measure of it. So, a great deal remains to be done through researchers to pinpoint all the components of effectiveness.

References

Amason, A. (1966). Distinguishing the Effects of Functional and Dysfunctional Conflict of Strategic Decision-Making; Resolving a Paradox for Top Management. *Academy of Management Journal*, Vol. 39(1), pp. 123-148.

Argyris, C. (1985). *Strategies, Change and Defensive Routines*. Boston: Pitman.

Beckhard, R. (1967). *Organizational Development: Strategies and Models*. MA: Addison Wesley.

Bennis, W.G. (1966). *The Concept of Organizational Health*. NY: McGraw Hill.

Cameron, K. (1978). Measuring Organizational Effectiveness in Institution of Higher Education. *Administrative Science Quarterly*, Vol. 23, pp. 604-627.

Cameron, K.S. and Whetton, D.A. (1981). Perceptions of Organizational Effectiveness of Organizational Life Cycles. *Administrative Science Quarterly*, Vol. 26, pp. 26-43.

Cameron, K. (1986). A Study of Organizational Effectiveness and Its Predictors. *Management Science*, Vol. 32(1), pp. 87-112.

Cameron, K.S., Bright, D. and Caza, A. (2004). Exploring the Relationships between Organizational Virtuousness and Performance. *American Behavioural Scientist*, Vol. 47(6), pp. 766-790.

Campbell, J.P. (1977). *Contributions Research Can Make In Understanding Organizational Effectiveness*: Kent State University Press.

Cheng, K., Wong, K. (1996). School Effectiveness in East-Asia. *Journal of Education Administration,* Vol. 34(5), pp. 98-115.

Chenhall, R.H. (2006). *Theorizing and Testing Fit in Contingency Research on Management*: Monash University.

Clinard, M.B., and Yeager, P.C. (1980), *Corporate Crime*. NY: Free Press.

Cummings, T.G. (1977), Methodological Critique of Fifty-Eight Selected Work Experiments. *Human Relations*, Vol. 30 (8), pp. 675-708.

Cunningham, J.B. (1977). Approaches to the Evaluation of Organizational Effectiveness. The *Academy of Management Review*, Vol. 2(2), pp. 463-474.

Cyert, R. (1963). *A Behavioural Theory of the Firm*. Prentice Hall. Eaglewood Cliffs. NJ.

Dennison, D.R. and Mishra, A.K. (1995). Toward A Theory of Organizational Effectiveness. *Organization Science*, Vol. 6(23), pp. 204-223.

Etzioni, A. (1988). *The Moral Dimension: Toward a New Economics*. New York: The Free Press.

Fey, C.F. and Denision, D.R. (2003). Organizational Culture and Effectiveness: Can American Theory Be Applied in Russia? *Organization Science*, Vol. 14(6), pp. 686-706.

Gbadamosi, G. (1995). An Evaluation of the Relationship among Communication, Commitment and Organizational Effectiveness, UNILAG: *Journal of Business*, Vol. 1(1), pp. 112-131.

Goldenberg, S.; and Kline, T. (1999). An Exploratory Study of Predicting Perceived Success and Survival of Small Business. *Psychol. Reports*, Vol. 85(2), pp. 365-377.

Gornitzka, A. (2000). *Analyzing Organizational Change in Higher Education.* Emerald Group Publishing Limited. UK.

Gregory, H. and Gaertner, K.N. (1984). Civil Service Reform in the Context of Presidential Transition in P. Ingraham and C. Ban, *Legislating Bureaucratic Change: The Case of Civil Service Reform*, Albany, NY: Suny Press.

Gun, J.A. and Holdaway, E.A. (1986). Perceptions of Effectiveness, Influence and Satisfaction of Senior High Schools' Principals. *Educational Administration Quarterly*, Vol. 22(2), pp. 318-319.

Harter, J.K. Schimdt, F.L. and. Hayes, T.L (2002). Business Unit level Relationship between Employee Satisfaction, Employee Engagement and Business Outcomes. A Meta analysis. *Journal of Applied Psychology*. Vol. 87, pp. 268-279.

Hoy, W.K. and Ferguson, J. (1985). A Theoretical Framework and Exploration of Organizational Effectiveness of Schools. *Educational Administration Quarterly*, Vol. 21(2), pp. 117-134.

Keeley, M.A. (1978). A Social Justice Approach to Organizational Evaluation. *Administrative Science Quarterly*, Vol. 22, pp. 272-292.

Klein, Jonathan I. (1992). A Theory of Partial Systems: Implications For Organizational Effectiveness. *Behavioural Science Journal*, Vol. 36(3), pp. 36-50.

Lewin, A.Y. and Minton, J.W. (1986). Determining Organizational Effectiveness: Another Look and an Agenda for Research. *Management Science*. Vol. 32(5), pp. 514-538.

Likert, R. (1967). *The Human Organization*. New York: McGraw-Hills.

Lotto, L.S. and Astuto T.A. (1984). Effective School and School Improvement: A comparative Analysis of Two Lines of Inquiry. *Educational Administration Quarterly*, Vol. 20 (3), pp. 41-68.

Mahoney, R.M., (1997). *Problems in the Measurement of Organizational Effectiveness*. Vol. (4).

March, J.G. and Sutton, R.I. (1997). *Crossroad-Organizational Performance as a Dependent Variable*. Vol. 8(6), pp. 698-706.

McCarthy, E. (1994), Work and Mind: Searching for Own. *Irish Journal of Psychology*, Vol. 15(25), pp. 1-29.

Miles, R.H. (1982). *Macro Organizational Behaviour*. Goodyear. Santa Monica.

Nobbie, P.D. (2003). Testing the Implementation, Board Performance, and Organizational Effectiveness of the Policy Governance Model in Nonprofit Boards of Directors. *Nonprofit and Voluntary Sector Quarterly.* Vol. 32 (4), pp. 571-595.

Nordhaug and Odd (1991), Organizational Effectiveness of Training, Aggregation and Transformation. *Scandinavian Journal of Management*, Vol. 67(2), pp. 111-121.

Osborn, N.R. and Hunt, G.J. (1974). Environment and Organizational Effectiveness. *Administrative Science Quarterly*, Vol. 19(2), pp. 231-246.

Pfeffer, J. (1977). Usefulness of the concept. In Paul S. Goodman and Johannes M. Pennings (eds.). *New Perspectives on Organizational Effectiveness*: San Francisco: Jossey-Bass.

Price, J.L. (1972). The Study of Organizational Effectiveness. *Sociological Quarterly,* Vol. 13, pp. 3-15.

Scott, P. (1995). *The Meanings of Mass Higher Education*. Buckingham. OUP.

Seashore S.E. and Yutchtman, E. (1967). Factorial Analysis of organizational performance, *Administrative Science Quaterly*, Vol. 12.

Sisman, M. (1996). *Effective School Management*. Eskisehir: Anadolu University Publications.

Steers, Richard M. (1977). *Organizational Effectiveness: A Behavioural View.* Santa Monica, CA: Goodyear.

Suchman, E.A. (1967). *Evaluate Research*. NY: Russel Sage Foundation.

Sundstrom, E., McIntyre, M., Halfhill, T., and Richards, H. (2000). *Work groups: From the Hawthorne Studies to the work teams of the 1990s*. Group Dynamics. Vol. 4, pp. 44-67.

Verma (1995). *A Study of Value Pattern Among College of Rohilkhand Region With Special Reference to Sense of Responsibility*, Ph.D. Thesis, M.J.P. Rohilkhand University, Bareilly.

Webb, R., Vulliamy, G., Hamalainen, S., Sarja, A., Kimonen, E., and Nevelainen, R. (2004). A Comparative Analysis of Primary Teacher Professionalism in England and Finland. *Comparative Education*, Vol. 40(1), pp. 83-107.

Yoo, J. and Brooks, D. (2005). The Role of Organizational Variables in Predicting Service Effectiveness: An Analysis of a Multilevel. *Research on Social Work Practice*, Vol. 15(4), pp. 267-277.

Yutchtman, E. and Seashore, S.E. (1967). Factorial Analysis of Organizational Performance. *Administrative Science Quaterly*, Vol. 12, pp. 377-395.

18

Elimination of Existential Anxiety and Identity Crisis through Advaitic Vedanta

A Comparison with Western Models

Navya Pande

Introduction

The study of self and identity has been a topic of research for more than a century. Cooley (1902) and James (1890) were among the first researchers to theorize about the self. Many psycho analysts—most notably Freud (1923/1961) and Erikson (1950)—wrote extensively about the self and its development. Many others like Allport (1962) have shown their curiosity by asking questions such as— "Who is the 'I' that knows the bodily 'me', who has an image of myself and a sense of identity over time, who knows that 'I' have propriate strivings? …I know all these things, and what is more, I know that I know them. But who is it who has this perspectival grasp? It is much easier to feel the self than to define the self" (Leary and Tangney, 2003). Freud explained development of self by explaining ego and its mechanisms while Erikson extended his concept by defining eight stages of psychosocial development each marked by the presence of one particular conflict or crisis (Erikson, 1950, 1956; 1970). However, for Erikson, the word 'crisis' is not just an emotional turmoil; it also has the meaning of 'opportunity' to deal successfully with corresponding stage (Muuss, Velder and Porton, 1996). Emphasizing more on adolescence, Erikson suggests that an individual must find an answer to the identity questions such as: "Where did I come from?", "Who am I?" and "What do I want to become?" James Marcia (1966; 1976; 1980) expanded upon Eriksonian theory by adding that the balance between identity and confusion lies in making a *commitment* to an identity. He has discussed four identity statuses, viz. identity diffusion, moratorium, foreclosure and identity achievement. Moratorium is the most conflicting status in which the individual tries to make a commitment but is unable to do that.

Self-identity is a complex multidimensional concept and has been explained as: "Who am I?" Individual forms "an integrated image of himself or herself as a unique person, which often includes ethnic identity" and what one is as distinguished from other persons, what one knows and believes, and what meaning one's existence has. Descartes found the self in the conscious experience of thinking "I think, therefore, I am" whereas John Locke (1975) identified the self with memory. He explained identity as the extension of consciousness backward in time. According to Locke, past experiences, thoughts, or actions that the person does not remember are not part of his identity. For him, identity and self-hood have nothing to do with continuity of the body or even continuity of mind. A person who remembers nothing of his/her past literally has no identity (Kihlstrom, Beer, and Klein, 2003). David Hume (2008) also established the connection between identity and memory, adding that the role of memory is to permit us to comprehend the causal relations among events.

Although the words "self", "self-concept" and "identity" are sometimes used interchangeably (Van Knippenberg *et al.*, 2004); most of the Western models separate "self" and "identity" from each other (Roeser, Peck, and Nasir, 2006). Self is the root through which self-concept and so called types of identities develop. 'Self-concept' and 'identity' have two common elements, viz. perceptual and social; the former being more concerned with 'self-concept' and the latter being more associated with 'identity'. Identity is often categorized into personal, social, cultural and ethnic (Schwartz *et al.*, 2005; Sneed, Schwartz, and Cross, 2006). Even personal identity is divided into different identities (daughter to Mr. X, wife to Mr. Y, mother to Ms Z, etc.) based on the different roles (Van Knippenberg *et al.*, 2004). Many theories of identity have been put forward which emphasize the social element more (Van Knippenberg *et al.*, 2004). Social identity theory states that a social identity is a person's knowledge that he or she belongs to a social category or group (Abrams and Hogg, 1990). Researchers point out that the social categories precede individuals. Individuals try to match their self-concepts with representative characteristics of a particular group. They obtain their identity from the categories or groups to which they belong (Turner *et al.*, 1987; Hogg and Reid, 2006; Young, 2009). Social categorization theory explains that when people adopt a social identity then there is a focus on intra-group similarities and intergroup differences on relevant dimensions. People stereo-type themselves in terms of prominent social categorization and this stereo-typing leads to an increased perceptual identity between self and in-group members and an increased perceptual oppositions between in-group and out-group members (Onorato and Turner, 2004). Another theory called the identity theory also holds the similar view and it states that people *identify* with their 'self' on the basis of the roles assigned to them by the structured society (McCall and Simmons, 1978; Stryker, 1980). In this theory, the core of an identity is the categorization of self into specified roles and expectations associated with it (Burke and Tully, 1977; Thoits, 1986). Due to this categorization and role expectations many times conflicts arise among various social groups and a wall is created between them.

The origin of any 'mental crisis' is always confusion borne out of ignorance (Touraine, 1971; Ayantayo, 2008). Studies identify two types of identity crisis, viz. '*motivation crisis*' and '*legitimation crisis*' (Baumeister, Shapiro, and Tice, 1985). The former occurs when the individual experiences a lack of guiding commitments (ignorance) but struggles to establish personal goals and values and the latter occurs when the person undergoes exploration of several identities but is unable to choose and be committed to one (confusion). The crisis can be ended by gaining the knowledge and ending the confusion. The crisis which Erikson and other Western scholars discuss is an outcome of role confusion (Erikson, 1950; 1956) and existential anxiety (Berman, Weems and Stickle, 2006). For some including Erikson, it occurs mostly in adolescence while some also report that it may occur at any stage of life (Pelletier, Verhoef, Khatri and Hagen, 2002; Fry, 2000). Existential anxiety involves apprehension about the meaning of life and death. Tillich (1952) defines existential anxiety around 3 related domains of apprehension. The first domain is fate and death. Anxiety about fate and death concerns the absolute threat to one's being in death and the relative threat to the self in our personal fate. The second domain is emptiness and meaninglessness. Anxiety about emptiness and meaninglessness concerns the fear that there is no "ultimate concern," and hence no ultimate importance in life that gives meaning to one's existence. The third domain is guilt and condemnation. Anxiety about guilt and condemnation involves perceived threats to one's moral and ethical identity.

Issues of self-play a role in many forms of psychopathology. People who are depressed tend to have negative views of self. Individuals with Schizophrenia often have difficulty representing key aspects of self at all

(Westen and Heim, 2003). The most blatant form of identity disturbance is found in dissociative identity disorder (Dell, 2002). Personal identity has been negatively associated with conduct problems (Schwartz, Pantin, Prado, Sullivan, and Szapocznik, 2005), drug and alcohol use (Bishop *et al.*, 2005; Jones, Hartmann, Grochowski, and Glider, 1989), and sexual risk taking (Hernandez and DiClemente, 1992; Schwartz, Mason, Pantin, and Szapocznik, 2008). Some research has also identified self-concept as a protective factor, along with family and school processes, against problem behaviour (e.g. Henderson, Dakof, Schwartz, and Liddle, 2006; Schwartz *et al.*, 2005).

The concept of identity has also been discussed in detail by various Indian philosophers such as Shankaracharya (Ramamoorthy and Nome, 2002; Rao, 2003) and Somdev (Acharya, 1996 in *The Sarva Darshana Samgraha*). Both of the aforesaid philosophers believe in the non-dualism (however, there are subtle technical differences in their approaches). In this paper we have explored Shankaracharya's approach. He clearly states (in a collection of *shlokas* titled *Atmabodha*) that he is a follower of '*Gyan Marga*' (path of knowledge) and those who are feeling the identity crisis and want to quench their thirst of existential issues would find solace in the knowledge stored in the rich *Vedantic* literature and not the skeptics who are often rigid and biased by their own reasoning. He well acknowledged the formerly discussed problems of categorizations and role-confusions. His following *shloka* sheds some light on this issue (Parthasarathy, 1971).

> *"Yathakaso Hrushikeso*
> *Nanopadhi gatho Vibhuh*
> *Tadbhedat Bhinnavat Bhati*
> *Tannase Kevalo Bhavet"*

Just as the all pervading *Akasa* (space) appears to be diverse an account of its association with various conditionings (*upadhis*) which are different from each other, the omnipresent truth appears to be diverse on account of its association with the various "*Upadhis*". The omnipresent truth becomes one after the various *upadhis* are destroyed. Whatever is above earth is sky (space). Then what is in a house is also space though we are distinguishing the house as drawing room, bed room, kitchen and bath room, or by constructing walls. The walls are man-made and due to worldly reasoning keep us in a belief that they are all different rooms though they are actually sky (space). Once the walls are removed, there is no room and no house. What is left is the sky. Similarly if man-made reasoning can be ignored, then we can see *Parmatma* or *Brahma* in every being. Here just thinking is not enough but one must be able to feel and believe this concept whole heartedly (Chinmayananda, 2003).

Very few scholars like Schwartz and Côté acknowledge this fact and suggest that it's time to put the pieces of the self-identity puzzle (categorizations) together, to identify commonalities between and among them (Schwartz, 2001; 2008; Côté, 2006) and thus create a larger and more coherent whole. Here, they are indirectly heading towards the path shown by Shankaracharya (though their perceptual approaches are different) who believes that—

> "*Satchidaatmani Anusyoote*
> *Nitye-Vishnow Prakalpitaah*
> *Vyaktayo Vividhassarvaa*
> *Haatake Katakaadivat*"

(All gold ornaments have different names but are basically of gold only) the single element which manifests itself in various forms (Chinmayananda, 2003). According to Shankaracharya, self and identity are inseparable; identity being only a projection and rather misinterpretation of self. Researchers try to solve the mystery of our true nature by exploring the 'identity' and categorising it into various parts (Côté, 2006; Côté and Levine, 2002) but, Shankaracharya clearly states that ideas such as caste, colour and position (social categorisations misinterpreted as identities) are imposed upon the *Atman* on account of its association with different *upadhis*, just as flavour, colour etc., are imposed upon water (Chinmayananda, 2003).

> "*Naanopaadhi Vasaadeva*
> *Jaati Varnaasra maadayah*
> *Atmanya aropitah thoye*
> *Rasa Varnadi Bhedavat*"

He not only explains the oneness between the self and the identity but also establishes non-duality between the self and *Brahma* by quoting *Aham Brahmasmi* from *Vedantic* epics (Parthasarathy, 1971). He emphasizes to develop a discriminative intellect (*Prajna*) to realize the transient and illusionary nature of imposed identities (*Upadhis*) and discover our true identity (*Brahma*). Human keeps on struggling to bring a balance in his life but is always entangled in the invisible cobweb of greed, attachment, anger, vanity, lust, etc. Moreover *Homo sapiens* is the most developed species so human is his sole judge himself. Due to his erroneous human reasoning, ignorance persists and he keeps on moving in the wrong direction. Our true nature (identity) is not visible just like the sun which is hidden behind the clouds. Once he realizes this fact and contemplates freely on his true nature, his '*pragna*' (*pure intellect*) develops and he realises that he is not the doer or an experiencer but the all pervading *Brahma* which is *satchidananda* (the absolute and eternal bliss).

> *"Samsarah Swapnatulyo hi*
> *Ragadweshadi Samkulah*
> *Swakaale Satyavatbhati*
> *Prabodhe sati Asadbhavet"*

This concept can be understood well by peeping into the subtleties of the lives of eminent persons such as Sri Aurobindo, Vivekananda, Pilot Baba, Pt. Sri Ram Sharma Acharya, etc., who abandoned all such impositions. They all realized about that 'single supreme identity' which is nothing but a spark of the omnipotent divine energy. It is reflected in their actions as well as in their writings. The lives of such persons were blessed with perennial well-being and sheer contentment. Contentment not only flooded their own lives but also drenched their disciples who became capable of overcoming all kinds of crises and existential anxiety by discovering their true 'self' (Paloutzian and Park, 2005). Many thinkers and researchers believe that spirituality helps people to get free by untangling the threads of imposed identities and this statement does not indicate towards and particular religion (Mulholland, 2012).

Remedies by Shankaracharya

Shankaracharya's path to come out with this crisis is *Gyan Marga* (path of knowledge) where a thinker by thinking and judging the reality to the surroundings can get out of the illusional identities and find out the true one.

First point is to identify the three bodies which are apart from our true nature. The logic is here that the one who witnesses the all three bodies is the true self and these bodies which have been witnessed could be object of this true self (Parthasarathy, 1971).

Anaadyavidya Anirvaachyaa
Kaaranopaadhi ruchyate
Upaadhi Tritayaadanyam
Atmaanam Avadhaarayet.

(*Avidya,* ignorance, has no beginning and is also quite difficult to define. This is also called *Karana Sareera* (Causal Body). So every living body has three forms of *sareera,* viz. *Sthoola* (gross body), *Sookshma* (subtle body) and *Karana* (causal body). The gross body and subtle body are products of *Avidya* and therefore, *Avidya* is called the causal body. *Atma* is none of these. It is the witness of its three bodies and never to be identified with them. *Atma* or self luminous consciousness, illumines the acitivites of the gross and subtle bodies. It is itself detached from all the bodies. Because of ignorance we think and attribute all the qualities of the three *Sareeras* to *Atma*).

Shankaracharya clearly says that the differentiation is not so easy. Rather it requires discriminative faculty (*prajana*) to be developed. Next he explains that all the five sheaths (*panchkosha*) seem to be so engrossed with our true nature that human being gets confused (illusion) by the very nature of these. So another way is to uncover the five sheaths and to identify the true identity.

Panchakosaadi Yogena
Tat Tanmaya Iva Sthitah
Suddhaatma Neelavastraadi
Yogena Sphatiko Yathaa.

Upanishads also lay emphasis to develop faculty of *pure intellect* through which the refined discrimination can be made and true identity can be revealed. Shakaracharya delineats this *pure intellect* as only way to get our true Identity.

Sada Sarvagato Apyatmaa
Na Sarvatra Avabhaasate
Buddhaaveva Avabhaaseta
Swaccheshu Pratibimbavat.

Ways to make our intellect pure is described in *Bhagvadgita*, Patanjali Yoga and various *upanishads*. The main theme of all these paths (*marga*) is to follow a *sattvic* life style and to abandon the *rajasic* and *tamasic* life style which illusions us.

Maharishi Raman also explains the same path to get the real identity by giving example of three states—dream, sleep and waking. He explains that in waking consciousness pleasure, happiness and suffering is observed but in deep sleep these become absent. Therefore, who witnessed that deep sleep experience of happily sleeping is *Ataman.* This implies that in waking states we get delusioned by wrongly identifying with *manas* or outer objects. So one of the remedy is also to get a clear discrimination between true and false by comparing these three states. As Shankaracharya explains in this *shloka*:

Raageechaa Sukha Duhkhaadi
Buddhow Satyaam Pravartate
Sushuptow Naasti Tannaase
Tasmaad Buddhestu Naatmanah.

Meditation is an important way to get out of these confusing identities. Many paths follow only this method. Buddhism considers mindfulness (clear non-judgmental awareness of the present moment) as the way to get rid of these confusing identities whereas *Rajyoga* emphasizes on contemplation and meditation to achieve the true identity. Similarly, Shankaracharya in the following *shloka* describes meditation as omnipotent instrument to get that true self which is beyond of all fears and sufferings.

Vivikta Desa Aaseeno
Viraago Vijitendriyah
Bhaavayet Ekam Aatmaanam
Tam Anantam Ananyadheeh.

(One should sit in a solitary place with a mind free from desires and controlling the sense organs, meditate with unswerving attention on the *Atma* which is infinite and one without a second).

A question can come in our mind that to what extent this practice of meditation to be continued. Here Shankaracharya elucidates that constant practice is required. Also, he states that those who have the genuine curiosity for finding the answer of the 'who am I' question and who persistently contemplate on the true nature of self by uncovering the worldly illusions; can only understand this path.

He explains the consequence of becoming self-realized (*Atma-bodha*) and eliminating the confusion between self and imposed identities in next *shloka*:

Jeevan Muktastu Tat Vidvaan
Poorvopaadhi Gunaan Tyajet
Satchidananda Roopatvaat
Bhavet Bhramara Keetavat.

(A *Jivanmukta,* i.e., one who has realized the *Atma* by long years of meditation/contemplation upon the divine nature of the *Atma* and has become completely free from ignorance (*Avidya*), even while he lives in his body, gives up the traits of the gross, subtle and casual bodies (*upadhis*) On account of his nature of *Sat Chit Ananda*, he verily becomes Brahma, like the worm which grows up in the mud nest for a long time and transforms into a wasp after contemplation over the form and nature of the wasp).

In this way *Advaitic Vedanta* explains the need of hour. Life style is changing each moment and due to the shallow nature of the materialistic desires, human beings face persistent crisis. The knowledge Shankaracharya or *Advaitic* system provides is eternal and has been present since a long time. Shankaracharya shows us the vast ocean of knowledge but to cleanse ourselves in its water and learn to swim and get free from all burdens—depends on us. It is our responsibility to know and follow the path so that we can not only we illuminate our life but also of others.

The main remedies seem to revolve around concept of *pure intellect,* constant practice of *meditation* and seeing through the fog of worldly things. Today humans are becoming more and more externally oriented but the knowledge provided by great thinkers support the development of inward orientation. Any crisis, any anxiety has a solution "inside" us and not in the worldly pleasures or the materialistic illusory techniques.

Bridging the Gap between Ancient Wisdom and Modern Scenario: Exploring Possibilities

Shankaracharya's *Advaitic Vedanta* provides us knowledge that attempts to create insight in us to understand the true nature of self. All the wisdom present in the scriptures is like the eternal constant greatest source of light which has the capability to illuminate our path towards self-realization. Ancient Indian knowledge has the capability to create a sound and highly effective approach to heal human psyche. It has already been acknowledged and accepted by great thinkers and philosophers not only in India but in the other parts of world also.

But, in today's scenario, we know that to accept and inculcate such great wisdom is not so easy task. As we know, the current lifestyle is marked by massive socio-cultural change globally. The youth are being misguided and blindly running in the rat race of worldly pleasures— ultimately getting disillusioned by everything they associate with their false identity and which they think might provide them happiness may it be money, love/relationships or beauty. They are getting education and gaining knowledge which is preparing them for searching happiness in appreciating the beauty of superficial ripples in the shallow river of false identity and materialistic achievements. In this process, individuals are losing touch with their inner true self. And then appears the real issue of existential anxiety and identity crisis. With the disillusionment, the eternal questions arise: "Who am I?", "How and where can I get happiness?", "Why everything is temporary?", "Who is controlling my life", "What is my real nature?" These questions are not uncommon. If any educated person takes some time out for himself and tries to open his inward eye he may easily find such questions pricking his consciousness leading to existential crisis which may later convert into psychological problems.

Not only is the present socio-cultural scenario challenging for applying the *Advaitic Vedantic* theory but also the existing psychological theories pertaining to dealing with existential anxiety or other self-related crises, are all Western. Even when we have highly valuable hidden treasure of ancient Indian wisdom, unfortunately no sound models which can accommodate with the current Indian/International scenario are yet being utilized in modern psychotherapy on a grand scale. A lot of work on Indian Psychology is going on (Bhugra, 1992; Gautam, 1999; Jeste and Vahia, 2007; Dalal and Mishra, 2010) but still there is a pressing need of devising new ways to bridge the gap between ancient wisdom and modern knowledge and culture.

If we have to utilize the knowledge provided by Shankaracharya in eliminating existential anxiety and attaining true nature of self, we must view *Advaitic Vedanta* in new light and devise new models which can be either accommodated with current ones or replace them. The aforementioned possibility seems to be a difficult choice but not an impossible one. Western Existential theory/therapy is also complicated and often didactic. It is also less popular but it is the only theory which deals with the existential issues so sensitively and together with Gestalt therapy, it has been a success in resolving psychological crises. Similarly, a new seed of *Advaitic Vedantic* wisdom can be planted and watered carefully in the congenial and fertile Indian soil. No psychological theory/model is perfect but if the ancient Indian wisdom is applied skillfully for enhancement of global psychological well-being and most importantly for Indian psyche; the resulting model might develop into a panacea for resolving existential issues, if applied aptly.

Learning lesson from *Advaitic Vedanta* in today's scenario is complicated due to its philosophical roots and the subtle nature but we should not forget that "we are human beings—the most wonderful creation of nature" and although we get distracted/deviated often and act erroneously; only "we" have the capability to rise above our animal nature and get connected with/get merged with the extreme source of energy—the supreme consciousness (Brahma). Only "we" have the capability to understand the illusory nature of this world and obtain eternal bliss.

Conclusion

The main aim of this paper was to present key points of Shankaracharya's knowledge system and try to merge them with current psychological concept of identity. Interesting aspect of Shankaracharya's theory is that he explains the issue of identity with many day-to-day examples and also provides us with cognitive remedies. Therefore, the researcher has tried to explore the concept. Further, qualitative studies can be planned to understand the existential issues being faced by individuals living in the current scenario and a model may be proposed which can work as a bridge between ancient Indian wisdom and modern psycho-sociological system.

References

Abrams, D., and Hogg, M.A. (1990). Social identification, self-categorization and social influence. *European Review of Social Psychology*, 1(1), 195-228.

Áchárya, M. (1996). *The Sarva-darsana-samgraha: Review of the Different Systems of Hindu Philosophy* (E.B. Cowell and A.E. Gough, Trans.). Delhi: Motilal Banarsidass.

Allport, G.W. (1962). The general and the unique in psychological science. *Journal of Personality*, 30(3), 405-422.

Ayantayo, J.K. (2008). Ignorance. The Bane of Inter-religious crisis in Nigeria: An Exposition. *Journal of Sustainable Development in Africa*, 10(2), 1-30.

Baumeister, R.F., Shapiro, J.P. and Tice, D.M. (1985). Two kinds of identity crisis. *Journal of Personality*, 53, 3, 407-424.

Berman, S.L., Weems, C.L., and Stickle, T.R. (2006). Existential Anxiety in Adolescents: Prevalence, Structure, Association with Psychological

Symptoms and Identity Development, *Journal of Youth and Adolescence*, 35, 3, 285-292.

Bernstein, D.A., Alison, C.S., Roy, E.I., Srull T.K., and Wickens, C.D. (1994) *Psychology*, 3rd ed. Princeton, W: Houghton Mifflin Co., 505, 90.

Bhugra, D. (1992). Psychiatry in ancient Indian texts: a review. *History of Psychiatry*, 3(10), 167-186.

Bishop, D.I., Weisgram, E.S., Holleque, K.M., Lund, K.E., and Wheeler-Anderson, J.R. (2005). Identity development and alcohol consumption: Current and retrospective reports by college students. *Journal of Adolescence*, 28, 523-533.

Burke, P.J., and Tully, J.C. (1977). The measurement of role identity. *Social Forces*, 55, 881-897.

Chinmayananda, S. (2003). *Atma-Bodha of Bhagawan Sri Sankaracharya*, Kessinger Publishing, LLC.

Cooley, C.H. (1902). *Human Nature and the Social Order*. New York: Scribner.

Côté, J.E. (2006). Identity studies: How close are we to developing a social science of identity? An appraisal of the field. *Identity: An International Journal of Theory and Research*, 6, 3-26.

Côté, J.E., and Levine, C.G. (2002). *Identity Formation, Agency, and Culture: A Social Psychological Synthesis*. Mahwah, NJ: Lawrence Erlbaum.

Dalal, A.K., and Misra, G. (2010). The core and context of Indian Psychology. *Psychology and Developing Societies*, 22(1), 121-155.

Dell, P.F. (2002). Dissociative phenomenology of dissociative identity disorder. *The Journal of Nervous and Mental Disease*, 190(1), 10-15.

Dutta, S.N. (2010). *Sankaracharya, His Life and Teachings: A Translation of Atma-Bodha* (1899), Kessinger Publishing.

Erikson, E.H. (1950). *Childhood and Society*. New York: Norton.

Erikson, E.H. (1956). The concept of ego identity. *American Psychoanalytic Association*, 4, 56-121.

Erikson, E.H. (1970). Autobiographic notes on the identity crisis. *Daedalus*, 730-759.

Freud, S. (1923). Certain neurotic mechanisms in jealousy, paranoia and homosexuality. *International Journal of Psycho-Analysis*, 4, 1-10.

Freud, S. (1961). The ego and the id. In J. Strachey (Ed. & Trans.), *Standard Edition of the Complete Psychological Works of Sigmund Freud* (Vol. 19, pp. 3-66). London: Hogarth Press. (Original work published 1923).

Fry, P.S. (2000). The Unique Contribution of Key Existential Factors to the Prediction of Psychological Well-Being of Older Adults Following Spousal Loss. *The Gerontologist*, 41, 1, 69-81.

Gautam, S. (1999). Mental health in ancient India and its relevance to modern psychiatry. *Indian Journal of Psychiatry*, 41(1), 5.

Henderson, C.E., Dakof, G.A., Schwartz, S.J., and Liddle, H.A. (2006). Family functioning, self-concept, and severity of adolescent externalizing problems. *Journal of Child and Family Studies*, 15(6), 719-729.

Hernandez, J.T., and DiClemente, R.J. (1992). Self-control and ego identity development as predictors of unprotected sex in late adolescent males. *Journal of Adolescence*, 15(4), 437-447.

Hogg, M.A., and Reid, S.A. (2006). Social Identity, Self-Categorization, and the Communication of Group Norms. *Communication Theory*, 16(1), 7-30.

Hume, D. (2008). *Personal Identity*. J. Perry (Ed.). University of California Press.

James, W. (1890). *The Principles of Psychology*. New York: Holt.

Jeste, D.V., and Vahia, I.V. (2007). Comparison of the conceptualization of wisdom in ancient Indian literature with modern views: focus on the Bhagavad Gita. *Psychiatry*, 71(3), 197-209.

Jones, R.M., Hartmann, B.R., Grochowski, C.O., and Glider, P. (1989). Ego identity and substance abuse: A comparison of adolescents in residential treatment with adolescents in school. *Personality and Individual Differences*, 10, 625-631.

Kihlstrom, J.F., Beer, J.S., and Klein, S.B. (2003). Self and identity as memory In M.R. Leary, & J.P. Tangney (Eds.), *Handbook of Self and Identity*, New York: The Guilford Press. 68-90.

Leary, M.R. and Tangney, J.P. (2003). The self as an organizing construct in the behavioural and social sciences In M.R. Leary, & J.P. Tangney (Eds.), *Handbook of Self and Identity*. (2nd Edition, 3-14), New York: The Guilford Press.

Locke, J. (1975). *An Essay Concerning Human Understanding*, Oxford: Clarendon Press.

Marcia, J.E. (1966). Development and validation of ego identity status. *Journal of Personality and Social Psychology*, 5, 552-558.

Marcia, J.E. (1976). Identity six years after: A follow-up study. *Journal of Youth and Adolescence*, 5(2), 145-160.

Marcia, J.E. (1980). Identity in adolescence. *Handbook of Adolescent Psychology*, 9, 159-187.

McCall, G.J., and Simmons, J.L. (1978). *Identities and Interactions: an Examination of Human Associations in Everyday Life*. New York: Free Press

Mulholland Jr, M.R. (2012). *The Deeper Journey: The Spirituality of Discovering Your True Self*: Downers Grove: Inter Varsity Press.

Muuss, R., Velder, E., and Porton, H. (1996). *Theories of Adolescence*. New York: McGraw-Hill.

Onorato, R.S., and Turner, J.C. (2004). Fluidity in the self-concept: the shift from personal to social identity. *European Journal of Social Psychology*, 34(3), 257-278.

Paloutzian, R.F. and Park, C.L. (2005). *Handbook of Religion and Spirituality*. New York: Guilford Press.

Parthasarathy, A. (1971). *Atma Bodha (Knowledge of the self) of Sri Shankaracharya*: Bombay: Bhartiya Vidya Bhavan.

Pelletier, G, Verhoef, M.J., Khatri, N., and Hagen, N. (2002). Quality of life in brain tumor patients: The relative contributions of depression, fatigue, emotional distress, and existential issues. *Journal of Neuro-oncology*, 57(1), 41-49.

Ramamoorthy, H. and Nome (2002). *Svatmanirupanam: The True Definition of One's Own Self*: Santa Cruz, CA: Society of Abidance in Truth.

Rao, S. (2003). *Adi Shankaracharya: The Voice of Vedanta*, New Delhi: Rupa Publications.

Roeser, R.W., Peck, S.C. and Nasir, N.S. (2006). Self and identity processes in school motivation, learning and achievement. In P.A. Alaxander, P.R. Pintrich and P.H. Winne, eds. *Handbook of Educational Psychology*, 2nd ed. 391-424, Mahwah, NJ: Lawrence Earlbaum.

Schwartz, S.J. (2001). The evolution of Eriksonian and, neo-Eriksonian identity theory and research: A review and integration. *Identity: An International Journal of Theory and Research*, 1(1), 7-58.

Schwartz, J. (2008). Self and Identity in Early Adolescence: Some Reflections and an Introduction to the Special Issue. *Journal of Early Adolescence*, 28, 5-15.

Schwartz, S.J., Mason, C.A., Pantin, H., and Szapocznik, J. (2008). Effects of family functioning and identity confusion on substance use and sexual behaviour in Hispanic immigrant early adolescents. *Identity: An International Journal of Theory and Research*, 8(2), 107-124.

Schwartz, S.J., Pantin, H., Prado, G., Sullivan, S., and Szapocznik, J. (2005). Family functioning, identity, and problem behaviour in Hispanic immigrant early adolescents. *Journal of Early Adolescence*, 25, 392-420.

Sneed, J.R., Schwartz, S.J., and Cross, Jr, W.E. (2006). A multicultural critique of identity status theory and research: A call for integration. *Identity*, *6*(1), 61-84.

Stryker, S. (1980). *Symbolic Interactionism: A Social Structural Version*. Menlo Park, CA: Benjamin/Cummings.

Thoits, P.A. (1986). Social support as coping assistance. *Journal of Consulting and Clinical Psychology*, 54(4), 416.

Tillich, P. (1952). *The Courage To Be*. New Haven: Yale University Press.

Touraine, A. (1971). Crisis and Conflict. *International Journal of Sociology*, 1, 3, 284-308.

Turner, J.C., Hogg, M.A., Oakes, P.J., Reicher, S.D., and Wetherell, M.S. (1987). *Rediscovering the social group: A self-categorization theory*. Oxford: Basil Blackwell.

Van Knippenberg, D., Van Knippenberg, B., De Cremer, D., and Hogg, M.A. (2004). Leadership, self, and identity: A review and research agenda. *The Leadership Quarterly*, 15(6), 825-856.

Westen, D. and Heim, A.K. (2003). Disturbance of self and identity in personality disorders. In M. Leary and J. Tangeney (eds). *Handbook of Self and Identity* (pp. 643-664). New York: Guilford Press.

Young, I.M. (2009). Five faces of oppression. In G. Henderson and M. Waterstone (Eds.), *Geographic Thought: A Praxis Perspective* (pp. 55-71). New York, NY: Routledge.

19

Health and Well-being as an Outcome of Proactive Coping

An Overview

Reeta Chauhan, Purnima Awasthi and *Saroj Verma*

The present review emphasizes the concept of proactive coping and its relation to health outcomes in the lives of individuals. This construct has emerged as a positive psychological construct which is conceptualized more broadly as an approach to life which helps individuals to think in more positive way and to act with all his/her resources during adversities. Review of studies indicates that preventive coping and proactive coping are different construct. Proactive coping generally enhances well-being but preventive coping does not. People who adopt proactive coping see future stress as challenges and they strive for life improvement and build up resources that assure progress and quality of psychosocial functioning. Rehabilitation literature emphasizes the proactive coping strategies and its beneficial outcomes. The mental and physical health outcomes studies revealed that proactive coping is an important self-regulatory behaviour which is highly associated with individuals' age, education, and gender. Some psychosocial and demographic factors highlighted in the present review and some interventions are also discussed in order to promote proactive coping and self-regulation.

Individual differences exist in developing health related behaviours and illnesses. Proactivity inclined individuals are generally engaged in anticipatory and preventive activities or regulate their behaviour (e.g. quit smoking to prevent lung cancer or using condom to prevent STD) in such a way which enhances their well-being and reduces or moderates the stress associated with illness or the stress related with other sources (Cunningham and De La Rosa, 2008). The proactive individual strives for life improvement and builds up resources that assure progress and quality of functioning. This article focuses on proactive coping and its effect on individual's health and well-being with the help of studies carried out in the field of health psychology, educational psychology, organizational psychology, and rehabilitation psychology.

Proactive Coping

The concept of Proactive coping was first introduced by Aspinwall and Taylor (1997) in the famous article "A stitch in time: Self-Regulation and Proactive Coping". This article was focused to the issue of coping with future stress. They defined proactive coping as individuals' ability to recognize future threats and to use strategies that may help to offset these problems at an early stage. Aspinwall and Taylor (1997) specify five stages in proactive coping such as resource accumulation, recognition of potential stressors, initial appraisal, preliminary coping efforts, and elicitation and use of feedback concerning initial efforts. They emphasized that individual differs on each stage of proactive coping on the skills and resources they have.

According to Proactive Coping Theory proposed by Schwarzer's (1999a) the proactive individual strives for improvement in his or her life and environment instead of mainly reacting to past or anticipated adversity. Proactive coping is autonomous and self-determined goal setting and realisation of goals. It deals with self-regulatory goal attainment processes and explains what motivates people to strive for ambitious goals and to commit themselves to personal quality management (Schwarzer, 1999). Schwarzer and Taubert (2002) proposed four kinds of coping strategies, i.e. reactive coping, proactive coping, anticipatory coping and preventive coping. Proactive coping can be distinguished from these similar construct on the basis of its temporal location in the coping process and the level of certainty it involves (Schwarzer and Taubert, 2002). Proactive coping takes place before anticipatory coping, which occurs immediately before an event. Additionally proactive coping occurs when the stressors to be encountered is less certain than the stressors that elicit reactive coping or anticipatory coping. However, proactive coping and preventive coping are quite similar with respect to their temporal position relative to a stressor and the level of certainty regarding those stressors, with proactive coping simply occurring in situation, whereby the upcoming stressor is slightly more certain.

Schwarzer and Taubert (2002) specify that proactive coping is based on preparing for possible positive appraisals of the future, whereas preventive coping is based on preparing for possible negative appraisals of the future. Therefore, proactive coping is defined by these authors to be "an effort to build up general resources that facilitate promotion towards challenging goals and personal growth," as opposed to preventive coping that aims "to build up general resistance resources that result in less strain in the future by minimizing the severity of the impact, with less severe consequences of stress, should it occur, or a less likely onset of stressful events in the first place (Schwarzer and Taubert, 2002, p. 27). In this conceptualization a proactive individual will tend to appraise stressors as challenges and worry less, whereas a preventive individual will tend to appraise stressors as threats and worry, more. Regardless of these appraisals and levels of worry however, it is proposed that proactive coping and preventive coping manifest in a similar set of skills. It can be recognized by the following three features as first, proactive coping integrates planning and preventive strategies with proactive self-regulatory goal attainment. Second, it integrates proactive goal attainment with identification and utilization of social resources, and third, it utilizes proactive emotional coping for self regulatory goal attainment (Greenglass, 2002, p. 41).

More clarification regarding these similar but different construct has been provided in studies. Gan, Yang, Zhou and Zhang (2007) studied the concept of proactive coping and preventive coping under the broad concept of future oriented coping. They tried to find out the mediating role of future oriented coping in student engagement and revealed that proactive coping fully mediated the relationship between stress and engagement while preventive coping partially mediated this relationship. Gan, Hu, and Zhang (2010) studied both the concept among freshman at a Chinese university regarding their adjustment. The result of the study suggests that only proactive coping plays an important role in university adjustment and they also proposed that proactive coping is a dispositional trait rather than a coping strategy.

Further Sohl and Moyer (2009) tried to differentiate between these conceptualizations. They compared how each operationalization of proactive coping relates to well-being. They revealed that the conceptualization of proactive coping as a positively-focused striving for goals predicted well-being whereas the conceptualization focusing on preventing a negative future was not found to be associated with well-being. Hu and Gan (2011) proposed that both constructs (proactive and preventive coping) are two sequential stages of a single process and are highly covariant. A study by Ouwehand, De Ridder, and Bensing (2001) with older adults revealed that people need to experience at least a slight feeling of threat in order to direct their attention to a potential stressor and to become motivated to engage in proactive coping. Simply in proactive coping stress is termed as "eustress" which consists of vital energy and productive arousal.

Measures of Proactive Coping

Proactive coping is a process, which is a set of skills with future and outcome oriented thinking. There are so many personality (internal resources) and contextual (external resources) variables which may influence the proactive coping processes (Aspinwall and Taylor, 1997). According to Aspinwall (2005) the individual differences, processes and skills collectively known as future oriented thinking, is an important concept in the field of health where one's belief about future outcomes are critical determinant of present behaviour. So it is evident that most of the studies related to gerontology and health assessed proactive coping with the help of measures based on Aspinwall and Taylor (1997) Theory. They argued that proactive coping primarily consists of various problems focused coping strategies such as planning, seeking instrumental support, and actively taking measures to prevent potential stressors. The studies related to intervention were combined with a self-management technique which is predicted by proactive coping for proximal and distal outcome. It is clear from the review that most of the time same set of authors were associated with studies carried out in the field of proactive coping.

The second conceptualization of proactive coping is based on Schwarzer's (1999a) theory. Proactive Coping Inventory developed by Greenglass, Schwarzer, Jakubiec, Fiksenbaum, and Taubert, (1999). This inventory is comprised 55 items and seven sub-scales, i.e. proactive coping, reflective coping, strategic planning, preventive coping, instrumental, support seeking, emotional support seeking, and avoidance coping with 55-items. Most of the studies used proactive coping subscale to assess its impact on health and well-being.

Proactive Coping and Health

According to new philosophy of health, proactive coping is viewed as essence of productive life and an important concept of quality of life. It is considered as integral part of the overall development of individuals. WHO (1984) defines health as the state of complete physical, social, emotional, psychological, economical, and spiritual well being, not simply the absence of illness. It has different dimensions within individuals' life such as physical, mental, social, spiritual, vocational and emotional. An individual's personal characteristics determine his/her health conditions. Studies indicate that individuals who are resilient and exhibit proactive behaviours enjoy good quality of life (Ouwehand, de Ridder, and Bensing, 2007). Psychosocial resources are important concepts in proactive coping which are utilized by a person during the process of proactive coping. Aspinwall and Taylor (1997) believed that individuals, who have well developed psychosocial resources, including a sense of personal control, high self-esteem, and optimism, are more likely to cope proactively and minimize the effects of stress, hence protects persons' health. Psychosocial resourcefulness is extensively regarded as a vital factor in optimal psychological functioning and linked well with psychological variables as optimism, self-esteem, self-confidence, internal locus of control, maturity, hardiness, self-acceptance, happiness, and self-actualization (Van der Merwe, 1997; Koenig, McCullough, and Larson, 2001). These indicators of psychosocial resourcefulness also have positive relationships with lifestyle, participation in physical activity and physical health (Van der Merwe, 1997).

Several Western societies are facing the challenges regarding the increasing number of elderly people because of increment in life span of individuals and lower birth rate. There is growing concern regarding maintenance of quality of life and rehabilitation of this population. Studies related to proactive coping and aging are sufficient in number in the field of rehabilitation, which focus on the relationship of aging with proactive coping and its effect on health and subjective well-being. These studies also help in better understanding of this particular construct in relation to functional improvement of elderly. Health can be considered as one of the most important resource for self-regulation, especially in older age. Preserving good health is often not an ultimate goal in itself, but a prerequisite to maintaining and pursuing numerous different types of personal goals that contribute to subjective well-being. These studies considered that coping is an essential aspect in successful aging. Different psychosocial resources and functional abilities declined as person grows older, so the successful management of these resources is necessary for a normative adult life. Fiksenbaum, Greenglass and Eaton (2006) examined the association between coping, social support, daily hassles, functional disability and physical and psychological health status among older adults. They reported that individuals who employed higher levels of proactive coping had better functional ability than those who employed less proactive coping. To the extent that elderly individuals engage in autonomous and self-determined goal setting and strive to commit themselves to personal quality management (proactive coping), they are more able to carry out everyday activities such as dressing, washing, shopping, and using the telephone. Thus, proactive coping positively affects independence in the elderly by contributing to the performance of more everyday activities. Proactive coping was also associated with fewer hassles, specifically fewer health problems. It appears that elderly individuals who employ coping strategies based on proactivity are less likely to experience daily stressors such as worries about health and well-being or not having enough money for personal needs. In another study by the same authors reveal that proactive coping negatively associated with depression, which is positively associated with functional disability among elderly (Greenglass, Fiksenbaum, and Eaton, 2006).

Ouwehand, deRidder, and Bensing (2006) examined as to what extent proactive coping is influenced by situation-specific features as well as by personal characteristics. It can be said that examining both the situational and individual influences provide a more complete picture of proactive coping behaviour. For this purpose they presented three vignettes to middle and older adults, in which each vignette representing a potential decline in an important resource such as health, social relationships and finance. It was found that proactive coping is highly variable within persons and the three situational factors, i.e. type of stressor, appraised threat and appraised control. Some people use more proactive coping in a health situation than in a financial situation whereas for other people, the pattern is just the opposite. It was also apparent that future temporal orientation was a significant, positive predictor of proactive coping i.e., those having a future temporal orientation has a positive impact on all four proactive coping.

Ouwehand, deRidder, and Bensing (2008) studied the individual differences in proactive coping strategies, i.e. the strategies people employ to prevent future stressors, among middle and older adults. They confronted the adults with three ecologically relevant issues, namely a potential decline in health, a potential change in social contacts, and a potential decrease in financial resources and examined to what extent differences in proactive coping with these situations were associated with five personality traits, namely future temporal orientation, goal orientation, dispositional optimism, self-efficacy, and aging anxiety. The result showed that future temporal orientation and goal orientation was significantly associated with proactive coping. In addition, a higher educational level was also important for explaining individual differences in proactive coping, but not regarding all types of potential changes. It seems that the impact of trait factors on proactive coping partially depends on the type of future stressor that is encountered and the skills that are necessary to deal with it effectively.

Pursuing and achieving personal goals influence subjective well-being. Successfully managing goal threats is an essential part of life. With aging, the balance between gains and losses becomes less favourable (Baltes and Baltes, 1990), which poses a threat to self-regulation processes with respect to goals. A potentially important strategy for postponing a decline in resources, which are important for goal achievement, is to handle such losses at an early stage and make efforts to prevent them or their consequences, in other words, to engage in proactive coping (Aspinwall, 1997; Aspinwall and Taylor, 1997). Ouwehand, deRidder, and Bensing (2008) examined that to what extent features of a potential goal threat (a potential loss in health) affect attention, planning and information-seeking, i.e. proactive coping in middle-aged and older adults. They reported that, time (until a potential goal threat will manifest itself) influences the amount of attention paid to signals that indicate the coming of the stressor as well as information-seeking about how to prevent the probable threat, whereas it did not affect planning. When a potential threat is likely to reveal itself in the short term, individuals paid more attention to danger cues and spent more time seeking information in comparison with when a potential threat would not reveal itself for a long time. It was also reported that control over the situation did not have an impact on proactive coping, but an interaction effect of time and control was found to be important in the group of participants who reported having a health-related goal. Furthermore, control affected how people evaluated their plans. People who had more control over the potential stressor were more motivated to carry out the plans they made for the future.

It is well-known that psychological factors are significant predictors of behavioural outcomes in rehabilitation patients. The way the patients cope with stress during their hospital stay plays an important role in their subsequent performance on outcome measures. Greenglass, Marques, de Riedder, and Behl (2005) examined the role of positive coping and mastery in rehabilitation setting. Result indicated that those individuals who used more proactive coping cover greater distance in two minutes than those who used less proactive coping. The relationship between proactive coping and functional independence was mediated by the perception related to

Getting on with life. A study on Israeli elderly persons for maintaining successful ageing shows that psychosocial resources (self-efficacy and social support) and proactive coping predicted successful ageing. It is found that elderly people can shape their quality of life in the presence of decline in health and functioning by using appropriate coping resources and coping patterns (Tovel, and Carmel, 2013).

Proactive Coping and Demographic Variables

Studies of proactive copings with demographic variable revealed that individual differences exist with age, gender and education level. The fact that men and women differ in their coping style is well established (Anshel, and Miesner, 2010). It is reported in the studies that men prefer more proactive coping while women depend on the other forms of coping. A study on the sample of German people assessing the distress related to Tinnitus revealed that women were more distressed than men and used less proactive coping strategies than men (Seydel, Haupt, Olze, Szczepek and Mazurek, 2013). Better individual resources empower individuals to cope more effectively with stress (Schwarzer, 2000). It has been found that older people use more proactive coping than younger people. Middle aged people whether male or female use less proactive coping than younger or older people. Studies regarding education showing inconsistent result for proactive coping. Those who were highly educated show more proactive coping than less educated people, whereas occupational status was not significantly associated with proactive coping competence. In addition, some evidence was found for the idea that people with lower socio-economic status have more current stress, which inhibits engagement in proactive coping. Better socio-economic status can be considered as important resource which a person can use when needed. People with a higher income have less physical health stress, which in turn is positively associated with competence (Ouwehand, de Ridder, and Bensing, 2009; Tomas, and Eva, 2009; Gautam, Punia and Yadav, 2013).

A study conducted on students to identify the gender age and learning context differences in university students' proactive coping and vulnerability to depression. This study slightly deviates regarding gender differences on proactive coping. It shows that female students are more able to proactively cope with the environmental demands than their male counterparts but on the other hand they were more susceptible to the depressive symptoms. The study also shows the similar finding with rest of the studies regarding age and proactive coping. Younger students show less proactive coping strategies and were prone to develop depressive symptoms than older students (Bagana, Negovan, and Vanea, 2012). A contrasting result regarding environment and proactive coping is provided by Bogadan, Rioux, and Negovan (2011). They assessed the place attachment, proactive coping and well-being in three different university environment (French University, Romanian private university and Romanian public university) and they found that student of Romanian public university scored higher on proactive coping than their two other counterparts.

Proactive Coping as Positive Psychological Variable and Well-Being

Studies with positive psychological variable indicate proactive coping to be associated with positive affect, satisfaction with life, optimism and social support. It is well-known that positive beliefs is associated with positive emotions and well-being and reduces mental health problems. The findings of a study on mindfulness indicate positive correlations between high levels of mindfulness, self-esteem, proactive coping and high satisfaction with life (Hinterman, Burns, Hopwood, and Rogers, 2012). Findings indicate that proactive coping enhances a perspective on life that involves a positive attitude towards future events in the form of optimistic expectancies and enhanced feelings of self-worth. A study by Chang and Sana (2001) suggested that optimism is significantly correlated with proactive coping which further associated with positive affect, satisfaction with life and less physical symptoms. Uskul and Greenglass (2005) examined the predictor of psychological well-being and found that optimism and proactive coping positively predicts to life satisfaction and negatively to depression.

Proactive Coping as Mediator and Moderator

A study on Chinese students revealed that proactive coping acts as a moderator on dietary intentions and planning. The students who scored higher on proactive coping would exhibit better dietary intention-planning-behaviour (Zhou, Gan, Knoll and Schwarzer, 2013). The study provides a base for development of interventions for improvement of dietary behaviours. Some studies used proactive coping as mediator as Davis and Brekke (2014) examined the mediating role of proactive coping for social support and role functioning among severely mentally ill individuals. They analyzed the impact of proactive processes on functioning of the severely mentally ill individuals. They included positive reappraisal and intrinsic motivation as proactive coping processes. A proactive coping orientation involves positively reappraising demanding or stressful situations as having value based on their perceived potential to promote growth (Folkman, 1997), an appraisal process that gives rise to intrinsically motivated goal-striving (Schwarzer and Taubert, 2002). Intrinsic motivation in itself is as goal-directed behaviour based on internally-driven rewards related to interest, meaning, and purpose (Ryan and Deci, 2000). They assumed that positively reappraising stressful circumstances as potential opportunities for growth give rise to intrinsic motivation, which is a theoretically proposed process underlying proactive coping theory (Schwarzer and Taubert, 2002) further contribute in positive role functioning. The result of the study indicated that social support and proactive coping may enhance the role functioning for a population with significant functional impairment (Bellack *et al.*, 2007). Results also suggest that social support from others represents an important coping resource that may promote proactive coping, which in turn mediates enhanced functioning for people with severe mental illness.

Proactive Coping, Self-Regulation and Intervention

Self-regulation is an important construct in health psychology. It focuses on the ways in which individuals direct and monitor their activities and emotions in order to attain their goals. Self-regulation and proactive coping both are part of coping mechanism of an individual. Both concept have their root somewhere in social cognition and are related to active coping processes of an individual, which focus on the motivational, cognitive and behavioural system. The difference is that the role motivation in proactive coping is found to be more positive than self-regulation. A moderately positive correlation between scores on the proactive coping subscale and self-efficacy was reported in previous studies, which suggests that self-regulation is one of the dimensions of proactive coping (Greenglass, 2002; Greenglass *et al.*, 1999). Zambianchi and Bitti (2013) analyzed the role of proactive coping with other variables in social well-being in emerging adulthood. They reported that proactive coping act as a positive predictor of social well-being in affect regulation. Studies linked to health behaviour show the importance of self-regulatory processes and proactive coping in maintenance of healthy behaviours.

Studies related to intervention are rooted in a framework of self-regulation and proactive coping theories and emphasizes an anticipatory planning and problem solving perspective. Aspinwall and Taylor (1997) conceptualizes proactive coping as a set of competencies which can be enhanced. Based on this conceptualization Bode, Ridder, Kuijer and Bensing (2007) planned a brief educational programme based on proactive coping theory for middle aged and older male and female participant. The programme included four sessions. The first session included the identification of the advantages of preparing oneself for future, second session included the recognition and handling of early warning signals, the third session included specification of strategies to reach their goal by mental stimulation technique, and in the last session participants evaluated the attempts to reach the individual goal. At last, feedback by trainers also provided. They used a prospective randomized control trial with an experimental group and a waiting control group and collected data at three point (base line, after completion of the programme and three months post intervention). The result of the study shows that after completion of programme participants reported higher level of proactive competencies. The stability of the intervention effects was also supported by the preservation of these effects three months after programme. Result suggested that concrete formulation of the individual goal can facilitate improvement of proactive competencies.

The aim of the second study, based on proactive coping theory, a self-management intervention to support patients recently diagnosed with type-2 diabetes, was to achieve sustained improvement in their self-care behaviours. The intervention emphasizes the crucial role of anticipation and planning in maintaining self-care behaviours. They also used a prospective randomized design. Two groups were formed. In first group recent screen-detected participant had included who received the intervention were compared with second group in which participants with usual care were included. They were examined on changes in proximal outcomes (intentions, self-efficacy and proactive coping), self-care behaviour (diet, physical activity and medication) and weight overtime (0, 3, and 12 months). The result indicated that intervention was effective in improving proximal outcomes and behaviour with regard to diet and physical activity, resulting in significant weight loss at 12 months. It was also reported that proactive coping was a better predictor of long-term self management (Toohlen, Ridder, Bensing, Gorter, and Rutten, 2009).

A study by Toohlen *et al.* (2009) assessed self-management techniques in group of diabetic patients, a booster session was added in the study. The booster phase included a how-condition and a why-condition. The how-condition was original, control condition repeating the protocol from initial phase and the why-condition challenged patient to focus on their higher order goals by asking to elaborate on one of their personal goals by repeatedly answering why-questions. The result revealed that participants improved on all psychological and behavioural variables during the initial phase and maintained these improvements over 12 months. But the booster phase yielded no further improvement (Kroese, Adriaanse, Vinkers, de Schoot and deRidder, 2014).

Silverman (2011) conducted two pilot study focused on the effects of music therapy on psychiatric patients' proactive coping skills. The result of the first study revealed that participants in the music therapy condition had higher proactive coping skills than participants in the psycho-educational control condition. Further in the second study the participants were compared for the effect of music therapy and psycho-education on the proactive coping skills. The participants in the music therapy condition reported slightly higher proactive coping than participants in the psycho educational control condition. This study shows that music therapy enhanced proactive coping skills among these patients.

Proactive coping has been emerged as a positive predictor of students' well-being. Being in the phase of late adolescence and emerging adulthood, they are more susceptible to health impairing behaviours (smoking, drinking alcohol, etc.) and stressed for future goals. Here we can emphasize the role of strong control on self and the ability to cope with life demands. Kadhiravan and Kumar (2012) planned an intervention for the students. The training programme was developed for the following skills: problem solving, decision-making skills, communication skills, interpersonal skills, and coping skills. The result indicated that developed training is effective in enhancing proactive coping of college students. Individuals who engage in proactive coping are better able to use personal and psychological resources to deal with future stressors (Schwarzer, 2002).

Conclusion

With the help of this article an attempt is made to present an overview of the studies carried out in the field of proactive coping. Review shows that it is a new and different construct from traditional coping, which has been used as a positive psychological variable. There are two different conceptualizations about this concept. Both have been outlined. Further, a glimpse of studies and measures, used in the studies carried out in the area of proactive coping has been provided, including the studies conducted in different field in relation to proactive coping.

Review indicates that proactive coping has emerged as a promising concept in different field of psychology, especially in field of health psychology. Individuals who use such type of coping have a vision and experience less stress because they may plan for their life goals. It can be seen that the interventions planned in the field of health psychology based on proactive coping provided fine and consistent results.

It is observed that this concept has been used for different samples with different conceptualization. Some studies used this concept in terms of dispositional tendency while other used it as a process through which different kinds of skills (e.g. communication skill) and resources (personal as well as social) can be acquired for goal achievement. There is a dearth of researches with regard to age differences as psychological proactive coping resources of different age groups will differ considerably. Further the need is also felt to consider the cultural aspects in investing the outcome of proactive coping in terms of psychological well-being.

References

Anshel, M.H. and Miesner, M. (2010). The approach-avoidance framework for identifying athletes' coping style as a function of gender and race. *Scandavian Journal of Psychology,* 51, 341-349.

Aspinwall, L.G. (1997). Where planning meets coping: proactive coping and the detection and management of potential stressors. In: Friedman, S.L., Scholnick, E.K., editors. *The Developmental Psychology of Planning: Why, How, and When do We Plan?* London: Lawrence Erlbaum Associates, 285-320.

Aspinwall, L.G. (2005). The Psychology of Future-Oriented Thinking: From Achievement to Proactive Coping, Adaptation, and Aging. *Motivation and Emotion,* 29, 4, 203-235.

Aspinwall, L.G., and Taylor, S.E. (1997). A stitch in time: Self-regulation and proactive coping. *Psychological Bulletin,* 121, 417-436.

Bagana, E., Negovan, V., and Vanea, M. (2012). Proactive coping and vulnerability to depression in university environment–gender, age and learning context differences. *Procedia-Social and Behavioural Sciences* 12, 30-39.

Baltes, P.B., and Baltes, M.M. (1990). Psychological perspective on successful aging: The model of selective optimization with compensation. *In Successful Aging: Perspectives from the Behavioural Sciences* (pp. 1-34). New York: Cambridge University Press.

Bellack, A.S., Green, M.F., Cook, J.A., Fenton, W., Harvey, P.D., Heaton, R.K., Laughren, T., *et al.* (2007). Assessment of Community Functioning in People with Schizophrenia and Other Severe Mental Illnesses: A White Paper Based on an NIMH-Sponsored Workshop. *Schizophrenia Bulletin,* 33, 3, 805-822.

Bode, C., Ridder, D.T.D. de, Kuijer, R.G., and Bensing, J.M. (2007). Effects of an Intervention Promoting Proactive Coping Competencies in Middle and Late Adulthood. *The Gerontologist,* 47, 1, 42-51.

Bogdan, C., Rioux, L., and Negovan, V. (2011). Place attachment, proactive coping and well-being in university environment. *Procedia Social and Behavioural Sciences,* 33, 865-869.

Chang, E.S., and Sana, L.J. (2001). Optimism, pessimism, and positive and negativity in middle-aged adults: A test of cognitive-affective model of psychological adjustment. *Psychology and Aging,* 16, 524-531.

Cunningham, C.J., and De La Rosa, G.M., (2008). The interactive effect of proactive personality and work-family interference on well-being. *Journal of Occupational Health Psychology,* 13, 3, 271-82.

Davis, L., and Brekke, J. (2014). Social support and functional outcome in severe mental illness: The mediating role of proactive coping. *Psychiatry Research,* 215, 1, 39-45.

Fiksenbaum, L.M., Greenglass, E.R. and Eaton, J. (2006). Perceived social support, hassles, and coping among the elderly. *The Journal of Applied Gerontology,* 25, 1, 17-30.

Folkman, S. (1997). Positive psychological states and coping with severe stress. *Social Science and Medicine*, 45, 1207-1221.

Gan, Y., Hu, Y., and Zhang, Y., (2010). Proactive and preventive coping in adjustment to college. *The Psychological Record,* 60, 643-658.

Gan, Y., Yang, M., Zhou, Y., and Zhang, Y. (2007). The two-factor structure of future-oriented coping and its mediating role in student engagement. *Personality and Individual Differences,* 43, 851-863.

Gautam, N.S., Punia, S., and Yadav, P. (2013). Proactive coping skills: Gender differential in different ecological settings. *Indian Journal of Health and Well-being,* 4, 1, 141-144.

Greenglass, E.R., Fiksenbaum, L., and Eaton, J. (2006). The relationship between coping, social support, functional disability and depression in the elderly. *Anxiety, Stress, and Coping,* 19, 1, 15-31.

Greenglass, E.R., Schwarzer, R., and Taubert, S. (1999). The proactive coping inventory (PCI). A multidimensional research instrument. [On-line publication]. <http://www.ralfschwarzer.de/> 3.02.13.

Greenglass, E.R., Marques, S., de Ridder, M., and Behl, S. (2005). Positive coping and mastery in a rehabilitation setting. *International Journal of Rehabilitation Research,* 28, 331-339.

Hinterman, C., Burns, L., Hopwood, D., and Rogers, W. (2012). Mindfulness: Seeking a More Perfect Approach to Coping with Life's Challenges. *Mindfulness,* 3, 275-281.

Hu, Y., and Gan, Y. (2011). Future oriented coping and job hunting among college students. *The Psychological Record,* 61, 253-268.

Kadhiravan, S., and Kumar, K. (2012). Enhancing stress coping skills among college students. *Journal of Arts, Science & Commerce,* 4, 1, 49-55.

Koenig, H.G., McCullough, M.E., and Larson, D.B. (2001). Handbook of religion and health. Oxford: Oxford University Press.

Kroese, F.M., Adriaanse, M.A., Vinkers, C.D., van de Schoot, and R., deRidder, D.T. (2014). The effectiveness of a proactive coping intervention targeting self-management in diabetes patients. *Psychology and Health,* 29, 1, 110-25.

Ouwehand, C., De Ridder, D.T.D., and Bensing, J.M. (2001). Proactive adaptation to ageing: An exploratory focus group study. Unpublished manuscript.

Ouwehand, C., De Ridder, D.T.D., and Bensing, J.M. (2006). Situational aspects are more important in shaping proactive coping behaviour than individual characteristics: A vignette study among adults preparing for ageing. *Psychology and Health,* 21, 809-825.

Ouwehand, C., de Ridder, D.T.D., Bensing, J.M. (2007). A review of successful aging models: Proposing proactive coping as an important additional strategy. *Clinical Psychology Review*, 27, 8, 873-884.

Ouwehand, C., de Ridder, D.T.D., and Bensing, J.M. (2008). The characteristics of a potential goal threat predict attention and information-seeking in middle-aged and older adults. *Motivation & Emotion*, 32, 90-99.

Ouwehand, C., de Ridder, D.T.D., and Bensing, J.M. (2008). Individual differences in the use of proactive coping strategies by middle-aged and older adults. *Personality and Individual Differences,* 45, 28-33.

Ouwehand, C., de Ridder, D.T.D., Bensing, J.M. (2009). Who can afford to look to the future? The relationship between socio-economic status and proactive coping. *European Journal of Public Health,* 19, 4, 412-17.

Ryan, R.M., and Deci, E.L. (2000) Self-determination theory and the facilitation of intrinsic motivation, social development, and well-being. *The American Psychologist,* 55, 1, 68-78.

Schwarzer, R. (1999). Self-regulatory processes in the adoption and maintenance of health behaviours. The role of optimism, goals, and threats. *Journal of Health Psychology,* 4, 115-127.

Schwarzer, R. (2000). Manage stress at work through preventive and proactive coping. In E.A. Locke (Ed.), *The Blackwell Handbook of Principles of Organizational Behaviour* (pp. 342–355). Oxford, UK: Blackwell.

Schwarzer, R., and Taubert, S. (2002). Tenacious goal pursuits and striving towards personal growth: Proactive coping. In E. Frydenberg (Ed.), *Beyond Coping: Meeting Goals, Visions and Challenges* (pp. 19-35). London: Oxford University Press.

Seydel, C., Haupt, H., Olze, H., Szczepek, A J., and Mazurek, B. (2013 distress depend on age and dur). Gender and chronic tinnitus: differences in tinnitus-related action of tinnitus. *Ear and Hearing,* 34, 5, 661-72.

Silverman, M.J. (2011). Effects of music therapy on psychiatric patients' proactive coping skills: Two pilot studies. *The Arts in Psychotherapy,* 38, 125-129.

Sohl, S.J., and Moyer, A. (2009). Refining the conceptualization of an important Future Oriented Self-Regulatory behaviour: Proactive Coping. *Personality and Individual Differences,* 1, 47, 2, 139-144.

Thoolen, B.J., de Ridder, D., Bensing, J., Gorter, K., and Rutten, G. (2009). Beyond good intentions: The role of proactive coping in achieving sustained behavioural change in the context of diabetes management. *Psychology and Health,* 24, 3, 237-54.

Tomas, S., and Sollarova, E. (2009). Proactive coping from the perspective of age, gender and education. *Studia Psychologica,* 51, 161-165.

Tovel, H., Carmel, S. (2013). Maintaining Successful Aging: The Role of Coping Patterns and Resources. *Journal of Happiness Studies,* 1-16.

Uskul, A.K., and Greenglass, E.R. (2005). Psychological well-being in a Turkish-Canadian sample. *Anxiety, Stress, and Coping,* 18, 269-278.

Van der Merwe, S. (1997). The relationship between physical activity and spiritual well-being with lifestyle and health. Potchefstroom (Unpublished Ph.D. thesis—Potchefstroom University for CHE).

WHO (1984). *Glossary of Terms used in "Health for All" Series*. Geneva.

Zambianchi, M., Bitti, P.E.R. (2013). The Role of Proactive Coping Strategies, Time Perspective, Perceived Efficacy on Affect Regulation, Divergent Thinking and Family Communication in Promoting Social Well-Being in Emerging Adulthood. *Social Indicators Research,* 1-15.

Zhou, G., Gan, Y., Knoll, N., and Schwarzer, R. (2013). Proactive coping moderates the dietary intention-planning-behaviour path. *Appetite,* 70, 127-133.

20

Child and Adolescent Mental Health Issues

A Practical Approach for Psychological Intervention

Neelam Verma

The importance of psychological well-being in children and adolescent, for their healthy emotional, social, physical, cognitive and educational development, is well-recognized. There is now increasing evidence on the effectiveness of interventions to improve children's and adolescent's resilience, promote mental health and treat mental health problems and disorders. The chapter organizes discussion of Disorder-Specific-Interventions targeted and mental health promotion including strategies related to fostering positive development among children and adolescents and modifying factors found to be correlated with such disorders. The chapter encompasses interventions based on clinical models and theories in clinical set-up, home based interventions for family members and community and school based interventions for class-room management of such problems. Intervention strategies will be based on specific disorder and its major demand for the type of intervention. Before discussing the treatment, it is essential to focus upon the assessment of such conditions using interview and other major assessments.

Psychological Assessment of Children and Adolescents: Major Assessment Tools

Following are the major assessment tools used for the evaluation of child and adolescent issues. Some of them are conducted to identify the problem and others are conducted to assess the severity of identified problem. Following are some of the tests commonly and widely used in clinical set-ups:

Measures to Assess Intellectual Functioning (Normals)

- Malin's Intelligence Scale for Indian Children (MISIC).
- Wechsler Adult Performance Intelligence Scale (WAPIS).
- Wechsler Intelligence Scale for Children (WISC).
- Raven's Progressive Matrices (RPM).

Measures to Assess Intellectual Functioning (Mentally Retarded)

- Seguin Form Board Test (SFBT).
- Vineland Social Maturity Scale (VSMS).
- Developmental Screening Test (DST).
- Gessell's Drawing Test (GDT).

Measures to Assess Cognitive/Neurological Functioning

- NIMHANS Index for Specific Learning Disability (SLD).
- NIMHANS Neuropsychological Battery for Children.

Checklists for Assessment of Clinical Disorders

- Child Behaviour Checklist (CBCL).
- Developmental Psychopathology Checklist (DPCL).
- Childhood Autism Rating Scale (CARS) for Autism.
- Conner's Abbreviated Rating Scale (CARS) for ADHD.

Projective and Semi-Projective Assessments for Diagnostic Purposes

- Children Apperception Test (CAT).
- Raven's Controlled Projection Test (RCPT).
- Draw-A-Person Test (DAPT).
- House-Tree-Person Test (HTP).
- Draw A Family Test (DFT).
- Picture Frustration Test (PFT).
- Rorschach Inkblot Test.

Above mentioned is the list of most commonly used tests for children and adolescents. The purpose of assessment is usually to make out a clear picture of the clinical conditions and plan most suitable intervention strategies.

Intervention for Learning Disabilities

Intervention for learning disorders requires paying specific attention on areas of deficit identified in SLD assessment. Based on that, the therapist identifies specific areas and makes a rehabilitative programme accordingly. Any learning disability usually involves basic deficits in reading, writing and arithmetical skills. Complementary skills may involve cognitive functions like attention, concentration and comprehension. Different exercises may be planned for each of the specific problem. Some basic exercises are given below:

Exercises to Improve Reading Skills: Students with reading difficulty may get frustrated while reading due to difficult pronunciation of words. For starting the reading rehabilitation it is better to use books and reading material that matches with child's level of interest and also their capacity. Therefore, easy vocabulary reading material may be beneficial to use in the initial stage of therapy.

Whole Word Approach: The whole word approach is a strategy to improve reading skill that involves selecting a word written in large alphabets on a flash card. Student traces the word with his or her finger and pronounces the word aloud. On the next level child repeats the word and frequently use that in stories. Tracing with finger is no longer required after some time and the words are also not presented on flash cards. The learned technique is generalized on new words and normal reading material.

Working on Phonetic Skills: This technique is based on the *Gillingham approach* that uses phonetic drill cards to implement the exercise. One letter is presented on a card and pronounced by the therapist, the child then repeats the name of letter. On the next level, therapist presents the sound of that letter and child learns accordingly. After the mastery has been done on a letter, therapist presents the letter and child is asked to produce the sound. On the next level the process reversed and therapist presents the sound without showing the card and child has to identify the name of the letter. Finally, the phonetic cues are practiced in written form to ensure the learning.

Reading Drills: There is an organized list of multiple letters selected for the procedure combined with their sounds. The technique works more or less like phonetic practices; yet the process is more organized and presented together rather than presenting one at a time. Major emphasis is placed upon learning to blend the sounds with specific letters. Regular drilling reinforces the sound symbol relationship.

Paired Reading: It involves reading at a rapid rate together by the therapist and the child. The child starts reading the text and therapist assists the child whenever required. The process involves not letting the child struggle with the spelling for more than 5 seconds and assist immediately. The process is repeated till there is at least fifty per cent progress or decrement in errors. Finally, the child may be asked questions to ensure that he has understood whatever has been read. This exercise simultaneously works on the comprehension skills. Initially, the amount of reading material may be kept less and increase gradually with progress.

Distar Reading Programme: This is a reading mastery programme which is highly structured, intensive and fast-paced. It mainly works on sequencing and decoding skills using symbolic games. The blending exercises are designed to improve understanding of synthetic relationship reinforcement during the programme. Consistent reinforcement is required for the child when s/he masters a particular skill.

Exercise to improve spelling skills: *Simultaneous Oral Spelling (SOS):* This technique is used to improve learning capacity for spellings. The same list is learned for three subsequent days and next list of five words or spellings is introduced after the period of three days only. It means, ten spellings are kept as a target for one week task. One word is shown to the child and s/he is asked to copy the word. While copying the word child is asked to say aloud each letter. When the child is done he is asked to cross check the spelling. When the target word is correctly reproduced for at least three times child is asked to write it from his or her memory without seeing the spelling. Word written from memory is again cross checked by the child and three trials of consecutive success are necessary to move on the next word. Same procedure is followed for other spellings too and proper steps and schedule is essential to follow.

Spelling Games: Spelling games such as anagrams, word building, and cross word puzzles etc. are available in the market. Anyone of them may be used as a play technique to encourage spelling learning. As rehabilitation strategy they work really good and child also enjoys them as they are presented in a game form. At home also, sets of square cards may be made at home and letters can be written on them by the child himself. Five sets are required because some spellings may have repeated words. Child can use them to learn spellings and parents can also participate in the game to encourage the child. Another form of the game may be used as a grid of letters with hidden words. The grid can be made easily at home and multiple sets can be used with different words. It has to be made by the parent otherwise child would already know the hidden words. Regular practicing of these exercises improves the skill to learn new words and spellings.

Writing Exercises: Writing exercises aims at improving written expression characterized by vocabulary, fluency, content and structure. In order to improve writing skills it is important to encourage spontaneous writing. Creative writing may be encouraged to ask the child writing personal thoughts and experiences in form of stories and poetries etc. *Vocabulary skills* can be improved by regular reading of news papers, magazines, dictionary, substituting words in a sentence along with crossword puzzles. *Fluency skills* can be taught in form of asking the child to make a meaningful sentence from jumbled words, sentence completion, and connecting two sentences together in a meaningful way and highlighting parts of speech in a sentence. *Content development skills* can be improved by using key words to build up a story, encouraging letter writing, leave applications, essays, and common thoughts. Process may also involve re-writing of wrongly processed/written stories. Diary maintaining may be encouraged to add into the skills. Finally, the *Structure Development Skills* are improved by minutely analyzing the punctuations and asking the child to find out wrong punctuations and also correcting them. Procedure may also involve asking the child to insert correct punctuations at adequate places, filling the blanks with adequate verbs and sentences.

Overall idea behind improving writing skills involves motivating children to write by thinking and organizing ideas into meaningful way, editing and self correcting them and finally re-writing them in organized form.

Basic Arithmetic Skills: Basic arithmetic skills are taught in three basic levels:

Concrete level of arithmetic skills involves teaching the child about numbers and counting by using concrete materials such as blocks, beads, small objects etc. on this level a row of objects may be made by the therapist and child is asked to count them in serial order. At a higher step child may be asked to give the therapist certain amount of objects and keep the rest with him or her and count them separately. When the child learns to count with this method objects are eliminated and the same procedure is implemented with the use of lines made on a paper. This is a very common way of teaching calculations to younger children. This level is known as *semi-concrete level.* Finally, the level shifts to the *Abstract level* and whatever has been taught with objects and lines is asked to practice at imaginary level.

Supportive Work with Families: Most of the times children with specific learning disabilities suffer from parent's harsh and punitive behaviours due to poor academic performance and low academic grades. Parents and other family members must be made aware of child's intellectual strengths and the specific part of their cognitive dysfunctions. Parents need to learn that criticizing and comparing the child with others may harm his or her self-esteem and inhibit the process of progress. They need to understand that intellectual functioning and disability are two different states of the child and they need to cooperate with the condition. High academic expectations may make them feel bad and the child too. Parents need to understand their cooperation may help the child to organize the schedule and improve the skills with regular practice. A collaborative alliance between parents, teacher and therapist can state the problems more clearly; thus more amenable to treat and use of contingencies for child even on small gains gives the best results.

Required Cooperation of Teachers: Since children spend major part of time in school teachers need to be cooperative enough to make the rehabilitation plan more effective. It is essential for the teacher to understand strengths and weaknesses of the child and accept them as they are. Comparing the child with other students and being judgmental may influence child's self-esteem in negative way. It is important for the teacher to have a positive interaction with child and help him organizing the activities and study schedule. Child should be given ample time to learn new skills and should be encouraged even for the small achievements. Home assignments may be short in length depending upon the capability of child. Small errors may be ignored while checking the test papers or rather than cutting the full marks child can be given at least half or one fourth credits. They can be taught relaxation to use in stressful conditions like before presentations and reading in front of the class. Improvements in accuracy, neatness and legibility are important to notice and given as feedback. Healthy peer interactions should be encouraged to improve social skills and comforting relationship among classmates. The child also requires consistent motivation to participate in the extracurricular activities like sports, annual function, music dance, etc.

Intervention for Autism and Other Pervasive Developmental Disorders

Pervasive developmental disorders possess a life time disability and there is no permanent solution of the condition. Improvements are possible with family interventions aiming at modifying behaviours through training and developing skills through consistent stimulation.

Psychoeducation: The first step towards treatment of autism should be educating family members about the clinical condition. Some very important aspects need to be explained to the family members while discussing the problem–

- It's a biological condition with genetic predispositions that are yet to be explored.
- It's a life-time disability and should not be associated and perceived as reaction to family stressors.
- They have difficulty doing joint activities, perceiving and showing affection due to clinical representation of symptoms.
- Communication difficulties are prominent in this condition that usually interrupt social situations.
- Rigidity to follow routines and inflexibility to adjust in new situation hampers peer relations.
- Through structured teaching they may be able to learn to communicate and become self-dependent.
- Degree of improvement depends upon the quality of teaching and competency of the teacher.
- They have all the rights to attend normal schooling as any other child; however, it is usually difficult to arrange for the teaching environment they require and pay special attention; it is, therefore, easier to arrange and centralize special education resources.

Delivering diagnosis is a crucial task and it has to be managed well by the therapist. It is essential to deal with the anxieties of the parents who are being informed about the disability of child which is not going to be cured anyway. Rather than focusing on the negative parts it is important to focus on the possibilities for future improvements.

TEACHH System: It's a structured teaching programme for autistic children and helps them learn according to their own skills. Autistic children have good visual processing abilities with excellent rote learning/ memory. Their activities should be planned accordingly keeping in mind their abilities and skills such as visualizing the steps of a task helps them to understand what they have to do in order to achieve success. Use of photographs may help them understand better than the verbal instructions. Based on child's strength and weaknesses plan of activities is decided and parents are required to follow the plan for at least about twenty minutes per day. Highly structured routines are good to be made and followed in distraction free environment.

Skills Training: Many of the children have low intellectual functioning and with significant language and communication delays. In order to train them to be able to perform self care activities and communicate demands following steps may be followed:

- Instructions can be given in pictorial form.
- Lengthy tasks may be divided into smaller parts in structured and sequential ways.
- Material of their interest should be identified and used in the training such as use of bright pictures, particular sounds, objects of child's interest etc.
- Adequate use of reinforcements is essential to encourage new skills to be learned.
- Generalization of skills may be taught by practicing them in different situations and reinforcing the child for the same.
- Interaction should be planned on particular intervals.

Working on Communication Skills: While dealing with the communication problems rather than focusing upon speech it is more helpful to work on developing information conveying skills. For doing so, sign language may be used and taught to the child. Training may involve modelling behaviours with frequent feedback and reinforcement on certain intervals. In order to do the same, first, opportunities should be sought where child interacts in a social situation, child's attempt to interact with others should be prompted and reinforced., Video aids and modelling may be helpful for doing so. Development of micro skills for improving social behaviours such as eye contact, social smile etc. can be taught with similar methods.

Management of Attention-Deficit/Hyperactivity Disorder (ADHD)

Management of ADHD may not be single directed and may require a multi-dimensional approach. Those who are having excessive hyperactivity may require medication initially and behavioural management may proceed simultaneously. Intervention of ADHD involves not only working with the individual; it is rather a mutual effort by clinician, family and school. Following are the major aspects that need to be involved for intervening this condition.

Involvement of Family: Psychoeducation: It is important to educate the family members about the clinical condition of child and also explain about the treatment process. Many times some children are in need of medication but the family members are apprehensive about the effects of drugs. In such conditions, psycho-educations help them to understand the need for treatment and also positively influences treatment adherence. For most of the children, home based intervention is planned that requires consistent assistance of parents to implement the intervention strategies. Educating the parents and family members facilitates the process and recovery of the child as well.

Use of Behavioural Techniques to deal with Behavioural Issues: Children with ADHD frequently display behavioural problems and they generally inhibit the therapeutic process. These children are likely to deny the home assignments and non-compliance to follow instructions. In such cases use of reinforcements to promote desirable behaviours and use of punishment for undesirable behaviours works really well. Based on conditioning methods it is necessary to make an association between desirable behaviours and rewards as the result of positive behaviour and similarly associating undesirable behaviours with unpleasant outcomes like withdrawing gains and time out. Behavioural methods are an important part of parent's management training and they need to be followed rigidly when dealing with such cases. The techniques target specific behaviours at a time and their progress is recorded using behavioural charting. The charting is basically done by parents and reviewed by therapist on every follow up.

School Based Management: In most of the cases of ADHD symptoms come to the notice by teachers. The condition appears pertinent in classroom behaviours and inhibits academic performance of the child; thus come to the notice of teacher. Since, the condition usually leads to difficulties in performing academic tasks, it is necessary for the teachers to know basic management of these children. In order to manage these children in classroom setting it is necessary for the teacher to understand child's condition and its genuineness. The teacher should be aware that the child is running through difficulties and needs support to tackle them. Punishing children with ADHD for not doing well in academics may adversely influence their self-esteem.

It is important to provide a quiet area to the child for doing assignments. Since these children are highly distractible and loose attention by small environmental stimuli their assignments can be planned as individual tasks, working in group and joint activities may not help them lot. Usually sitting next to the window seat, sitting on the back benches, and any sitting area where visual or auditory distracters are available should be avoided. Since they have an automatic arousal condition, they can be allowed to take small seat breaks. Seat breaks should be planned in a structured manner such as asking the child to collect assignments of other children, distributing test papers, rubbing the black board, writing the day, date and topic to be taught on the black board, etc. The tasks assigned to control roaming behaviour are usually presented as duties and child may be rewarded to reinforce the desirable behaviours. Attention is a major target for this condition and many times assignments are incomplete due to the same reason. Children usually fail to finish tasks by the required time or unable to copy from the black board due to visuo-spatial/motor disturbances. To deal with this problem child can be seated with a study-buddy who can help out to complete assignments and assist the child. Tasks can be divided into smaller goals and step by step working should be emphasized. Due to poor attention and impulsivity their comprehension may be affected; therefore, instructions should be given in small statements and only when the child is motivated to learn. Long assignments should be avoided and tasks taking long hours to complete may be dropped. Written instructions may be paired with oral instructions to improve comprehension. Teacher has to be vigilant as their attention loses many times while doing a task, in such a condition teacher may aware the child by cuing or providing signals that the child is being distracted. Minor impulsive behaviours may be ignored; however, misbehaviours must be dealt with warning the child first and using time out if non-compliance occurs. Acknowledging positive behaviours is necessary to reinforce them and increase their frequency. On decided intervals report may be given to parents and therapist and also, their feedback should be taken. A mutual effort benefits them the most and increases the prognosis.

Same management styles given for school can be adapted at home also to help the child completing assignments and other academic tasks. Parents can combine them with rewards and punishments when required.

Cognitive Retraining Techniques to Enhance Attention

Children with predominant attention deficit improve significantly with both manual and computerized cognitive retraining techniques. The treatment aims at improving cognitive functions and majorly attention. Techniques to improve attention may be presented in play form so that they become more enjoyable for the child and they cooperate for the process. As manual cognitive retraining techniques letter cancellation tasks, colouring under the margin tasks, maze tasks, spot the difference tasks, matching and sorting games are good to use and have been found to be effective in research trials. Computerized activities have also shown good results and found to be effective to enhance attention skills. As a treatment modality, computerize cognitive retraining involves use of video games involving speed and motor functions. Computerized activities may not be affordable for every client, therefore, the manual techniques can be used effectively.

Social Skills Training: Since, the behavioural problems are very much correlated with hyperactive children, they usually influence the peer relations adversely. Academic problems caused by poor attention and hyperactive behaviours also interrupt the social functioning of child and disturb relationships with classmates. Impulsivity and visuo-spatial problems in ADHD may interrupt social conversations due to impulsive reactions without listening the other person and inability to judge distance while talking. Role playing exercises helps the child to learn body language, voice change messages, importance of eye contact during social conversations along with maintaining adequate distance while talking to others. The child also learns to identify best solution for a problem among all the available alternatives. Step by step learning is emphasized and adequate problem solving skills are worked on. Finally, the individual learns to implement previous strategies in current situation to solve a problem.

***Self-Instruction Training*:** Self-instruction training helps child to deal with the internal speech deficiency and cope in the overt situations. Self-instruction training helps them to patiently listen inner instructions and follow them gradually. At initial stages child says the instructions a loud and they are gradually produced into soft whisperings. Finally, they turn into inner speech/instructions and used in overt situations. The training involves use of instructions to specify task demand and clarify the goal. Usually the practice starts with smaller goals and gradually the complexity increases. The technique is effective to improve problem solving and also impulsivity. Self-awareness helps the child to better understand and cooperate for the treatment.

Managing the Disruptive Children: Treating Conduct and Oppositional Behaviours

Family Based Interventions: Psycho-education: Aim of psycho-education is to bring into the notice of parents that disruptive behaviours are somehow learned from the environment and family functioning plays an important role in developing these conditions. They need to understand that how family dysfunctions lead to disruptive behaviours and how they can be well tacked by the parents. Modification required in child's behaviour need modification to some extent in parental behaviour too. Parents are usually taught to pay attention on the child and praise the positive behaviours. They are also asked to observe impact of ignoring minute problem behaviours and decreasing their frequency. Positive and healthy interaction patterns are encouraged and use of rewards and time out is taught. Rewards for not doing disruptive things and controlling anger usually show gradual improvement in positive behaviours. Time out in initial state may escalate the level of aggression; however, aggression decreases gradually and steady improvement is seen after some time. Use of supportive play also enhances the quality of relationship between child and parent; thus likely to show improvement with joint efforts made by them. They are taught to identify antecedents of certain behaviours and modify them to the extent they are possible. They need to learn not only pin-pointing negative behaviours but praising positive behaviours too. Also, the use of adequate contingencies for target behaviours is taught and monitoring of target behaviours is done to see the progress of therapy.

Working Through Parent's Own Conflicts: Many times parent's own conflicts and stressful life conditions make it difficult to understand the need for treatment and their cooperation for the process. In such conditions, they are taught to deal with their own stress and be prepared for the treatment of child. Other type of intervention may involve keeping the adolescent with foster care where he or she is socialized by using rewards and negotiations by foster parents.

Sometimes, parents may require marital counselling to overcome marital difficulties and as a treatment especial attention is paid on these issues because they seem to be important in improving the conduct behaviours. Major focus is to improve quality of parent child interactions and thus improving the quality of life. If stressors would be low, problems will decrease automatically.

Working with the Child: Teaching Social Skills: It is assumed that disruptive behaviours are learned by the environment and faulty learning patterns may lead to disruption of behaviours in form of poor social skills. By working on the social skills, individuals are taught to deal effectively with the stressful social situations and take appropriate decisions.

Cognitive Skills Training: The training aims at improving selection of adequate stimulants from the environment and improving emotional processing skills. They are taught to work on choosing adequate alternatives to make healthy reactions towards aggressive conditions. Cognitive skills training may not be effective alone; however, it works best with the parent management training.

Dealing with Stealing Behaviours: In order to deal with stealing behaviours it is important for the parents and family members to keep a check on every suspicious object or anything that does not belong to the child. They should avoid searching the places in child's absence; however, it is important to note availability of things that have not been provided by the family members. Using time out can again be effective and it may result in decreased stealing behaviour in future. Parents are supposed to listen to the child when s/he admits fault and praise for admitting fault thus doing a positive behaviour. Wrong behaviours should be warned once, praised if they stop and time out should be used if they continue even after warning. The child can be given some alternative way of earning to gratify genuine demands. Token economy has been found to be most effective for such cases as they increases the likelihood of performing more desirable behaviours and tokens work as incentive and reinforcement for them to continue doing such behaviours.

Behavioural Contracting: Behavioural contracting is a method to deal with the problematic behaviours in most fairways. Both the parties, i.e. child and parents express their demands to the opposite party and both of them decide cost of not being able to fulfil each other's demands. Parents usually express their demands to the children and children keep the demand for gains. Decided gains should be in limit, affordable and usually set by the parents not by the therapist. With each behavioural progress their gains are provided and gains are withdrawn with each undesirable behaviour. The programme gradually teaches the child an association between desirable behaviour and positive outcomes along with negative results of undesirable behaviours. Continuing the programme generally decreases the problem behaviours and increases the likelihood of performing desirable behaviours.

Treating Tics and Habits

Psychological approaches to treat habits and tics have been found to be effective in research trials. Mostly behavioural techniques have been used to modify the behaviours; however, some sort of cognitive preparation also helps individuals to be aware of tic behaviours and control them effortfully. Some of the techniques to control tics and habits are described below:

Psycho-education: The primary goal of offering psycho-education to the parents is to convey that tics are basically involuntary and are not caused by mental conflicts of the child; they rather induce stress in the child when they have to face embarrassment caused by them in social situations. Many times harsh and punitive behaviour of parents increases the tic behaviours.

Awareness Training: Through awareness training, individual can understand the correlation between specific environmental factors and tics. There are four major components of awareness training compiled in certain steps. First component involves recording of tic's frequency and listing the associated environmental variables. The recording involves tic behaviour being performed (shoulder shrugging), duration of observation (30 minutes), situation in which the behaviour is being performed (while watching TV) and consequence (stopped doing the behaviour when pin-pointed). Second component of awareness training involves response description. Response description requires child to elaborate tic behaviours in front of the therapist by using mirror or video tape recording. This description helps the child to get more aware of the tic behaviours and motivate to stop them. Third component of this training incorporates response detection where the child is made alert immediately before the occurrence of tic. Therapist alerts the child prior to occurrence of tic. Finally, the fourth component involves making the child aware of the environmental situations in which tics are likely to occur frequently such as while watching TV, while studying etc. the whole process needs cooperation of parents and most importantly the child. This awareness training helps the individual to understand the severity of tics and need to control them. Frequent feedbacks about lowering frequency of tic behaviours may work as a motivational factor for the child to make efforts to stop such behaviours.

Competing Response Training: Competing response training involves performing an incompatible response immediately before the urge to perform tic or immediately after the tic has occurred. The competing responses has to be opposite of the tic behaviour and should be associated with the tics. Competing responses are predefined and has to be performed each time the tic behaviour occurs. Some of the competing responses may involve opening the eyes wide when eye blinking occurs or about to occur, taking deep breath through nose and keeping the mouth closed while thumb sucking or urge to perform thumb sucking etc. for controlling tics muscles can be asked to make as stiff as possible so that the tic does not occur at all. A hierarchy should be made on the basis of severity of tics and most frequent or most severe behaviours/tics should be tackled first. Gradually, all other tics can be covered at every sitting over the period of sessions.

Contingency Management: At the starting of this procedure both therapist and child can review the feelings associated with tics. Obviously the tic behaviour have some satisfactory effect on the child due to which s/he continues performing them, still there are conditions of embarrassment when they occur in social situations. Therapist and child discuss the inconvenience caused by tics and positive aspects when tics are not performed. It helps the therapist to boost individual's motivation and work effectively on reducing them. In order to carry out contingency management it is necessary to identify the contingencies that will be associated with desirable and undesirable behaviours. Children may be rewarded for tic free periods or when they cooperate for therapeutic tasks. Use of token system has been found to be most effective in such cases; however, verbal appraisals also work well in these conditions. Reinforcing the children decreases the frequency and severity of tics and simultaneously they learn to understand the difference between embarrassing conditions in presence of tics and convenient social behaviours in absence of tics.

Contingent Negative Practice for Involuntary Tic Behaviours: Some of the tics may be reduced by forcefully performing them every time they occur. The procedure involves voluntarily engaging in tic behaviours rather than fighting with the urge to perform them. The child performs them forcefully every time they occur for about 30 seconds. The implication behind this strategy is that practicing them forcefully increases the voluntary control over them due to desensitization and habituation. For example, the child is asked to purposely practice eye blinking for 30 seconds whenever s/he blinks his/her eyes. Habituation of response occurs with this practice and desensitization increases the voluntary control over the behaviour.

Relaxation Training: Tic behaviours are somehow associated with stress and tension of the individual and it has been found that relaxation procedures may effectively work to reduce frequency and severity of tics. Deep breathing exercises, progressive muscle relaxation, imaginary exercises and visualizations have been found to be the most practiced exercises for these cases. Relaxation procedures may not be recommended for every case; however, those who suffer from anxiety and stress due to tics in social situation may be benefited most.

School Based Management: Tic behaviours many times influence child's academic performance, thus, school staff must be aware of treating such students with most adequate strategies. Contingencies may be given as similar by the parents in form of rewards or verbal appraisals. Basic cooperation of teachers is required to deal with academic problems of the child occurring due to tics. Their support and cooperation helps the child to adjust well in the school environment and it also prevents them from awkward situations. More importantly manipulating educational environment helps those most. The educational environment may be manipulated in form of setting reasonable goals like decreasing the length of assignments, increasing the time limit to finish a task etc., by providing them directions and repeating them, sequencing task in a particular order, highlighting significant words etc. and most importantly providing alternative methods of learning. Children with vocal tics may be given liberties while oral presentations and tests. Making the school staff aware with child's difficulty may increase the support system and child can effectively perform in academics.

Intervention for Enuresis

Retention Control Training (RCT): This technique is based on the assumption that many children have low bladder functioning capacity. This training is basically a kind of exercise to enhance capacity of the bladder. The child is asked to take extra amount of water so that the bladder fills to its maximum capacity. Urination is asked to delay for some time and child holds the pressure of urine. After a decided interval child is allowed to urinate. Initially, the duration to retain urine may be less and increase gradually as the training progresses. Retention control training directly enhances volume-control skills of the bladder and indirectly nocturnal incontinence.

Sphincter Control Exercise: This technique strengthens the sphincter muscles and this increases the strength and capacity of bladder to hold urination. In this exercise the child is asked to start urination and stop the stream of urine in between and again continuing voiding of urine after few seconds. The process is asked to repeat and practice every time the child has to urinate. Repetition of exercise combined with rewards and reinforcements motivates child to cooperate for the process and also decreases the frequency of voiding.

Kegel Exercise: The kegel exercise involves purposely manipulating muscle to prematurely terminate urination by contracting the muscles of pelvic floor. The exercise has been introduced as stream interruption while voiding. The exercise requires initiating urination and terminating it completely. In this exercise, urination is not continued after intervals; rather it involves permanent termination of urination. The exercise may be difficult to perform every time; however, can be practiced at least once a day. This exercise has physiological base and its regular practice decreases the frequency of urination.

***Urine Alarm*:** This technique involves a moisture sensitive switching system that switches every time the child urinates and an alarm is associated with the wetting condition. The condition implements as every time the wetting occurs the alarm rings immediately. Different kinds of alarms are available and many of them can be directly attached with children's lower or trouser. The mechanism relates to conditioning method where bladder sensation is the conditioned stimulus and wakening is the conditioned response. The ring and wakening associate with aversive stimulus; thus decrease the frequency of incontinence. After regular practicing of this exercise, the child either completes urination in toilet, or terminates it for adequate time or stop urinating at the time alarm rings.

***Paired Association*:** The technique requires pairing or combining stream interruption exercise and kegel exercise together. To combine them together and practice, the parent stands outside the toilet and sounds the alarm and child practices the kegel exercise inside the bathroom. The child is rewarded accordingly for cooperating and achieving desirable effects. Since the technique is practiced in wake state, efficacy of urine alarm may increase during night time.

***Cleanliness Training and Use of Rewards*:** The cleanliness training requires child to avoid bed wetting by following above mentioned exercises and rewarding them for following instructions adequately. While training them for cleanliness they are required to take responsibility of their behaviour and manage at their own. In order to be responsible they have to change their bed-sheets and lowers every time they perform bed wetting. In progressive conditions, they may be asked to wash them at their own or simply dip and rinse them in water. Tokens may be given for dry nights and they can be rewarded for desirable behaviours.

***Over-Learning*:** This exercise is practiced to increase bladder capacity during sleeping hours. The technique is used when there is some amount of progress and child has achieved at least 14 dry nights. The child is asked to drink 2 ounces of water prior to 15 minutes of bed time. If the child remains dry for two consecutive nights, amount of water increases. The amount of water increases until the child consumes number of ounces obtained by adding two to his or her chronological age. If the child remains dry for 14 consecutive nights, process can be terminated.

Dealing with the Anxious Children: Management of Separation Anxiety and Attachment Disorders

Most of the approaches to deal with attachment and separation anxiety issues among children have been found to be based upon the family intervention. Since both the conditions relate to attachment and separation from primary caregiver, it is essential to work with the family system itself to deal with the problem. Most of the literature concerning these particular clinical conditions revolves around the family therapy and parenting styles. Other approaches like art and play therapy have been found to be complementary to use with family based interventions.

Family Based Intervention: Reason to work with family is to work on attachment patterns and improving parent-child ties. The basic reason for their anxiety is insecurity felt in the absence of the attachment figure that can be dealt by following certain rules of behaving with the child. Consistent responding to the child is also necessary to give him the idea that the problems are being noticed and responded in certain ways.

- Setting limits is important and loving boundaries are essential to make. Make the child feel that you are countable whenever they need you; however, facing the difficulty is important to learn coping.
- Misbehaviour of a child when anxious indicates that s/he does not know how to handle a stressful situation. Ruling and dominating the child in that state may aggravate the stress. Being calm and relaxed in that state gives the impression to the child that stress can be managed without being hyper.
- Making predictable routines helps the child to adjust in brief modification of schedules.
- Giving expressions of love and affection by holding the child develops more secure attachment patterns.
- Allowing the child to express their emotions make them feel comfortable to share feelings and emotions; thus enhances the quality of relationship.

Using Play and Art as Treatment: It has been explained psycho dynamically that joint activities of art and play improve the quality of relationship by enhancing the quality of time spent together. While playing parents are supposed to observe the child and let him or her take a lead of the play. Parents are directed not to comment on negative behaviours adopted during play or criticize them. They are rather directed to pin point positive behaviours displayed during play and reinforcing the child for doing so. Play material may be used as clay, puzzle games, story narration exercises etc. It has been seen that anger can be expressed by scratching and smashing the paper. Doing joint activities works like a repairing and healing process to improve relationship between child and the caregiver.

Treating Child Abuse and Neglect: Child abuse and neglect is a major issue in current psychological paradigm; however, evidence based treatments are yet to be explored and documented. Since, the condition of maltreatment, abuse and neglect is mainly associated with family circumstances it is important to treat both children and family members separately. Particularly in cases of neglect, parents play a major role and interventions need to focus on smoothening family functioning.

Intervention with the Survivors: Major aim of these programmes is to stimulate child's cognitive abilities specifically in cases where family dysfunctions have been a cause of emotional abuse and neglect. The process aims at modifying negative beliefs related to abusive condition and de-valuating self. Usually such conditions evolve negative thoughts in children and they might suffer from low self-esteem. These issues may be targeted in either individual or group therapy. The aim of such treatment is to provide an understanding of surviving condition and make it clear to the survivor's mind that it was not created by them and they are not worthless. They can be taught the assertive ways of dealing with such conditions and keeping their views without being violent. They are taught that they can speak in-front-of adults and they have every right to do that. Difference occurred in the personal relations caused by abuse may be dealt, however, they can take long time.

The child may be presented with family stressful conditions and harsh behaviour of parents as a stressful response to that condition. The procedure helps at modifying child's belief about the hostile parenting and giving them a genuine background for doing such behaviours. Inter-personal skills training may help children and parents to understand each other's condition and react in every healthy way possible. Relaxation training may be effective to deal with child's anxious states related to abuse.

Intervention with Parents: Major aim of such programmes is to work on improving parenting skills and teaching them to deal with personal difficulties like anger, mood swings and drug abuse. Many times they may find it difficult to understand child's developmental processes and react in undesirable way. Therefore, as a first step, they need to understand child's developmental process and understand their needs changing with the development. Sometimes, there may be personal issues that can interrupt the interactions and child may suffer from abuse in form of parental anger out-bursts, mood swings etc. in such cases, parents are taught to develop emotional regulation skills. Cognitive techniques allow parents to learn control over impulsive reactions and manage stressful conditions. As a behavioural modality they may be taught to identify triggering conditions of stress and avoiding them by using relaxation and distractions. Negative states may be delayed with the use of such techniques and parents can overcome their anxieties. Methods can be taught in individual setting or may be conducted in a group. Group based treatments may help the parents to learn alternative ways of reacting in a stressful condition by discussing the problem with other group members. When a general topic is discussed in group it generally gives an idea to the other group members how the problems should be tackled in healthy ways without neglecting the child. Parents can learn how to negotiate with children and how to use power in a healthy way. It helps them improving parent-child interactions, improves disclosure patterns, encourages sharing behaviour and protect from abandonment.

Many times parent's own conflicts such as marital discord and stressful relations result in abusive conditions. In such cases, it is important to identify the target issues and help the couple to resolve them in order to improve the interactions with child. They are taught to identify their conflicts and resolve them at their own level. They need to learn why these issues are important and how they are interrupting their child's emotional life. Usually interventions aimed at improving harmonious relationship between couples decrease the level of parental stress and helps in improving child's condition.

Dealing with Survivors of Sex Abuse: The therapy with sexually abused children involves facilitation of intense and complex feelings caused by abuse. Positive changes are important to bring and promote protective and supportive relations with non-abusive parents. Assertiveness is necessary to learn to prevent further conditions of abuse. Individual therapy may be used as a supportive treatment to allow ventilation of negative feelings caused by sexual abuse. Play, drawing, story writing may be effective form of ventilation and exhaling the stressful emotions. Individual therapies for such cases may have a disadvantage as these children may be pre-occupied with isolated condition where abuse took place and they may replicate the abuse on isolated condition of therapy. There may be apprehension about being alone with the therapist especially if the therapist is of opposite sex. It may inhibit the process and progress may be delayed. Group therapy may have an advantage in such conditions. Group sessions aim at collecting children with similar abusive conditions and help them ventilating their mixed feelings of distress. Many times children may be confused between a sexual gratification need and emotional support need and they may give wrong clues to their peers. At this level, normal heterosexual relationships are important to discuss. They need to be told about the vulnerable conditions of further abuse and deal with them effectively using role plays.

There may be times where parents may be guilty about the event when sexual abuse took place and they were not available for the child. Therapy should target these issues and they can be offered help to learn how to be supportive and protective for the abused child.

Treatment of School Refusal: Returning Children Back to School

The major techniques to treat school refusal involve cognitive and behavioural procedures. Since in most of the children refusal relates to separation anxiety it is necessary to identify the thoughts related to that condition and modifying those thoughts using both cognitive and behavioural techniques.

Behavioural Methods: Important techniques for behavioural procedures involve hierarchy building of anxiety situations resulting in avoidance behaviours. Since many times the anxiety manifests in somatic arousal, these procedures help to mediate the anxiety and relaxed states.

Graded Exposure: At the first step, anxiety inducing situations are identified. A comprehensive table is made to compile them together. On the next level the child is asked to rate them on the basis of most anxiety provoking and least anxiety provoking situations. Therapist must explain the child how to do this. Once the child is done, a hierarchy of situations is made starting from least anxiety provoking to most anxiety provoking situation. Relaxation is also taught to the child so that it can be used when anxiety increases during the exposure. Usually deep breathing and muscle relaxation exercises are common to use. Exposure begins with imagined form following step by step procedure. At a time, only one situation is practiced and it is necessary to teach the child relaxation and coping strategy before staring the procedure. The child is asked to raise his finger when anxiety increases. Suggestions to relax and cope in the situation are presented by the therapist and once the child is comfortable to tolerate the anxiety, process can move to the next level of hierarchy. Gradually, when the child learns to cope imaginably conditions are implemented on real life situations. The imagined form of exposure is known as *in-vitro* exposure and the real form is known as *in-vivo* exposure.

Parent Management Training

Parent management training is a strategy that seeks to work upon modifying behaviours using behavioural management techniques and limit setting. Following are the main components of this method:

Establishing Commands: Many times children who refuse school to gain attention try negotiating commands and change the rules set by the parents. In this condition, a list of commands is made in order to eliminate negotiation. Parents are taught to deliver commands with assertiveness rather than delivering them as requests.

Scheduling Routines: Scheduling routines usually helps to set goals for the day. Morning routine is the most important part for school refusal behaviours, thus need to be emphasized most. Scheduling a more rigid and strict schedule limits non-compliance behaviour. Including rewards with school attending behaviour promotes smooth transition of the behaviour as attending school.

Use of Rewards and Punishments: It includes identifying positive and negative behaviours associated with school refusal. Usually giving rewards for positive behaviours and not paying attention on negative behaviours (e.g. somatic complaints) works well with such cases. Use of contingencies and behavioural contracting helps to promote desirable behaviours.

Cognitive Behavioural Treatments: Use of cognitive behavioural methods includes identifying negative thoughts related to anxiety situations resulting in school refusal. Condition can be associated with school objects such as presentation anxiety, anxiety of being judged that usually result in avoidance or escaping behaviours. Once the therapist has identified the negative thoughts one of them can be targeted to work upon. Targeting negative thoughts includes challenging and questioning in order to refute them. Common questions used to refute negative thoughts may be asking the client to prove chances of imagined resultant condition, or asking about the worst that can happen as a result of doing behaviour which is being avoided. Overall the goal of modifying cognitive schemas is to help the client to get rid of the irrational cognitions and confront in to the real world.

Role Playing: Role playing helps the client to understand the consequences of facing the anxiety provoking situations. It also prepares the client to act adequately in a particular situation and builds up confidence to perform those activities that are being avoided.

Play and Art Techniques: In very young children, use of playing and other art work can work effectively as a treatment modality. Children who have negative schemas about school can be dealt effectively by using play and art material. Use of play therapy can be combined with story narration involving positive thoughts and statements about school. Primary target of such activities is to modify negative thoughts related to school objects and converting them into joyful experiences. The technique not only helps those who have attended school for some time and later started refusing but may also help to prepare a child who is going to attend school for the first time ever. Use of various art techniques in form of craft work, drawing, painting, dancing etc. builds self-confidence in the child and work effectively for those cases who avoid attending school due to performance anxiety.

School Based Intervention: School has to take part in the treatment process as the primary object of refusal is school and the anxieties are associated with school itself most of the time. Comforting child in school environment, helping him/her to interact with other children, protecting from bullying behaviour of other classmates are major tasks that can be easily dealt by the teacher. Giving children a free yet scheduled environment, exploring their strengths and praising them for the same, allowing and promoting asking behaviour to resolve queries, involving the child in extra-curricular activities according to interests and skills work best in these conditions. An interactive approach of combining the clinical procedures with school based programmes may give best results to treat school refusal.

Treating Suicide Issues among Children and Adolescents

Suicide conditions among children and adolescents are a major issue for health practitioners in current scenario. Since, the issue is highly sensitive it has to be dealt with adequate sensitivity from the part of professionals. Major techniques that have been found to be effective in suicidal cases are discussed below:

***Cognitive Behaviour Therapy (C.B.T.)*:** Cognitive behaviour therapy has been found to be most rational treatment for treating suicide among adolescents. The reasons for the same could be identified as: It deals with negative cognitions associated with suicidal attempts, behavioural skills are taught to the client to overcome hazards that lead to suicidal behaviours, it has been found to be effective in clinical conditions that strongly relates to the self-harming behaviours and suicidal tendencies like depression, impulse control disorder, borderline personality disorder etc.

Steps to Carry Out the Treatment

Before starting CBT with children and adolescents, it is necessary to give them some information about the process and cross check their understanding by asking relevant questions. Since CBT requires cognitive sophistication of clients to be effective, it is important that clients' cognitive level matches the therapeutic requirement. Since the procedure is being used with children and adolescents, it is essential to educate the family also as they are usually helpful in implementing the therapeutic programme. Also, many times attitude of family members may be a predisposing factor for suicidal behaviours of the client; in this case, explanation of the process would help them to understand the genuineness of the problem.

Enhancing Problem Solving Skills process involves encouraging the client to identify problems that can be resolved. On the next level, the client is asked to identify the possible options to solve the problem and brain storm to choose the best one which is rational and logical in every lieu of that situation. It is important to help the client identifying the solvable problems because the problems that do not have any solution may induce the depressive feelings themselves and it may worsen the condition. For the problems that are difficult to deal should be dealt differently and client may be prepared to cope with them by enhancing coping skills. In order to solve a problem usually the previously used methods are reviewed and client is guided to solve the problems in the similar way. In between while planning the strategies to overcome hazards, it is essential to keep them checking in real situations and exploring the facts of the strategy that how it works. Keeping a progress record would usually help the clients to understand that how the learned strategies are working for them.

Charting of Thoughts or Self-Monitoring is done to elicit possible relationship between the emotions, events and thoughts associated with them. Usually record keeping by the client facilitates the process; however, if the clients find it difficult to keep a diary or record they may be asked verbally about the mentioned things like what was running in their mind, when they were coming for the session. Their answers may be explained them and they can be told the occurrence of automatic thoughts in a particular situation. It is important because the suicidal behaviours are usually governed by some automatic thoughts that are negative in nature. Identification of these thoughts is important for modifying them.

Refuting Irrational Beliefs and Cognitive Restructuring is the next step. The thoughts are challenged and the likelihood of them being true is discussed with the client. While challenging the thoughts opposing factors of client's beliefs are presented by the therapist. The process helps the client to see that how the automatic thoughts are influencing his/her cognitions and on what basis they seem to be illogical or irrational.

***Dialectical Behaviour Therapy (DBT)*:** This techniquewas originally developed for individuals with borderline personality disorder. In recent years its efficacy has been tested for treating suicidal children and adolescents and it has given tremendous results. The therapy proceeds with identifying basic conditions where suicide has been attempted and searching for other better alternatives. Since individuals who attempt suicide are highly sensitive by emotions and give extreme reactions in conflicting situations. Use of DBT with suicidal adolescents mainly focuses upon change and acceptance. The process of change is derived from the behavioural medicine/treatments like skills training, contingency management etc. and the process of acceptance focuses upon accepting the reality as it is without being judgmental. Change perspective incorporates the spiritual contents taken from eastern spiritual traditions. A major part of DBT involves working on mindfulness and teaching individuals to live in the current moment. The practice includes asking patients to concentrate and feel whatever they are doing in the current moment. The treatment procedure enhances client's motivation and they get more aware of their capabilities of accepting and changing. To progress the treatment usually chain analysis is used to identify links between the stressful conditions leading to problem behaviour or suicide attempt. On the next level alternative methods to react in stressful conditions are explored and used to reach better outcome as healthy reactions to frustrating and conflicting situations. The therapy aims at decreasing conflicts and increase understanding of normal and pathological behaviours in stressful conditions. Techniques learned during therapy are implemented in real life situations and family members participate in the procedure to implement them effectively. A skill training as a part of DBT focuses on improving emotional regulation, mindfulness, interpersonal effectiveness, distress tolerance and finding healthy alternatives to react in stressful conditions, i.e. problem solving and decision-making. Telephonic consultation is also an important part of this treatment as most that suffer from the condition face feelings of breakdown in certain situations and find unable to cope with them. Therapeutic process of DBT generally is a lengthy process; however, when used with adolescents with suicidal tendencies 12 weeks effective programme has been adopted in most of the trials.

***Inter-Personal Therapy (IPT)*:** Interpersonal Therapy was originally developed for treating depression and has been found to be effective as treatment modality. Since suicidal cases possess strong underlying depressive symptoms; therefore, the efficacy of IPT is not questionable. The process works at improving problem solving skills and simultaneously working on socio-occupational functioning. The client is made to learn about the bipolarities of situations and building strength to choose the best alternatives in stressful times. The process focuses on identifying precursors of conflicting situations; client's associated feelings and emotions about them and basic reactions during that time. Task of therapist is to make the client aware of his or her strengths of identifying alternative solutions and using them in times of need. The motive is to channelize emotions in healthy directions and improving overall functioning of the individual. In many cases, depressive symptoms found to be decreased significantly and improvement was noted in overall functioning of the individual.

***Family Based Interventions*:** Family conditions and stressful events of family have been found to be a major precursor of depressive trends among adolescents. The aim of family based interventions is to decrease familial conflicts and encourage positive interactions among family members. The intervention starts with psycho-educating the family members about client's condition and possible factors associated with family functioning. Therapist aims at modifying crude interaction patterns and developing a healthy atmosphere. Many times high expressed emotions among family members may exaggerate the conditions and adolescents may indulge in repeated suicidal attempts. To prevent this condition, it is important to deal with critical, hostile and emotional over-involved behaviours of family members and protecting the clients with related issues. Suicidal youth is difficult to handle and it is necessary for the family members to provide a soothing environment. It is important for them to understand the conflicts of the client that may relate to hormonal imbalances, peer pressure, maladjustment in school etc. it is important to make transparency in the relationships so that a healthy relationship can be encouraged between child and family members. Many times when there is nobody to share the pain, ultimate condition is to end life to get rid of all the problems of life.

***Group Therapies*:** Group based treatments aims at building strength to overcome aggression and impulsivity in healthy ways. The process is conducted in its original form, i.e. a group of members with similar problems and almost similar age. Interactions are encouraged to discuss personal feelings, thoughts and usual reactions in stressful conditions. Group discussions stimulate the thinking and many clues may be obtained by discussing different alternatives adopted by different group members. The target is to identify most general conditions in which adolescents attempt suicide, the most common feelings associated with those conditions and most frequent reactions given by them. On the next level, group members discuss the alternative responses that had been used by them in some situations or the other. Major aim is to learn about channelizing emotions in positive ways and delaying the anger outbursts.

Psychological Management of Adolescent Substance Abuse

Most of the time substance taking behaviour starts with experimentation continues with temporary pleasurable effects and finally ends up with life destroying outcomes. Substance abuse initiation among adolescents has been found to be associated with peer pressure, fear of isolation and rejection among group members, curiosity to explore the effects, correlating use of alcohol and cigarette as status symbol, to overcome depression and loneliness and escape from stressful life events. Many times at the time of initiating substance intake adolescents think that only weak individuals get addicted and they won't slip into that condition.

Intervention strategies involve motivation enhancement to leave the drugs, group settings to discuss effects of drug abuse and most importantly maintaining the will power to get rid of the condition. Some of the effective treatment approaches are:

Motivation Enhancement Therapy: The goal of motivation enhancement therapy is to assess the inner will of the client to leave substance and maintaining it to achieve success. Those who enter the therapy with some sort of motivation are more likely to get desirable effect; however, those who have been brought by the family members by force may not get that much benefit. Still, most of the involuntary clients get benefit at some point or the other. The therapy starts with the assessment of client's level of motivation. Some may be slightly motivated and perceive the issue to be problematic, still are not ready or convinced for the treatment. Some may be very enthusiastic for treatment and have set goals and plan for management but unable to implement them. Those who have set goals have high chances of implementing them with structured routines and consistent encouragement by the therapist and family members. If the will power persists, they usually achieve success and if not they may have a relapse of condition. Those who manage to maintain the motivation and do not lose hope achieve the abstinence; however, those who are discouraged by the temporary problems and withdrawals fall in the cycle of relapse and rehabilitation.

Enhancing Coping Skills: When an individual is undergoing therapy it is important to work on maintaining the motivation to enhance skills to cope with craving. It is essential to identify the cues that promote substance intake such as company of friends, club meetings, parties into pubs etc. and take precautions. These are the high risk situations in which substance intake occurs and even motivated clients are unable to resist in these circumstances. Skills need to be enhanced to identify high risk situations and master the alternative behaviours rather than consuming substance. It is important for the clients to be assertive and make a bold statement for denying the use of substance. If the situation seems unavoidable it is better to move out from there or suggest alternatives to others also to do something creative. They can identify the time slots where craving increases and activities can be pre-planned to fill the gaps. Activity scheduling improves the daily functioning and engages the clients in more healthy acts.

Improving Inter-Personal Relationships: Many times individuals with substance abuse face great difficulties at home even after undergoing treatment. The cause of treatment is most of the time high expressed emotions of family members in form of hostility and critical behaviours. Receiving treatment is not sufficient for the client to improve. They also require support of family members to achieve progress in the therapy and be abstinent. Generally, the critical comments are passed on the client regarding deterioration in academic performance, bad friend circle, wasting time and money etc. It has been seen that sometimes this critical attitude results in relapse in the condition and stress caused by the family atmosphere can provoke the substance taking behaviour. In order to improve personal relations and build up social support it is important for both family members and the client to indulge in joint activities as much as possible. Family outings can be planned for the same or a specific time slot can be allotted where all the family members are supposed to sit and share their views. Adolescents can also be encouraged to attend group meetings organized for the same problems where everybody share views about impacts of substance taking and how they get rid of the problem.

Relapse Prevention Training: Relapse prevention training is a cognitive-behavioural method based on learning theory. It aims at helping the client to explore and identify resulting positive and negative conditions of substance abuse. Its association with antecedents and consequences is asked to explore and finally they are taught to identify alternative solutions for those conditions. As a cognitive modality they are asked to be prepared cognitively to leave drugs and as behavioural method they are taught to implement the attributed alternatives to prevent themselves from the negative consequences of their use. Confrontation of thoughts is encouraged to prevent substance abuse.

Assertiveness Training: Assertiveness training is a behavioural method to improve social skills of the patient. Many times adolescents find unable to assert in front of their friends and are at high risk of abusing the drugs again. To prevent them from this condition they can be given assertiveness training about how to be vocal in a situation and how to say no. In fact, more than telling them how to say no, work is done to teach them why to say no. They are taught the difference between being assertive and aggressive and use of bold statements to say no to drugs. Certain statements can be practiced in sessions using role plays such as *"Thanks very much but I don't drink", "it's not worth the risk", "no thanks, I don't want to drink and look like a fool falling all over", "no thanks I have to drive", "I'm planning to participate in the school concert, you can come if you want".*

Combined use of Therapies: Many times a combination of effective treatments may be used. Those who suffer from anxiety and withdrawal symptoms may require relaxation training to overcome the symptoms. Different relaxation modes may be used for that such as diaphragmatic breathing, progressive muscle relaxation, visualization etc. Sometimes, individual and group treatments are combined along with family therapy. Sometimes, when adolescents recover, there may be feelings of guilt related to the losses and problems occurred in the family, in such cases, guilt feelings need to be handled with support. Ventilation of thoughts may be allowed on certain occasions to make the mind free of stressors. School also needs to cooperate with such adolescents and encourage them for new life to be started. Client may be encouraged to participate in extracurricular activities to enhance self-esteem and make the social support available for them.

References

Berman, A.L., Jobes, D.A., Silverman, M.M., (2006). *Adolescent Suicide Assessment and Intervention.* 2nd ed. American Psychological Association. Washington, DC.

Carr, A. (1999). *The Handbook of Child and Adolescent Psychology; A Contextual Approach.* Hove and New York. Brunner Routledge, Taylor and Francis Group.

Cepeda, C. (2010). *Clinical Manual for the Psychiatric Interview of Children and Adolescents.* American Psychiatric Publishing. Inc. Washington DC., London, and England.

Hersen, M. (2002). *Encyclopedia of Psychotherapy.* Vol. 2. Elsevier Science. USA.

Hirisave, U., Oommen, A., Kapur, M. (2002). *Psychological Assessment of Children in the Clinical Setting.* 1st ed. Publication no. 48. Vinayaka Offset Printers. Bangalore 76.

Proulx, L. (2003). *Strengthening Emotional ties Through Parent-child-Dyad Art Therapy.*

Salsman, N.L., Arthur, R. (2011). Adapting dialectical behaviour therapy to help suicidal adolescents, *Current Psychiatry.* Vol. 10, No. 3.

Schroeder, C.S.; Gordon, B.N. (2002). *Assessment and Treatment of Childhood Problems; A Clinician's Guide.* 2nd ed. New York. London. The Guideline Press.

Viskochil, J. *School Refusal Behaviour from Terminology to Treatment,* University of Utah. (year could not be found)

Wagner, B.M. (2009). *Suicide Behaviour in Children and Adolescents.* New Haven and London. Yale University Press.

Watson, T.S., Gresham, F.M. (1998). *Handbook of Child Behaviour Therapy.* New York, London. Plenum Press.

21

Primary Prevention and Empowerment of Teacher Trainees within the Classroom Setting

Anjali Bhatia

While some amount of stress is inevitable and even desirable for productivity and problem-solving, protracted stress can lead to serious physical, emotional and behavioural consequences. Teacher trainees are under heightened stress because of their dual roles as present students and in-training teachers. They also have to balance work and home responsibilities. The investigator explored how coping skills training imparted during class hours to teacher trainees could facilitate them to handle their own stress as well as that of their future students. The trainees, both male and female, were aged between 21 and 39. An eclectic approach, integrating theatrical and narrative along with regular psycho therapeutic perspectives was adopted. The investigator was supportively involved with the trainees in her role as teacher and mentor. Among the stressors identified for the sample were—study pressures, family conflicts, unrealistic expectations, lack of language fluency, uncertainty about future employment, daily commuting and financial constraints. Based on her observation of the students, the investigator found that coping skills training brought a positive attitudinal change in them as regards their own and others' mental health and psychosocial situation. The implications of this study for mental health and empowerment of the class community are discussed. Intervention of this kind may be viewed as a means of primary prevention, wherein problems are forestalled before they occur.

Stress has been defined as "a demand (environmental and/or internal) made upon the adaptive capacities of the mind and body (Fontana, 1989). If the individual's adaptive capacities can meet the demand, then the situation may be perceived as a challenge with the prospect of successful problem-solving. This may be called emotional excitement or emotional prostress (D'Zurilla and Nezu, 1989). When demand exceeds or overwhelms capacity, the individual can suffer from physical and mental debilitation that results in burnout, that is, he or she is emotionally spent and deprived of productive energy; stress has turned into distress (Neenan and Palmer, 1996). Stress can have both immediate and long-term psychological, physiological, and behavioural effects.

The task of a therapist is to help stressed individuals to identify, challenge and change those patterns of thinking that produce emotional disturbance and problem-solving interference in the face of environmental stressors; this process of cognitive change enables the individual to develop an enduring emotional and practical problem-solving outlook (Abrams and Ellis, 1994).

However, in those cases when a therapist or other mental health professional is not available, it becomes a concern of any significant other in the individual's environment, who has knowledge and understanding of mental health and stress-related issues, to facilitate such change through available means. Primary prevention attempts to forestall a problem from occurring altogether. With urbanization and industrialization, society today seems colder and harsher. Individuals are less self-reliant and, therefore, turn to the government and a variety of professionals to meet their needs. However, not everyone with a mental disorder or adjustment problem is able to receive treatment from professionals. Early intervention may, therefore, be a better measure for preventing mental disorders altogether wherever and whenever possible.

Objectives of the Study

The investigator has been observing during her teaching experience that a majority of Indian students, irrespective of the course of study they are pursuing, are not equipped to cope with the challenges of life. They are prone to stress, burnout and frustration. The commonly-cited causes of such stress are high expectations of parents; an insensitive school system that focuses exclusively on marks, irrespective of the impacts on mental health; increasing competition for jobs; and breakdown of traditional systems of familial and social support. The consequences can range from emotional disorders to violence and aggression.

The scenario is more complex in the case of students training to be teachers; that is, teacher trainees. Not only are they are they being fitted for a school system where many of their idealistic perceptions of the teaching profession are likely to be disturbed; but they will also witness the emotional distress of students who are adversely affected by this system. As teachers, they are expected to mould healthy human beings. But their own work pressures and professional constraints may restrict them from doing so.

In such a scenario, training in coping skills is urgently needed for teacher trainees. It is expected that this will facilitate them for handling their own stress as well as that of their students. The investigator wished to explore how coping skills training imparted in the classroom in a inconspicuous way during the course of lectures, could equip the trainees with coping strategies for not just the course but for all areas of life functioning.

The objectives of the present study are:

- To identify the causes of stress among teacher trainees.
- To impart training in coping skills to teacher trainees.
- To facilitate the participants to develop personal coping strategies.

Design: The present study may be called exploratory and "intuitive" rather than quantitative. The investigator was not objectively detached from the participants but rather supportively involved in her role as teacher and mentor. Her approach was broadly humanistic and psycho-social. She was aided in this exploration by the course curriculum which included components such as guidance and counselling, mentoring, and therapeutic approaches. This made it easier to introduce mental-health related issues in the classroom.

Sample: The sample consisted of 60 teacher trainees, both male and female, enrolled in the B.Ed. programme of a private university. Their ages ranged from 21 to 39. Some were fresh graduates while others had considerable work experience. Many of them were married and had children.

While none initially appeared to be suffering from significant psychological distress, the investigator was concerned about the possible impact of stressors (as outlined in the previous sections of this paper) on the long-term mental health of the trainees.

Tools: The investigator incorporated within the classroom setting, several exercises and practices directed towards self-exploration of the students. The purpose of these exercises was to—

- Lower defences.
- Encourage questioning.
- Develop insight.
- Achieve catharsis.

Method

Exercise 1: Dream Disclosure

Duration—2 sessions of 50 minutes each

The teacher asked to trainees to write down their unfulfilled dreams anonymously on a piece of paper. The papers were then collected and in turn, each participant was to pick up one randomly, read out the contents, and then speak aloud how they would have responded had this been their dream. Participants were instructed to respond immediately, with no more than a minute allowed for thinking about their response. This was done to encourage spontaneity and discourage psychological defences. Emphasis was laid on possible courses of action they would have adopted.

Observations: A common unfulfilled dream that emerged was not being able to pursue one's chosen vocation. Since the participants were all teacher trainees, it raised the question of what constraints inhibited them from pursuing their chosen goal, and their motives in pursuing their present course.

Exercise 2: The Unsent Letter

Duration—2 sessions of 50 minutes each

Participants were instructed to write a letter to anyone whom they wished. The letter could be angry, regretful, joyous or grateful; in short, they were to express their feelings towards any person, force or situation in their lives. As in the dream disclosure exercise, the participants did not put their names at the end. Once all the letters were collected in one place, each participant had to choose one randomly and reply aloud as if it was addressed to them.

Observations: Some addressed their letters to their parents, some to friends and some to themselves. A few even addressed them to God. A considerable emotional expression of resentment and dissatisfaction was observed, along with an outflow of gratitude, forgiveness and expectation. Overall, this exercise was seen to be cathartic and leading to better group cohesion.

Exercise 3: Narrative Techniques

Duration—3 sessions of 50 minutes each

The word 'narrative' refers to the stories of people's lives. Narrative approaches to counselling accept people as the experts in their own lives. They assume that people have many skills, beliefs, values, and abilities that will assist them to reduce the influence of problems in their lives. By telling their story, people can find meaning in contradictory events, accept alternate truths, and shape happy endings.

Participants in the narrative exercise were asked to write down their lives, or particular phases of their lives, as stories in the third person. After initial reluctance, some participants were able to relate incidents from their lives that they thought formed a complete story. The task was now to thread the entire life into one story with purpose and coherence. 'Personification' as a narrative device was adopted, wherein conflicts were to be depicted as characters in the story, enabling the participant to externalize the problem.

Observations: There was a defensive attitude in the participants about sharing their personal stories in class, which gradually reduced as the teacher explained the significance of the narrative approach. Gradually, they were able to plunge into the exercise with enthusiasm. Most found this exercise challenging, but by the end of the session they were willing to re-write their life stories to find meaning.

Exercise 4: Psychological "Homework"

Duration—No fixed session, continued throughout the academic term

The investigator supplemented classroom activities with "psychological homework". Participants were encouraged to keep a diary of their thoughts, feelings and self-development. Some who voiced individual problems were recommended relaxation and concentration techniques to de-stress. They were also given access to the teacher after class hours to discuss their problems in an informal manner.

Insight and *self-questioning* were developed by administering personality questionnaires and emotional intelligence inventories to the trainees during practical sessions.

It must be noted here that the above were not projected to the participants as professional help. It was made clear to them that the teacher was using her knowledge of psychology to provide advice and support for their adjustment. Those who expressed a need to seek professional help were given references to a mental health professional.

Observations: The investigator found that the above programme brought about a positive attitudinal change in the participants as regards their own and others' mental health and psychosocial situation. They were able to lower social inhibitions, discard perfectionist beliefs, accept divergent views and develop individualized coping strategies.

Results and Discussion

Based on the investigator's observations during the above programme of coping skills training, the causes of stress among the trainees were found to be:

- ***Study Pressures***: The course curriculum in the university was strenuous, demanding 6-7 hours of classroom study plus preparation after hours. A semester system, with a continuous assessment pattern, put a lot of pressure on the trainees.
- ***Family and Marital Conflicts***: In some cases arising from or aggravated by, the study pressures of the trainees: As stated earlier, many of the trainees were married with children. An interesting anomaly was that many trainees' families (in-laws) wanted them to pursue the B.Ed. course so that the family income could be enhanced; but at the same time shied away from providing help in household duties to ease the pressure on the trainee. Balancing family responsibilities with study was proving to be a cumulative burden. In some cases, there was no role conflict but still there were underlying family issues adding to their stress.
- ***Unrealistically High Expectations from Oneself***: Some trainees had been scoring consistently well throughout their academic career. However, because many subjects in the B.Ed. curriculum were completely new for them, and the teaching and examination system somewhat different from the traditional universities they had so far studied in, some trainees experienced a drop in their

performance. Others had been performing in the average to low range before joining the course, but were eager to score well in B.Ed. to enhance their professional opportunities.

- **Lack of Fluency in the Language of Study:** English was the medium of instruction for the course. As most of the trainees were native Hindi speakers, and many had carried out their entire education in the Hindi medium, they faced a major problem in understanding basic concepts and expressing themselves adequately.
- **Lack of Job Security:** Many trainees had been employed prior to joining the course. The B.Ed. programme was a step to enhance their qualifications and employability. However, given the employment scenario in the country, they were not sure whether their previous employers would take them back after the year-long professional break. Others were concerned that the time and finances invested in the programme may not lead to immediate employment after completion of the course.
- **Daily Long Commutes:** The University was located in the outskirts of the city, which involved a daily commute of two hours for those living in the city. This considerably reduced the amount of time available for rest and recreation.
- **Dissatisfaction with one's Career Choice**: The investigator found that some trainees had been compelled to take up the B.Ed. programme under family pressure, financial needs, or confusion about their own career options. Almost none of them had received any career counselling in their entire academic career. This pointed to a dire need for providing career assessment and counselling at the secondary and higher education levels.
- **Financial constraints:** The B.Ed. programme is a professional course with a high fee structure. To this could be added the expenses of commuting, books, and other study materials. For some trainees, this expenditure put a strain on their finances and reduced their budget for other activities.

One notable finding that emerged was that the participants, who held belief in a higher power, were able to cope better under stress. They found it beneficial to recall incidents in their life when this Power had sustained them under difficult circumstances. Moreover, the more such instances they recalled, the more responsive they were to the coping skills training. The investigator, therefore, suggests that a transpersonal perspective may be useful while working with stress-related problems. The central concept in Transpersonal Psychology is a sense of self-identity which is deeper or higher, broader, and more unified with the Whole. The root of the term, transpersonal or literally "beyond the mask," refers to this self-transcendence. Faith in a Higher Entity that is a source of power and strength has been an inseparable part of the Indian ethos. With Indian students, therefore, this approach may even work with those individuals who are otherwise feeling too "hemmed in" by circumstances, to re-appraise their life situations in a more positive manner.

Implications for Mental Health and Community Empowerment

If one takes the classroom as a community, then one can view these exercises as a means of empowerment within the community. *Empowerment* can be defined as "an intentional, ongoing process centred in the local community, involving mutual respect, critical reflection, caring, and group participation, through which people lacking an equal share of resources gain greater access to and control over those resources" (Zimmerman, 2000).

Mutual respect emerges when participants gather the courage to share their painful emotions and experiences in front of their classmates and accept the solutions emerging from the process. *Critical reflection* skills develop when expression of feelings leads to an understanding of the causes wherein those feelings sprung from. *Caring* and *group participation* stem from the realization that many others are in the same predicament and that by simply sharing one's experiences, a more closely-knit class community can develop.

The "resources" in this context refer to opportunities that have been denied to many participants. Even though the majority comes from the average to above average socio-economic classes; conservative family backgrounds and gender restrictions have inhibited many of them from realizing their potential as fully functional individuals. Stereotyped notions of women being suited only for certain professions (such as teaching); the role conflict arising from the demands of the study course and family life; lack of awareness about career choices; and a process of socialization that encourages denial of feelings, have all contributed to self-defeating habits and low motivation to change. Self-expression ranges from fluent and creative in some members to rigid and conformist in others.

Resources here also refer to access to mental health services. Not a single trainee from the sample had ever visited a mental health professional in their lives, even though many of them reported intense feelings of depression, despair, anger and even suicidal impulses.

How was the class community able to alleviate this resource poverty? The teacher (who was part of the community) communicated her understanding and knowledge related to mental health, to the students. As stated earlier, this was no substitute of professional help but it initiated the process of getting help, by identifying the need for it. Moreover, self-disclosure of emotional imbalances in a group setting lowered the barriers of doubt or shame that restricted individuals from taking professional help. Accepting that one had missed opportunities due to social conformity, helped group members to shed defences and identify means of self-expression.

While classroom innovations can be no substitute for professional counselling, the teacher can use these skills and exercises to develop a broad understanding that helps prevent problems before they occur. It is thus a means of *primary prevention.*

References

Abrams, M. and Ellis, A. (1994). Rational emotive behaviour therapy in the treatment of stress. *British Journal of Guidance and Counselling*, 22 (1), 39-50.

Duffy, K.G. (1998). Community psychology. In S. Cullari (Ed.), *Foundations of Clinical Psychology* (pp. 348-365). Allyn and Bacon.

D'Zurilla, T.J. and Nezu, A.M. (1989) Clinical stress management. In A.M. Nezu and C.M. Nezu (Eds.), *Clinical Decision-making in Behaviour Therapy: A Problem-Solving Perspective.* Champaign, IL: Research Press.

Fontana, D. (1989). *Managing Stress*. London: Routledge.

Neenan, M. and Palmer, S. (1996). Stress counselling: A cognitive-behavioural perspective. *Journal of the International Stress Management Association* (UK Branch), 8 (4), 5-8.

22

Challenges and Interventions

Vision for the Future

Aradhana Shukla

Mental health conditions, which include behaviour and mental health problems, e.g. depression, anxiety disorders (post-traumatic stress) and disruptive behavioural disorders (like attention deficit, hyperactivity, mood swing, substance use, suicidal behaviour and aggressive/disruptive behaviour) are the most important causes, upon which adjustment of youth and adults is based. The adjustment problem is most common and worldwide problem that has trapped the adolescents but the adults are totally detached from it, is not true. It means that adjustment problem has covered all. There are many factors that lay their negative but significant impact on the person's mental health and all factors, in sum, deteriorate the behaviour and this behaviour appears in terms of adjustment deficit.

Countries in the WHO European Region face enormous challenges in working conditions but in Indian condition the position of mental health is not well. We, the Indians face many more plateforms than any one because inteperations relation are tested rather more rudely and need more power to be more adequate than others. So, there are many challenges before us and we have to resolve them not only for us in particular but also for the social welfare in general. In the current social setting we need to pay attention on many challenges and it is the duty of a civilized citizen, health care professional and government. These challenges, in case, properly understood and meet out, can foster mental health because they are aimed to:

- Review the provision of mental health services.
- Promote debate on aims and ambitions of mental health services.

- Consider how to make mental health services fit for the purpose to deal with challenge 20-30 years ahead.

In addition to this description behaviour of daily life conditions also plays an important role. It has also observed that the persons who show do disruptive behaviour proves as burden for them and for their surroundings. This condition play a vital role in the development and behavioural constraint.

Burden: Mental health is currently one of the biggest challenges facing by every country in the region with mental health problems effecting at least one in four people at some time in their lives. The prevalence of mental health disorders is very high in Europe. Of the 870 million people living in the European region, at anyone time about 100 million people are estimated to suffer from anxiety and depression, over 21 million to suffer from alcohol use disorders; over 7 million from Alzheimer's disease and other dementias. About 4 million from schizophrenia, 4 million from bipolar affective disorder and 4 million from panic disorders. Moreover, cardiac discare is the next but not least problem that is almost conditions, amongs from deteriorative health related circumstances and affect it more after the attack.

Neuropsychiatric disorders are the second greatest cause of the burden of disease on the region after cardiovascular diseases. They account for 19.5 per cent of all Disability Adjusted Life Years (DALYs-years lost to ill health and premature death). Depression alone is the third greatest cause, accounting for 6.2 per cent of all DALYs Self-inflicted injuries are the eleventh leading cause of DALYs, accounting for 2.2 per cent. Alzheimer's disease and other dementias are the fourteenth leading cause of DALYs. Accounting for 1.9 per cent. The number of people with these disorders is likely to increase further as the population ages.

Neuropsychiatric disorders also account for over 40 per cent of chronic disease and are the greatest cause of years lived with disability. Depression is the single most important cause. Five of the highest fifteen contributors are mental disorders. In many countries, mental health problems account for 35-45 per cent of absenteeism from work.

One of the most tragic results of mental health problems is suicide. Nine of the ten countries in the world with the highest rates of suicide are in the European region. The most recent available data show that about 1,50,000 people of whom 80 per cent are male, commit suicide every year. Suicide is a leading and hidden cause of death among young adults, second only to traffic accidents among those aged 15-35 years.

Stigma and Discrimination

Too often, the widespread sigma attached to mental health problems jeopardizes the development and implementation of mental health policy. Stigma is the main cause of discrimination and exclusion as it affects people's self-esteem, helps to disrupt their family relationship and limits their ability to socialise and get housing and jobs. It also contributes to the abuse of human rights in some large institutions.

Detrioration in Mental Health

Now the problem of mental health have been ravelled before the government and it is thought that mental health is very important for each and every citizen and it must be watched and cared regularly. It is fundamental to the quality of life enabling the people to experience the life as meaningful and to be creative and active as well. Public health (whether physical or mental) reinforces life style conducive to mental well-being. Mental health enhancement needs to teach the whole population, including people with mental health problem and their career. It may be hoped that development and implementation of effective plan to promote health will enhance mental health for all.

Prevention of Harmful Stress and Suicide

It is often seen that care based in community has been shown to offer a better quality of life and great satisfaction for service users and their families than traditional hospital care. It is the height of carelessness that the hospital are nearby to be closed and private nursing homes, multi-specialty centres or super specialty centres have taken their place. So far as the matter of rich class is concerned they do not have any problem to spend the money. They get admitted in these super especially hospitals/ referrals to be cured but what does the poor do? He experiences harmful stress and sometimes becomes as much despaired that he commits the suicide. So it is the responsibility of government to open such types of more medical care centres and provide state level facilities to the poors so that they cannot be deprived of the treatment.

In addition to this debate we also feel that although the condition of physical health care is relatively better and government is paying attention on it but the conditions of mental health care system is very poor. On the one side mentally ill patients consider finally as marginalized and he does not want to share him with others. But after feeling severity when he consults the doctor, he does not avail the facilities which he has to. The social cause of mental health problems are manifold, ranging from individual causes of distress to issues that affect a whole community or society. They can be induced or reinforced in many different setting including home, education and workplace. Marginalized and vulnerable group such as refugees and migrant population and people who are unemployed, imprisoned or left out having different sexual orientation, have disabilies or are already experiencing mental health problem can be at particular risk.

Poor Mental Health Services

In many instances, care based in the community has been shown to offer a better quality of life and greater satisfaction for services users and their families than traditional hospital care. Across the region, bed numbers are falling and institutions are being closed down, but the pace of change is uneven. Institutional care still dominates in most parts of the region. In a quarter of European countries, mental health services are not available in the community. In some countries, over 50 per cent of all patients are treated in large mental hospitals. Indeed, more than two-third of all mental hospital beds in Europe are in psychiatric hospitals. In some countries 85 per cent of the money devoted to mental health is spent on maintaining large institutions. In over one-third, treatment for severe mental health disorders is not available from family doctors and there are no mental health training programmes for family doctors or other primary health care professionals. One-fifth of countries do not make the three essential psychotropic drugs (amitriptyline, chlorpromazine and phenytoin) available in primary health care. One-fifth also do not have a therapeutic drug policy or an essential drug list. The quality of care depends heavily on the quality of the workforce. The significant variations between countries in the number of mental health professionals arouse concern with psychodist psychologies and nurses.

Treatment Gap by the Person Concerned or by the Doctors

Not only in India but also in Western countries most of the people feel that there is a vast gap between treatment suggested and treatment done. It has been largely opined that when a person reported his mental problem then he received less attention and no care by the psychiatrist or psychologist. Studies of European countries reveal that only 44 per cent get treatment.

Delivery of Mental Health Services in the Community

Research and service delivery in primary health care settings have received maximum attention across the country. Mental health priorities in primary health care (Mehta, Joseph, and Verghese, 1984) highlight the need to train primary health care workers in (a) health education on the prevention of psychiatric illness and strengthening the mental health indices; (b) identification of psychological problems; (c) ability to understand the criteria of referral; and (d) ability to function as a resource. Only 50 per cent follow-up was reported in such clinics in primary health care settings; the best follow-up was for epilepsy, while the worst follow-up was for psychosocial or neurotic problems. In his report, Sriram (1990) specially highlights the need for therapy from a public health perspective in view of the widespread prevalence of neurotic conditions in the population. A 50 per cent follow-up of neurotic and somatising patients was reported by Kulhara, Chandiramani, Mattoo, and Varma (1987) and Sen (1987) argued that a large number of those with psychosocial problems could be treated without drugs by using psycho-social techniques. Thus, there is a sizeable population which, according to Sen (1987), fails to fit into the Western diagnostic classificatory systems and these disorders are an outcome of the reaction to stressors produced by the social and cultural demands of the patients. Thus, it is important to understand the etiology of illness from a different enthnographic intuitive perspective.

Mental Health Delivery through Satelite Clinics

Narayana Reddy, Channabasavanna, Gourie-Devi, Das, Prabhu, Shariff, Kaliaperumal, and Reddamma (1986) proposed the delivery of mental health care through satellite clinics. Satellite clinics were introduced in four taluk headquarters at a distance of 50 to 115 km from NIMHANS, Bangalore by multidisciplinary neuropsychiatric teams. In these clinics, 33.2 per cent cases epilepsy, 5.7 per cent of mental retardation, 22.7 per cent of psychiatric illness and 26.4 per cent of other neurological illnesses were examined. Community involvement enhanced awareness about mental illness.

Mental Health Delivery through the Training of Professionals

An attempt was made to implement the national Mental Health Programme (Narayan Reddy, Channabasavanna and Srinivasa Murthy, 1986) by training professionals and health planners from the different states of the country, and primary health care personnels at the state level.

Training Lay Volunteers

Training lay volunteers as resource persons to counsel individuals with minor psychiatric problems and refer those with serious problems has been implemented for over a decade in Bangalore (Kapur, 1992).

Training of School Teachers

Kapur (1992) further developed several programmes related to school mental health. These included sensitizing teachers to the mental health problems of children and training them to counsel children identified as disturbed. In addition in collaboration with other workers, several strategies for the management of psychiatric disorders in the school setting have been evolved (Kapur, 1992). Some of the programmes have been evaluated in terms of process and outcome. These approaches are welcome to the extent that they alleviate the distress of psychiatrically disturbed individuals. However, their effectiveness can only be assessed through their short and long term outcomes and their cost benefit analysis.

One of the best illustrations of "interventive" epidemiology in community mental health was the collaborative study of severe mental morbidity (ICMR & DST, 1987). This four centre study conducted in Bangalore, Baroda, Calcutta and Patiala, not only considered the prevalence of mental illness but also evaluated the intervention strategies. The intervention was carried out by involving multipurpose workers and doctors of the primary health centres in the study areas, by training them in the identification and management of severe mental illness and epilepsy along with their routine health care tasks. The PHC team was effective in identifying and managing 20 per cent of the psychotics and epileptics in the community. A simple and crude costing exercise was carried out. The study highlighted the urgent need for "health service research" into the operational aspects of primary health care.

An update on community mental health in India and the USA, published as the proceedings, provided major insights into the area. The proceedings of the Indo-US Symposium on community mental health (Srinivasa Murthy and Burns, 1992) offered a comprehensive overview of the state of the art information in six major areas: (a) mental health planning and policy development at the national level; (b) integration of mental health with primary health care; (c) development of models using para-professionals and non-professionals; (d) family and social support systems in the case of the mentally ill, (e) alternative patterns of care for the mentally ill; and (f) mental health services for special groups such as children, adolescents and elderly. The proceedings highlighted that the development of community mental health programmes was a continuing process in a multi-dimensional arena, wherein mental health disciplines could contribute to the promotion of mental health, prevention of mental disorders and care of the mentally ill.

Ayurveda and Allied Healing Traditions

Ayurveda focuses equally on preventive, curative and promotive aspects of mental health. It is a holistic approach which aims at harmony between the body, the mind and the soul. In most of the Indian medical systems such as Ayurveda, Unani or Siddha a combination of rituals, exercises, diet and medicines is prescribed based on certain principles. Similarly, in the yogic sciences, an integrated approach has been advocated. The eight steps of Patanjali exemplifies a scientific approach to an individual's efforts at self-actualisation and deals with all aspects of human existence in relation to the environment. These are *yama*, *niyama*, *asana*, *pranayama*, *dharana*, *dhyan*, *Samadhi* and *prathyahara* and the three stages of mediation. The holistic approach is characterized by a focus on well-being which goes beyond the curative dimension, and is achieved by maintaining harmony between the body, the mind and the environment. An individual can effect changes only through practice and will power.

In the Indian conceptualization ill health and well-being are understood at different levels of an individual's mental, physical and spiritual life with forces from the environment interacting with the individual to produce health or ill health. Consequently, the treatment has to be complex and holistic. Western methods tend to be anchored exclusively on one aspect or the other in a simplistic fashion in search of scientific respectability, while the eastern holistic approach requires far more complex ways of evaluation.

Indigenous Folk Healing Tradition

In developing countries healing practices are available to most people which are rooted in their cultures. The techniques vary depending on individual practitioners. Healers prescribe rituals (often of tantric-type), prayers, environmental manipulation and a host of other culturally acceptable supportive measures. The salient feature is that the healer and the healed have the same idiom of communication. However, only a few empirical studies have been conducted so far. The process of healing, which occurs instantaneously, is called "miracle" or "faith healing". This warrants an ethnographic study of the relationship between the healer and the healed.

Research needs to be undertaken on effectiveness of dialogues between religious healers/mystics and their clients who face stress and problems in coping with neurotic, somatising disorders, hysterias including possession states provided by treatment healers "possessed" by gods or demons who bless, curse, exercise or give an oracle, alleged miracles or faith healing; astrological consultations, and healing practices offered at the shrines of different religious groups. Another topic of interest is the way in which these healers offer solace in irremedial situations.

Thus, research should have practical implications for the researcher and subjects alike, with theoretical anchors and indigenous origin of a holistic nature, and ecocultural specificity for contemporary Indian society.

Personalization

Co-production in terms of service development and service delivery should in principle be the default for all patients receiving mental health services in the future, regardless of diagnosis. The early training of all health and social care staff, and their continuing professional development, should include as a core principle the need to provide patients with a personalized service, and to involve them, and their family and careers, as equal partners in decisions about mental health service design and service delivery. This means that we will need to recruit a workforce for the future that has a truly participative and listening approach to patient care, as well skills helping people who ay lack capacity to make decisions.

This message also applies to national and local commissioners of mental health services across the UK, whom we would like to see review their commissioning processes to ensure the engagement of service users, families and carers.

Self-Management

Mental health services need to build service users capacity to safely self-manage their conditions. This will involve training service users both in their own care (whether it is, for example, adherence to prescribed medication, managing a comborbid physical health problem, self help psychological therapy or improving diet and exercise regimes) as well as establishing ongoing monitoring and support that ensures people are self managing their condition effectively. There may be an important role for peer support in this process.

Mental Health in Primary Care

GPs of the future need to become leaders in mental health care. This does not mean they need to become mental health specialists, but it does mean that they need to know a such about mental health as they do about physical health.

In the future mental health services should be primary care led, with specialist interventions and expertise easily accessible in primary care settings. This will involve professionals on both sides of primary and secondary care working together in a more collaborative way, alongside patients and family and careers. However, the very language of "both sides" is unhelpful. What in effect we would like to see is a merging of primary and secondary care services so that the distinction (and many of the problems that arise from people being moved from one box to the other) becomes much less evident.

Crisis Care and Community Support

People want good, local expert community support, both when they are in need of crisis care and in helping them to cope with the problems and challenges of daily living. There are good examples of such services in the UK, but they are patchy and under pressure from both demand and financial constraints. If mental health services in the future are to meet people's needs in these areas, then local commissioners across the UK need to learn from these models and discuss with mental health service users and their careers how they can be implemented.

The quality of future research could improve if the following measures are adopted:

1. Studies ought to be thematically linked, with more collaborative work amongst individuals and centres which are multidisciplinary in nature.
2. Increased communication amongst researchers.
3. Studies that focus on interactions between the individual and his environment.
4. Studies that are marked by ecocultural sensitivity.
5. Longitudinal and naturalistic studies.
6. Development focus in the study of age, gender and context of mental health and illness.
7. Focus on special populations at risk for mental and physical health.
8. Research with interventional focus rather than purely out of scientific curiosity.

References

Gupta, I.D. Gautam, S. and Kamal, P. (1992). General practitioners attitude towards psychiatric disorders and psychiatric patients. A survey of Jaipur city, *Indian Journal of Psychiatry*, 34, 140-144.

Indian Council of Medical Research and Department of Science and Technology (ICMR & DST, 1987). *Collaborative Study on Severe Mental Morabidity,* New Delhi ICMR and DST.

Kapur, M. (1992), School mental health in India. In S. Malhotra, A. Malhotra & V.K. Varma (Eds), *Child Mental Health in India*, Delhi; McMillan India Ltd.

Kulhara, P., Chandramani, K. Mattoo, S.K. and Varma, V.K. (1987). Pattern of Follow up visits in a rural psychiatric clinic, *Indian Journal of Psychiatry*, 29, 189-195.

Mehta, P., Joseph, A., and Verghese, A. (1984). Mental health priorities in primary health care. *Indian Journal of Psychological Medicine*, 7. 439-447.

Narayan Reddy, G.N. Channabassavanna, S.M. Gourie-Devi, M, Das, B.S. Prabhu, G.G. Shariff, I.A., Kaliaperumal, G.G. and Reddamma, K. (1986). Extension of mental health services by satellite clinics as a model. *NIMHANS Journal* 4, 71-75.

Sen, B. (1987), Psychiatric phenomena in primary health care: Their extent and nature. *Indian Journal of Psychiatry*, 29, 33-40.

Srinivasa Murthy, R. and Burns, B.J. (Eds). (1982) *Proceedings of the Indo-US Symposium on Community Mental Health.* Bangalore: NIMHANS.

Sriram, T.G. (1990), Psychotherapy in developing countries: A public health perspective. *Indian Journal of Psychiatry*, 32. 138-144.

Verghese, A. (1988), Family participation in mental health care. The Vellore experiment. *Indian Journal of Psychiatry*, 30, 117-121.

Index